D0771216

UNIVERSITY LIBRARY
LOMA LINDA, CALIFORNIA

Eukaryotic Gene Regulation

Volume II

Editor

Gerald M. Kolodny, M.D.

Harvard Medical School
Beth Israel Hospital
Boston, Massachusetts

CRC Press, Inc.
Boca Raton, Florida

Library of Congress Cataloging in Publication Data

Main entry under title:

Eukaryotic gene regulation.

   Bibliography: p.
   Includes indexes.
   1. Genetic regulation. 2. Gene expression.
I. Kolodny, Gerald M. [DNLM: 1. Cells.
2. Genes. 3. Genes, Regulator. QH450 E87]
QH450.E94   574.87'322   80-13873
ISBN 0-8493-5225-8 (v. 1)
ISBN 0-8493-5226-6 (v. 2)

   This book represents information obtained from authentic and highly regarded sources. Reprinted material is quoted with permission, and sources are indicated. A wide variety of references are listed. Every reasonable effort has been made to give reliable data and information, but the author and the publisher cannot assume responsibility for the validity of all materials or for the consequences of their use.

   All rights reserved. This book, or any part thereof, may not be reproduced in any form without written consent from the publisher.

   Direct all inquiries to CRC Press, 2000 N.W. 24th Street, Boca Raton, Florida, 33431.

© 1980 by CRC Press, Inc.

International Standard Book Number 0-8493-5225-8 (Volume I)
International Standard Book Number 0-8493-5226-6 (Volume II)

Library of Congress Card Number 80-13873
Printed in the United States

FOREWORD

The control of gene expression in eukaryotic cells is of fundamental importance in understanding development, regeneration, aging, genetic diseases, and cancer.

Our ability to treat many human diseases is limited by our lack of knowledge as to why one cell type expresses one gene pattern and another cell type expresses another. For example, adult epithelial cells divide, whereas adult neurons do not. If the genes for cell division could be turned on in neurons, one might be able to repair spinal cord injuries by regenerating new functional neurons. Kidney transplantation might give way to kiney regeneration. Diabetes following pancreatitis might be cured by regenerating new islets cells.

The regulation of gene expression is also an important component of the mechanism of normal human development. Anomalies in development involve these regulatory pathways and attempts to understand, prevent and repair these anomalies would be strengthened by an understanding of how gene control is achieved.

The cause of cancer and its many manifestations is at present unknown. Since many of its manifestations, including its control of cell division, appear to represent abnormal patterns of gene expression, studies of the regulation of gene expression will provide important insights in the understanding and treatment of cancer.

This volume attempts to present some of the recent work on regulation of gene expression in eukaryotic cells. It is, however, purposely limited to an examination of nuclear transcriptional events. Gene regulation at the post nuclear and translational level is not covered and the reader is referred to other excellent reviews on this subject now available.

There is an attempt in the following chapters to review those components of the nucleus which may have gene regulatory functions and to explore how each of them may be contributing to gene regulation. These components include chromatin, RNA, RNA polymerases, histones, nonhistone proteins and hormones. We have not included salts, lipids, and polysaccharides simply because they are probably too limited in their structural and chemical complexity to offer more than the most gross specificity.

I wish to acknowledge the support, advice and editorial help in the preparation of this volume from Terri Weintraub, Barbara Perris, Sandy Pearlman, and Benita Budd Segraves of the CRC Press.

THE EDITOR

Gerald M. Kolodny, M.D. is Director, Division of Nuclear Medicine, Beth Israel Hospital, Boston, Massachusetts and is on the faculty of The Committee on Cell and Development Biology, Harvard Medical School.

Dr. Kolodny graduated in 1958 from Harvard College, Cambridge, Massachusetts, with a B.A. degree in chemistry and obtained his M.D. degree in 1962 from Northwestern Medical School, Chicago. After finishing training, he was a postdoctoral fellow in the Biology department of The Massachusetts Institute of Technology, Cambridge, and then a research associate at the Huntington Laboratories of Harvard University.

Dr. Kolodny is a member of American Society for Cell Biology, Tissue Culture Association, American Association for the Advancement of Science, Society of Nuclear Medicine, Radiation Research Society, Association of University Radiologists, Radiological Society of North America, American College of Radiology, American Medical Association. Among other awards, he has received the Advanced Academic Fellowship of The Picker Foundation and Picker Scholar Award.

Dr. Kolodny has published more than 50 research papers in the fields of cell biology and biochemistry. His current major research interests include RNA metabolism and the control of eukaryotic gene transcription.

CONTRIBUTORS

Trevor J. C. Beebee, Ph.D.
Lecturer in Biochemistry
School of Biology
University of Sussex
Falmer, Brighton
ENGLAND

Peter H. W. Butterworth, Ph.D.
Reader
Department of Biochemistry
University College, London
London, ENGLAND

Ronald F. Cox, Ph.D.
Consultant
Nuclear Enterprises, Inc.
San Carlos, California

John H. Frenster, M.D.
Clinical Associate Professor
Department of Medicine
Stanford University
Stanford, California

Georgiy P. Georgiev, D. Biol.
Head, Laboratory of Nucleic Acid
 Biosynthesis
Institute of Molecular Biology
Academy of Sciences, U.S.S.R.
Moscow, U.S.S.R.

R. S. Gilmour, Ph.D.
Senior Scientific Staff
Beatson Institute for Cancer Research
Glascow, SCOTLAND

Gerald M. Kolodny, M.D.
Division of Nuclear Medicine
Harvard Medical School
Beth Israel Hospital
Boston, Massachusetts

Alexey P. Ryskov, D. Biol.
Senior Scientific Staff
Laboratory of Nucleic Acid
 Biosynthesis
Institute of Molecular Biology
Academy of Sciences, U.S.S.R.
Moscow, U.S.S.R.

Ian R. Phillips, Ph.D.
Postdoctoral Fellow
Department of Biochemistry and
 Molecular Biology
University of Florida
Gainesville, Florida

Klaus Scherrer, Dr. Sci. Technol.
Directeur de Recherche
Centre National de la Recherche
 Scientifique
Institut de Recherche en Biologie
 Moleculaire
Universite de Paris
Paris, FRANCE

Elizabeth A. Shephard, M.Sc.
Research Assistant
Department of Biochemistry and
 Molecular Biology
University of Florida
Gainesville, Florida

Gary S. Stein, Ph.D.
Associate Professor
Department of Biochemistry and
 Molecular Biology
University of Florida
Gainesville, Florida

Janet L. Stein, Ph.D.
Assistant Professor
Department of Immunology and
 Medical Microbiology
University of Florida
Gainesville, Florida

R. Tsanev, Ph.D.
Professor
Bulgarian Academy of Science
Institute of Biochemistry
Sofia, BULGARIA

TABLE OF CONTENTS

VOLUME I

VOLUME II

Chapter 1

EUKARYOTIC DNA-DEPENDENT RNA POLYMERASES: AN EVALUATION OF THEIR ROLE IN THE REGULATION OF GENE EXPRESSION

Trevor J. C. Beebee and Peter H. W. Butterworth

TABLE OF CONTENTS

I. CONTROL OF GENE EXPRESSION AT THE LEVEL OF THE RNA POLYMERASE

Any temptation to believe that the regulation of gene expression in nucleated cells might lie primarily at the level of transcription has its origin in the precedents established for prokaryotic systems. Simple DNA sequence (where sequences are represented in the chromosome once or only a few times), multiple structural genes often existing within one transcription unit, very rapid turnover of messenger RNA (mRNA), and concurrent transcription and translation limit the scope for regulation to occur at any point other than at the level of transcription in prokaryotes. On the other hand, eukaryotes contain amounts of DNA grossly in excess of that required to code for cellular proteins, and the DNA is extremely complex (in terms of the multiplicity of sequence repeats); a large proportion of the primary gene transcripts, constructed within the nucleus, never reaches the cytoplasm; there is a spatial separation of transcriptional from translational events which requires the transport of information from the nucleus to the site of protein synthesis. Thus, the potential for regulating the expression of specific sections of the chromosome can be dictated by any number or all of these steps in this highly organized process. With the current state of our knowledge and the limited but rapidly developing technology, one must exercise real caution in ascribing primary regulatory significance to any one of these phenomena.

This chapter concerns one stage in the overall process of expression of genetic information in eukaryotic cells: the role of DNA-dependent RNA polymerases in the controlled expression of specific (classes of) genes. The real question is whether any RNA polymerase exerts a direct regulatory influence in any system. To invoke this enzyme as being directly involved in control processes, variable initiation specificity, elongation rate, or termination efficiency must be defined in terms of some structural modification of the enzyme itself.

A. Prokaryotic Precedents

In bacterial systems, not all potential control mechanisms satisfy these strict terms of reference. In general terms, two categories of regulatory mechanism are prevalent: positive and negative control, both of which operate at the level of transcription (reviewed by Lewin[1]). Both mechanisms require the binding of a control element to DNA in the proximity of the RNA polymerase binding site: a positive control element interacts with DNA at a site adjacent to and promotes the recognition of this site by the polymerase (for example, the cyclic-AMP binding protein which facilitates the binding of the polymerase to the lac promoter[2]); a negative control element binds to the DNA at a site which prevents the movement of the RNA polymerase from the promoter into the region containing the structural genes, e.g., the binding of repressor to the operator of the lac operon.[3] Neither of these control proteins interacts directly with the RNA polymerase, and therefore, they do not satisfy the criteria for control operating directly on the enzyme.

However, there are at least three other possible control mechanisms which, under certain conditions, may be operative in bacterial cells. There is ample evidence that different RNA polymerases bind to and transcribe from different promoters; that is, they have different template specificities. Following infection by the phage T_7, the host *Escherichia coli* RNA polymerase transcribes a limited portion of the phage genome (the "early" genes); one of the early gene products is an RNA polymerase which recognizes the promoters for the "late" phage genes.[4] A more subtle situation is displayed in the modification of the *Bacillus subtilis* RNA polymerase following infection by phage SP01;[5] expression of viral genes results in the binding of virus-coded proteins to the host polymerase which promote the transcription of specific sections of the phage genome. Perhaps the most challenging mechanism of control which has been proposed for prokaryotes is that of Travers[6] which suggests a role for auxiliary factors which associate with the RNA polymerase mediating the recognition of specific classes of promoters, e.g., those for ribosomal RNA coding sequences. While positive and negative control elements are involved primarily in the "fine" regulation of expression of small groups of genes under coordinate control, these alternative mechanisms dictate a "coarse" form of control, where gross changes in cellular function are to be expressed.

Although this brief survey of prokaryotic control systems begs the criticism of superficiality, it serves to place in perspective different systems of control which may be operative at the level of transcription of genetic information in bacteria.

B. The Eukaryotic Problem

We are faced with a much more complex problem when attempting to rationalize the types of mechanism regulating gene expression in nucleated cells. From a single fertilized egg, the complete organism develops through embryogenesis into a complex array of different cell phenotypes. As phenotype changes during this process, the patterns of gene expression must be changed. Ultimately, the adult phenotype is maintained through subsequent generations. It is conceivable that the "fine" contol of cellular processes may still be achieved by mechanisms similar to those operating in bacterial cells through the transient association of regulatory proteins with the chromosome. However, during replication, when associated proteins must be released from the chromosome, the opportunity arises to replace or maintain a complex array of regulatory factors which direct the expression of phenotype. This group of proteins are normally referred to as "nonhistone" proteins, whereas the histones (which form the protein core of the nucleosomal particle[7]) have a predominantly structural role in the organization and packaging of the chromosome.

If discussion is restricted to the differentiated eukaryotic cell, it is known that, in general, 50 to 80% of the genome is made up of sequences represented only once (or a few times) in the chromosome: the unique or nonrepetitive sequences. The remainder of the genome (excluding satellite DNA) is composed of "moderately repetitive" sequences (see Lewin[8] for review). While there are some notable exceptions (such as the coding sequences for histones), most structural genes exist as single copies in the haploid genome. Current models of the organization of DNA sequence suggest the interspersion of unique with repetitive regions and invoke a regulatory function for the latter.[9] However, the *modus operandi* for these putative regulatory sequences is still far from clear: it is conceivable that they constitute multiple recognition sites for the binding of RNA polymerase and/or regulatory factors (of the "positive" or "negative" control type) or sequences which, when transcribed, constitute processing enzyme cleavage points. The fact that only a small proportion of the genome (up to 10%) may be transcribed at any time confers a major role on proteins which restrict the access of the RNA polymerase to the chromosome. Almost invariably, the initial RNA transcripts are considerably longer than the sequences which ultimately appear in the cytoplasm, the latter representing sequences complementary to only about 2% of the genome.[9] The generation of mature RNA by progressive cleavage of the primary gene transcript is, of course, a potential regulatory step. In the case of stable RNA species (rRNA and tRNA), the structural relationships and the cleavage steps required to generate mature RNAs are comparatively well characterized (extensively reviewed by Perry[10]), and there is some experimental evidence to suggest that control is exercised during these processes.

However, the precursor-product relationship between rapidly synthesized, high molecular weight, nuclear (HnRNA) and mRNA has been a contentious issue for more than 10 years[11] and has only recently received unequivocal experimental support. A high proportion of HnRNA is turned over within the nucleus. From a detailed comparison of total nuclear HnRNA and messenger populations of single cell types, HnRNA has been shown to be as much as five- to tenfold more complex than mRNA and contains repeated sequences. The evidence suggests that repetitive and nonrepetitive sequences are interspersed in the region of the HnRNA molecule 5′ to the mRNA component (assuming that message is located at the 3′ termini of these molecules).[12] During the maturation process, these 5′ sequences may have a role in the (controlled) selection of RNA to be transported from the nucleus to the cytoplasm; some of the repetitive sequences may form regions of secondary structure which may be recognized by processing enzymes[13] or which link remote portions of the HnRNA molecule[14] so that the sequence which appears in the cytoplasm is made up of noncontiguous sections of the primary gene transcript.[15] The opportunity now exists to examine in detail the relationship between the structure of the macromolecular precursor of a specific mRNA and subsequent processing events: Bastos and Aviv[16] have identified a precursor for the globin mRNA in both mouse Friend cells and mouse spleen some seven times larger (27S, approximately 5000 nucleotides) than the mature 10S message (approximately 750 nucleotides) together with a partially processed molecule (15S, approximately 1600 nucleotides). The 27S species has a halflife of only 5 min, but it is still uncertain whether this molecule represents the primary gene transcript or some partially processed intermediate. It should also be pointed out that even the mRNA is oversized with respect to the absolute coding requirement for globin (430 nucleotides): this excess in length is a common feature of those mRNAs which have been purified.[8] These phenomena, as well as further posttranscriptional events such as poly-A addition,[17] "capping" of mRNA precursors[18] and translational controls[19] all have regulatory potential and will be discussed in detail elsewhere in this volume. Our purpose in summarizing the complexity of the eukaryotic genome and the proposed structure and processing of primary gene transcripts is to draw attention to the fact that transcriptional controls are only part of a much more complex picture of regulation. It also serves to illustrate the problems inherent in any attempt to diagnose a direct role for the RNA polymerase per se in regulating the expression of specific coding sequences.

Transcriptional controls operate primarily at the level of the initiation of RNA synthesis. Considerable work is possible (and will be discussed later) on the initiation of the synthesis of rRNA and tRNA because detailed information is available on the precise structure of the primary gene transcript and the DNA sequences which code for them. From the foregoing discussion, it is apparent that, for mRNA, often (if not invariably) the structural gene may be separated from the RNA chain initiation site by a sequence many times longer than the message itself. The information necessary to enable us to study the factors which regulate the expression of a specific structural gene at the level of initiation of RNA synthesis will be contained in the DNA sequence

5′ to the initiation site for the precursor molecule: this remains a considerable challenge for the future. In the meantime, using suitable hybridization techniques, it is possible to identify the transcription (in vivo or in vitro) of coding sequences for stable RNA species or mRNA. However, the conclusion that a sequence is transcribed does not necessarily mean that it will be processed to a biologically active form. One of the simplest examples of this is in the resting peripheral lymphocyte where the 45S precursor of 18S and 28S rRNA is synthesized but, in the maturation process, the 18S sequence is degraded.[20]

For all these reasons, studies on the regulation of RNA synthesis in eukaryotes at the level of the RNA polymerase remains a somewhat phenomenological art!

II. THE STATUS OF THE DNA-DEPENDENT RNA POLYMERASE IN NUCLEATED CELLS

The extent to which our understanding of the process of RNA synthesis in prokaryotes has developed over the last few years has been dramatic. This has been due largely to the ease with which the RNA polymerase may be isolated and purified from bacteria in large amounts. A heteromultimeric enzyme is involved in the expression of all types of RNA in the exponentially growing bacterial cell. The classical description of this multimer presents it as being made up of at least four types of subunit (B′, β, σ, and α_2) having a molecular weight of about 500,000 daltons. Even in the case of the well-characterized *Escherichia coli* enzyme, it has been argued that what is isolated and finally purified is the "most stable assembly" of polypeptide chains: efforts to achieve a homogeneous enzyme by classical protein purification techniques may eliminate certain less stable interactions which may be crucial in the selective expression of different classes of coding sequence.[21]

Although techniques were available 20 years ago for the study of transcription in vitro in animal cell nuclei, the general observation was that the RNA polymerase activity was (to all intents and purposes) exclusively associated with the chromosome as a transcription complex: the so-called "aggregate" enzyme.[22] This conclusion was probably conditioned by the types of experimental system used which was usually derived from rat liver! Had the problem been approached using rapidly dividing eukaryotic cells, it is likely that the whole development of this area of investigation might have taken on a rather different complexion. However, using the "aggregate" nuclear enzyme system, evidence appeared in 1966 which suggested that a multiplicity of polymerase activities was present in eukaryotic cells.[23] With the advent of techniques which "solubilized" the aggregate enzyme activity, the concept of multiplicity was confirmed, and three classes of enzyme were identified according to (1) their sequential elution from DEAE-Sephadex® (types I, II, and III)[24] and (2) their differential sensitivity to amanatoxins (class A [or I] were insensitive to α-amanitin concentrations up to $10^{-3} M$; class B [or II] were inhibited by concentrations in the range 10^{-9} to $10^{-8} M$, and class C [or III] were inhibited by intermediate concentrations in the range 10^{-5} to $10^{-4} M$).[25] Neither of these two classifications is without ambiguity: we shall adopt the former and, as far as possible, relate published work to this system of nomenclature.

Several reviews of the multiplicity, structure, and function of these eukaryotic enzymes have been published recently.[26-29] In the brief synopsis of this vast area of experimental effort which follows, we examine the principles underlying the progress which has been made to construct a general picture of the machinery of RNA synthesis in nucleated cells. Conceptually, this area has been dominated by the notion that polymerase activity exists primarily as a nucleoprotein complex. This may be the case in cells with a low mitotic index (such as liver and thymus, probably the two most heavily studied systems). Whether the same situation pertains in rapidly dividing cells whose metabolic state resembles more closely that of bacteria remains an open question.

A. Isolation and Purification of Eukaryotic RNA Polymerases

The common approach to the isolation of RNA polymerases is to resolve nuclei from whole cells or tissues. While giving rise to a formidable initial protein purification, this technique may select for polymerase which is tightly bound to the chromosome and, thus, may eliminate a large proportion of other polymerase pools (see below). In general terms, there are two techniques which are used to solubilize polymerase activity from nuclei: (1) by sonication in high-salt concentrations (0.3 M ammonium sulfate) or (2) by incubating nuclei in media containing Mg^{++} and low-salt concentrations.[30] The wide variation in detailed application of these techniques has been summarized elsewhere.[26] The precise mechanism by which these procedures gives rise to "soluble" polymerase activity is somewhat obscure. Treatment with high salt probably releases large amounts of protein from the chromatin, and sonication will then fragment the DNA.[31] The absolute dependence of the low-salt extraction procedure on the presence of Mg^{++} implies that chromosome fragmentation by nucleases is probably the primary phenomenon. Whether either of these procedures actually dissociates transcription complexes is not clear. A certain amount of evidence is accumulating (our own unpublished observations) to suggest that this is not the case: even after extensive purification of activities released from chromatin by either of these two techniques, the enzymes appear to remain bound to very short DNA fragments. The implications of this will be discussed below.

The initial resolution of multiple RNA polymerases is best accomplished by salt gradient elution from DEAE-Sephadex®, coupled with an assessment of α-amanitin sensitivity. In certain instances, it has been shown that the sequence of elution of different classes of enzymes is not invariant, and, in some lower eucaryotes, there is a decreased sensitivity to α-amanitin. This subject has been reviewed elsewhere.[28,29] Experience has shown that extensive purification procedures are required to yield homogeneous enzyme preparations.

B. Localization of RNA Polymerase Activities in Eukaryotic Cells

By carrying out simple cell fractionation techniques and making use of differential sensitivity to α-amanitin, the intracellular distribution of polymerase species has been studied. In approaching this problem, it must be recognized that an enzyme which is not associated with nuclear chromatin may still be contained within the nucleus or may be free to diffuse between the nucleus and the cytosol. Such a pool of polymerase activity may be diagnosed, even in the presence of enzyme bound to and transcribing chromatin: that which is "bound" to the chromosome (actively elongating RNA chains in vitro) can be blocked by high concentrations of actinomycin D, while that which is "free" or soluble will continue to be able to transcribe the synthetic template poly-d[A-T];[32] for reasons which are described in detail elsewhere[29] it is desirable to titrate the mixed system with actinomycin D to attain total suppression of the "bound" RNA polymerase. Although this technique will define the existence of a pool of "free" enzyme within a cell fraction, it is difficult to quantitate the relative size of this pool by this procedure alone as the transcriptional efficiency by polymerases of poly-d[A-T] varies between enzyme species.

Virtually regardless of the cell type, nucleoli contain only form I RNA polymerase.[33] The question arises as to whether this is the only location of this enzyme, and, on this point, information is scarce. The answer is probably conditioned by (1) the type of cell under scrutiny (having either a high or a low mitotic index) and (2) the technique used to isolate organelles. In our experience, nuclei which have been prepared by homogenization of rat liver in isotonic sucrose contain no pool of "free" polymerase I;[34] however, if homogenization in hypertonic sucrose is used, nuclei are found to contain "free" polymerase I,[34,35] and the data suggest that nuclei may be leaky with respect to the pool of "free" enzyme. It is unlikely that the pool of "free" enzyme is very large in rat liver as Seifart et al.[36] failed to identify significant quantities of type I polymerase in their analyses of a postnuclear supernatant, whereas another species of polymerase (III) was present. On the other hand, in the extranuclear fraction of HeLa cells,[34] mouse plasmacytoma,[37] and phytohemaglutinin- (PHA) stimulated periperal lymphocytes (unpublished data),[185] a considerable "free" pool of polymerase I was apparent. The comparison between these rapidly dividing cells and hepatic tissue may indicate a difference in the status of any polymerase depending on the growth state of the cells.

The situation with respect to type I polymerase serves to emphasize several important criteria which need to be considered if an overall view of RNA metabolism is to be appreciated. Firstly, any species of enzyme need not be (and, in fact, is not) restricted to a single locus in the cell: the cycle of reactions involving chain initiation and termination requires that enzyme be both bound to the chromosome and free at some time and, in the latter state, may equilibrate with an extrachromosomal pool; secondly, in restricting one's attention to a single locus, a part of the overall process may be overlooked; thirdly, by extracting the enzymes from whole cells, one obtains a complex of enzymes derived from more than one pool, and it is questionable at the moment whether it is possible to identify components of these pools in the mixture.

What has been said here with respect to polymerase I may equally well apply to both polymerases II and III. Both of these species exist as nucleoprotein complexes in the nucleoplasm. Using the poly-[dA-T]/actinomycin procedure, "free" pools of these enzymes have been recognized in rat liver nuclei prepared in hypertonic sucrose.[34] That there may be a considerable pool of "free" polymerase III is indicated by the common finding of this enzyme in the postnuclear supernatant of rat liver,[36] mouse myeloma,[37] and many other cell types.[28]

There is enough evidence available to suggest that the classical definition of intracellular distribution of these enzymes (I, nucleolar; II, nucleoplasmic; and III, nucleoplasmic and cytoplasmic) is too restrictive and should be extended to account for two pools of any one polymerase (at least). It is not yet practical to define the sizes of the pools of any single polymerase species, but it may be anticipated that at appropriate time during the cell cycle, the balance between that which is involved in the synthesis of RNA ("bound" enzyme) and that which constitutes the "free" pool may change. This situation and other factors regulating the "level" of polymerases in eukaryotic cells will be dealt with in depth in the section below concerned with control mechanisms.

C. Structure and Microheterogeneity and Eukaryotic RNA Polymerases

The analysis of the subunit structure of the nuclear RNA polymerase activities has confirmed that higher organisms contain three structurally distinct enzyme species (mitochondrial and chloroplast RNA polymerases will be omitted for this review). In general terms, all these enzymes bear a marked structural relationship to the well defined E. coli holoenzyme in being heteromultimers having molecular weights in the region of 500,000 daltons; each contains two large subunits (in excess of 100,000 daltons), which appear to be characteristic for each class of enzyme, and a number of smaller subunits (less than 100,000 daltons). Each class of enzyme is probably genetically distinct although there is immunological evidence that there may be some sharing of antigenic determinants: in yeast,[38] three small polypeptide chains appear to be common to types I and II polymerase, and there is evidence of a similar phenomenon in calf thymus[39] and in mouse plasmacytoma.[40] This whole subject is reviewed extensively

Table 1
THE SUBUNIT MOLECULAR WEIGHTS OF CLASS I, II, AND III RNA POLYMERASES FROM MURINE PLASMACYTOMA MOPC 315

Class I			Class II				Class III		
Common subunits	I_A	I_B	Common subunits	II_O	II_A	II_B	Common subunits	III_A	III_B
			(o)	240					
			(a)		205				
(a) 195									
			(b)			170			
							(a) 155		
			(c) 140						
							(b) 138		
(b) 117									
							(c) 89		
							(d) 70		
(c)	60	—							
							(e) 53		
(d) 52									
							(f_1) 49		
			(d) 41				(f_2) 41		
							(g)	32	33
(e) 29			(e) 29				(h) 29		
			(f) 27						
			(g) 22						
(f) 19			(h) 19				(i) 19		
			(i) 16						

Note: The molecular weights ($\times 10^{-3}$) of the subunits of each class of mouse myeloma MOPC 315 RNA polymerase is presented: those for classes I and II are derived from Sklar et al.[47] and for class III from Sklar et al.[40] Different RNA species within any one class of polymerase contain a number of "common" subunits, and microheterogeneity is defined in terms of the presence, absence, or variation in the molecular weight of one subunit only.

elsewhere.[21,27,28] Our review will concentrate on current concepts of microheterogeneity within polymerase classes. The subunit structures of mouse myeloma polymerases is summarized in Table 1.

1. Class I RNA Polymerase

Two species of form I RNA polymerase (I_A and I_B) have been described in a wide variety of systems.[29] The problem here is to distinguish between the possibilities that the two species are both physiological forms of the enzyme or that one may be derived from the other as an experimental artifact. The multiplicity of form I polymerases has been diagnosed chromatographically on DEAE-Sephadex® and phosphocellulose. In our experience, their order of elution is reversed on phosphocellulose, and, in constructing a common nomenclature between laboratories, we have taken this into account.[29] The two forms differ in their subunit composition. When extracted by the high-salt, sonication procedure from rat liver nucleoli, the I_A enzyme is composed of six subunits of molecular weight 195K, 128K, 60K, 44K, 26K, and 19K;[41] form I_B is identical, save that the 60K subunit is missing. Similar data arise from studies on enzymes purified from calf thymus[42] and the mouse plasmacytoma.[40] There is some question as to whether both species are physiological forms of the enzyme: from a detailed analysis of the high-salt, sonication procedure,[34] it was shown that the conversion of I_A to I_B occurs, the extent of interconversion depending on the precise extraction conditions. When rat liver nucleoli were extracted by the low-salt incubation method, quantitative extraction was achieved which comprised only form I_A (although there was an apparent reduction in the molecular weight of the largest subunit from 195K to 175K, presumably by limited proteolysis[41]). In nucleoli, most (if not all) of the form I enzyme is in the form of a transcription complex; form I polymerase isolated from the cytoplasm of HeLa cells[34] and an extranuclear fraction of *Xenopus* ovaries[34] has chromatographic properties similar to I_B polymerase, although a subunit analysis of this enzyme has not been carried out to confirm true I_B structure as defined above. These findings have led us to conclude that the complete enzyme (I_A) is the transcribing form and I_B may constitute the unbound pool of this class of enzyme. Similar conclusions have been reached by Matsui et al.[43] More evidence is required before we can be certain that intracellular pools of this (or other) species of polymerase differ structurally, but the present evidence of experimental interconversion indicates that caution must be exercised before coming to this conclusion. In general, it has been difficult to demonstrate differences in the catalytic properties between the purified I_A and I_B enzymes.

2. Class II RNA Polymerase

Multiple species have been identified in form II enzymes isolated from a variety of eukaryotic cells. The difference between them lies in the molecular weight of the largest subunit: the form II enzymes from mouse plasmacytoma all contain subunits of molecular weight 140K, 41K, 30K, 25K, 20K, and 16K and a large subunit of 240K, 205K, or 170K (forms II_O, II_A, and II_B, respectively).[37] Biochemically, these forms are indistinguishable, and it cannot be discounted that the differences may arise as proteolytic artifacts.[44,45] Therefore, in mammalian systems, the physiological significance of form II heterogeneity remains unresolved. A potentially interesting situation has been shown to exist in certain plants. Two forms of type II RNA polymerase have been identified in germinating soybean which again differ only in the molecular weight of the largest subunit: in ungerminated embryos, the enzyme (II_A) is in a soluble form and has a 200K subunit; as germination proceeds, the enzyme becomes bound to the chromatin template, and, following extraction, the largest subunit is found to be reduced to 170K.[46]

3. Class III RNA Polymerase

While heterogeneity in type III enzymes has been demonstrated in a number of systems, the structural differences between enzymes of this class seem to be subtle. In the only well-characterized instance, the mouse plasmytoma (MOPC 315), a reduction in the molecular weight of one subunit (from 33K to 32K) appears to be the only recognizable distinction between forms III_B and III_A.[40] Again, one must be cautious concerning the physiological significance of this microheterogeneity. It may be relevant to point out that in initial cell fractionation experiments on these cells, Schwartz et al.[37] showed that forms III_A and III_B were concentrated in the nucleus and the cytoplasm respectively.

D. The Function of Each Class of Eukaryotic RNA Polymerase

The involvement of each class of RNA polymerase in the expression of different classes of genes has been implied from studies of the intracellular localization of the enzymes and from following the effects of α-amanitin on the synthesis of RNA species in vivo and in vitro. It is not our intention to duplicate the extensive reviews which already exist, but attention will be drawn to a number of pertinent pieces of recent work.

As nucleoli contain only form I RNA polymerase, a role in the expression of ribosomal RNA coding sequences was ascribed to this activity. Studies on the α-amanitin sensitivity of RNA synthesis by form I enzyme in isolated nuclei and nucleoli provided evidence of this.[48-50] Recently, the hybridization characteristics[51] and fingerprint analyses[52] of in vitro transcripts by the endogenous nucleolar form I enzyme both confirm the expression of rRNA coding sequences by this enzyme.

It is generally accepted that form II transcribes HnRNA (the putative precursor of mRNA) in its nucleoplasmic locus, and extensive studies both in vivo and in vitro using α-amanitin support this view.[28] Much of this evidence is circumstantial, but direct confirmation has emerged from a number of different approaches to the problem. Mutants have been produced in Chinese hamster ovary cells[53] and a BHK cell line[54] which contain an α-amanitin-insensitive form II RNA polymerase. Whereas the expression of polyoma virus genes in infected mouse 3T3 cells is inhibited by α-amanitin in the growth medium, somatic cell hybrids between these infected cells and the α-amanitin-resistant BHK cell mutant results in the α-amanitin-insensitive expression of polyoma functions.[54] This implies the direct involvement of form II polymerase in the transcription of viral messenger RNAs. Furthermore, SV40 can be isolated from infected mammalian cells in a form which contains polymerase II as a transcription complex.[55] An alternative approach has been to raise antibodies to form II polymerase of *Drosophila melanogaster*[56] and to show that these antibodies bind in the chromosomal interband regions and puffs which are known to be transcriptionally active in the larval salivary gland, adding further weight to the conclusion that form II is involved in mRNA synthesis.

Having established that polymerase III was inhibited by high concentrations of α-amanitin, 5S and pre-4S genes were shown to be transcribed by this enzyme in mammalian nuclei[50] and chromatin.[57] Furthermore, this enzyme has been implicated in the expression of viral 5.5S and cellular 5S and pre-4S RNA in adenovirus-2 infected HeLa cells[58] and 5.5S and 5S RNA synthesis late in productive infection of KB cells by adenovirus.[59]

E. Selective Transcription by Eukaryotic RNA Polymerases In Vitro

Functions for each class of RNA polymerase have been established, but the problem of reproducing selective expression of specific coding sequences in vitro has been intractable. There are a number of obvious reasons for this. The vast complexity of the eukaryotic genome has tended to restrict attention to those sequences which are heavily reiterated (particularly those for the stable RNAs, tRNA and rRNA). Even in these cases, attempts to reproduce in vitro the in vivo function of the different RNA polymerases has been complicated by our inability to isolate intact DNA duplex, devoid of single-stranded breaks ("nicks") which constitute pseudopromoters for the polymerases. Small bacteriophage DNAs provided the answer to these problems in studies of bacterial polymerase specificity, but animal viral DNAs have not proved to be the solution in the eukaryotic case. The reader is referred to Chambon's review article[28] where these difficulties are discussed in depth. We shall concentrate on recent experiments concerning the transcription of rRNA and 5S RNA coding sequences in vitro using purified RNA polymerases I and III respectively.

The work of Van Keulen et al.[60] and Van Keulen and Retel[61] on the transcription of rRNA coding sequences by the purified form I enzyme from yeast deserves careful scrutiny. Throughout their experiments, they use an enzyme prepared from whole cells of exponentially growing *Saccharomyces carlsbergensis*. The following facts are established:

1. Using heterologous templates (such as phage DNAs), transcription occurs only from "nicks".
2. Symmetrical transcription tends to occur at high enzyme to DNA ratios and is exacerbated by the presence of Mn^{++} in the reaction medium.
3. The yeast form I polymerase transcript of homologous, high molecular weight DNA in the presence of 5 mM Mg^{++} gives rise to a predominantly asymmetric product up to 3×10^6 daltons in size.
4. It is shown that up to 85% of this transcript is ribosomal RNA, the largest species corresponding to the known 42S rRNA precursor, and contains the 5' terminal, nonconserved spacer; there is no evidence that spacer sequences not transcribed in vivo are copied in this in vitro system.

It can be concluded, therefore, that in these experiments, the form I polymerase carries out correct initiation and termination events which must be the criteria for the definition of polymerase specificity.

Within these data lie the answers to many of the problems which have dogged the demonstration of enzyme specificity in vitro. High molecular weight, intact DNAs are inevitably a prerequisite. The use of Mn^{++} as the divalent metal ion obscures polymerase specificity, and it is clear from the data presented that the *E. coli* RNA polymerase is no substitute for the homologous enzyme. The requirement to use low enzyme to DNA ratios in order to demonstrate selective transcription is supported by similar observations[62] which arose from studies in our own laboratory which indicated selective expression by form I RNA polymerase[63] of ribosomal cistrons in a system derived from *Xenopus laevis;* as it is probably impossible to obtain high molecular weight DNA with no "nicks", there may be some salvation in the appealing argument that, in DNA excess, the high affinity of the polymerase for its "promoters" may be dominant, while excess enzyme tends to transcribe from "nicks". It is also worth bearing in mind that both of the pieces of work cited here make use of enzyme extraction protocols which either select for polymerase not bound to the chromosome or enzymes taken from whole cells (which will be a mixture of enzyme derived from all potential pools).

A rather different approach has been adopted to examine the specificity of polymerase III. In *X. laevis,* the 5S genes are tandemly arranged and interspersed with non-transcribed spacer regions. Parker and Roeder[64] have studied the transcription of these genes in chromatin derived from stage 1 oocytes by homologous class III and I_A RNA polymerases and class II mouse myeloma enzyme and the *E. coli* RNA polymerase. Using a 5S *X. mulleri* DNA probe (produced in a recombinant plasmid), they show that purified polymerase III stimulates 5S synthesis 10- to 50-fold and 5S RNA accounts for between 30 and 50% of the total RNA synthesized (i.e., 3000-fold above random); the product was preferentially transcribed from the sense strand and was very similar in size to 5S RNA from the cells. However, there was evidence that spacer sequences (not transcribed in vivo) were copied to a significant extent by the exogenous enzyme, implying incorrect chain termination. None of the other eukaryotic enzymes (homologous or otherwise) stimulated 5S synthesis, and the *E. coli* polymerase, though giving rise to some 5S sequence, transcribed the antisense strand also. These conclusions have been generally borne out by Yamamoto et al.[65] from the in vitro transcription of HeLa chromatin by HeLa polymerase III. However, Parker and Roeder[64] extended their studies to the in vitro transcription of *Xenopus* native DNA (rather than chromatin) but failed to show convincing selective expression of the 5S sequences by polymerase III. Part of the reason for this may be the state of intactness of their DNA template (not stated) and the fact that these experiments were carried out at saturating enzyme concentrations. Bearing in mind the criteria for selective transcription in vitro from Van Keulen and Retel's work (see above), it may be too early to conclude that "chromatin-associated proteins are required for the selective and asymmetric transcription of the 5S RNA genes in amphibian oocytes" by polymerase III[64].

The diagnosis of selective transcription by an RNA polymerase is determined by our ability to define correct initiation and termination of RNA synthesis. For polymerases I and III, this is possible because the structure of the in vivo primary gene transcripts (and, in some cases, the gene themselves) are known. The problem is very different for polymerase II. The comfortable (!) hypothesis that the coding sequence for a protein lies at the 3'-terminus of a macro-molecular mRNA precursor is beginning to look a little old fashioned at the time of writing (December 1977). Until a coherent model is available, describing the nature of messenger RNA precursors, it is going to be difficult to pursue this problem further. In the meantime, the fact that a DNA sequence is transcribed in vitro by the form II RNA polymerase (be it in the form of "native" DNA or chromatin) cannot be taken as indicative of ipso facto polymerase specificity as the structure of the DNA or the arrangement of its associated proteins may dictate which sequences are expressed. This is not to deny form II the property of 'specificity'. The consistent observation that this enzyme does not transcribe ribosomal cistrons[61] or 5S rRNA sequences,[64] under in vitro conditions where preferential expression of these genes is achieved by other enzymes, is evidence (albeit negative) that form II initiates RNA synthesis at discrete DNA loci. The problem is that we lack the criteria to distinguish between correct and random initiation events at the moment.

In conclusion, attention should be drawn to an underlying theme in the foregoing discussion. Circumstantial evidence from a number of laboratories where some degree of transcription selectivity has been demonstrated in vitro (with polymerases I and III) hints that the source (and, hence, the nature) of the enzyme may be a critical consideration: the usual enzyme extraction procedures which tend to select for chromatin-bound polymerases may, by analogy with the prokaryote transcription system, give rise to a "core enzyme" fundamentally unable to initiate transcription correctly. This argument may be particularly pertinent to the form II RNA polymerase where the conditions for optimal activity of the purified enzyme (high-salt concentrations, Mn^{++} and a single-stranded DNA template) may be described charitably as being somewhat unphysiological!

III. THEORETICAL BASIS FOR THE REGULATION OF RNA SYNTHESIS AT THE LEVEL OF THE RNA POLYMERASES

Before discussing the experimental data which relate to the control of gene expression at the level of RNA synthesis, the theoretical basis on which such regulation might be founded will be considered. In the light of current knowledge of the multiplicity, structure, and functions of eukaryotic RNA polymerases, there would appear to be a limited number of mechanisms by which control could be exerted at the enzyme level. Later, the experimental evidence from many laboratories will be examined in an attempt to determine whether data are available which provide a clear indication that any or all of these potential control mechanisms operate in vivo.

It seems to us that three major ways can be envisaged in which polymerase molecules could be involved in regulatory processes. The mechanisms proposed below are discussed in relation to quantitative, rather than qualitative, changes in the rates of transcription of particular genes but would apply equally to the extreme cases of qualitative switches, where such occur.

A. Gross Alteration in the Amount of Active Enzyme

This implies a change in the number of RNA polymerase molecules (of any particular class) being made available for transcription, a situation which could be created either by *de novo* synthesis (or degradation) of enzyme or by activation (or inactivation) of previously existing molecules from or to a totally inert state. This model requires that either *de novo* synthesis of polymerase may constitute a potential regulatory event (under conditions where there is no change in the rate of degradation of the enzyme) or a regulatory gene coding for a polymerase degradase could be invoked. The controlled synthesis or degradation of a single polypeptide component of these multimeric polymerase molecules could equally well satisfy this concept of control; in this instance, the subunit whose expression is regulated may function as an allosteric effector, in the absence of which "core" polymerase is totally inactive. The existence of multiple species of RNA polymerase gives rise to the possibility that the *de novo* synthesis of enzymes (or allosteric effectors which are required for their activity) could be controlled at the level of transcription as the mRNA for one RNA polymerase (or a subunit thereof) is transcribed by another class of enzyme. Of course, regulation could also be applied at other well-characterized posttranscriptional events.

The overall effect of this type of mechanism is to alter the concentration of active RNA polymerases and, therefore, to modify the potential for the number of RNA initiation events per unit of time. Another implication is that there must be, in the case of stimulation of RNA synthesis, a capacity for more initiation events to occur, i.e., the gene dosage cannot be rate-limiting and the gene must not be previously saturated with RNA polymerases.

B. A Change in the Catalytic "Efficiency" of Active Polymerase

The possibility must be considered that the rate of RNA synthesis could be altered by changing the properties of already active RNA polymerase molecules. This implies a finer control than that exhibited by the first mechanism proposed above and could theoretically be exerted at virtually any stage of the transcription process. In practice, this would presumably depend upon which stage was rate-limiting under the particular circumstances. In situations of polymerase limitation, increased efficiency of promoter association and/or initiation would perhaps be most effective in stimulating RNA synthesis. In situations of gene-dosage limitation, where cistrons are packed with polymerases, an alteration of the elongation rate may serve the same purpose. In both cases, the basis for such control could reside either in the interaction of some low molecular weight effector or a novel polypeptide with the polymerase or in the covalent modification of the polymerase, e.g., phosphorylation. However, the important distinguishing feature of this type of regulation is that there is no change in the number of active RNA polymerase molecules, only their ability to carry out the different stages in RNA synthesis has been modified.

By invoking factors which affect the rate of RNA synthesis in either a positive or a negative mode, certain mechanistic limitations have been imposed. Any modification of initiation which increases the efficiency of the process will have immediate and progressive effects depending on the number of polymerases so modified (assuming a polymerase-limited situation). The same should be true of negative initiation factors. A different situation, however, must be envisaged for elongation factors since, during linear transcription of a cistron, the rates of polymerase movement (assuming saturation of the cistron with polymerase) will presumably be limited by the slowest molecule. Thus, for a positive elongation factor to function, the polymerase pool would need to be saturated with it. Perhaps more interestingly, a negative factor might function if only one polymerase per cistron was affected by it.

Within the strict terms of reference for this review, it must be acknowledged that it is going to be difficult to differentiate between the type of effector molecules discussed above which interact directly with or modify the active RNA polymerase and other regulatory phenomena which elicit a similar response but which do not involve any structural modification of the enzyme involved (such as the interaction of the cAMP-binding protein with a site on the lac promoter which facilitates polymerase binding[2]). In the case of factors whose putative role is to modify elongation rates, due consideration must be given to the importance of posttranscriptional events. Such processing appears to be ubiquitous in eukaryotes for all types of RNA and usually occurs immediately after (or possibly even during) the termination of transcription. Furthermore, processing is probably a major point of regulation itself. Thus, interpretation of altered elongation rates may be complicated by the possibility of feedback effects directly consequent on rates of termination and processing. Careful observations will always be necessary to determine where the rate-limiting regulatory step is actually located.

C. Modulation of RNA Polymerase Specificity

The mechanisms described above were conceived in the context of the expression of discrete genes and not in relation to the genome as a whole. Although some classes of genes, perhaps all, may be subject to large quantitative variations in their rates of transcription, an even more complex situation arises when considering the regulation of genes relative to one another. This must more closely approximate to the problem faced by the living cell, but unfortunately there is, as yet, little information on the true complexity of the phenomenon. We have only limited data on the degree to which individual gene sequences are regulated in relation to others and the extent to which controls are applied to "batteries" of genes to create particular viable phenotypes rather than to large numbers of structural genes independently. The mechanisms described in Sections III. A and B might easily apply to groups of genes transcribed by the same RNA polymerase, and effectors might exist capable of influencing the activities of more than one type of enzyme when coordinate regulation is required. However, the multiplicity of the eukaryotic RNA polymerases is sufficient only to obtain a coarse control of the major classes of RNA and not the variety of messenger RNA populations exhibited, for example, by the various cell types in differentiated organisms.[66] Indeed, it seems likely that only one of the major RNA polymerase classes (type II) is involved in the vast majority of messenger RNA synthesis in eukaryotes. Messenger RNA populations in animal cells within the same organism vary both qualitatively and quantitatively between cell types, with distinct abundance classes differing by orders of magnitude in their relative occurrences in the cytoplasm.[67,68] Could regulation of these phenomena be exerted at the RNA polymerase level?

Even assuming that batteries of genes, rather than individual sequences, are controlled coordinately, it is clear that specific recognition events must be involved at some stage in the processes of activation or repression. The precise number of activity states which need to be invoked to explain the diversity of cell types in complex differentiated eukaryotes is impossible to compute accurately, but if the intermediate conditions which presumably occur during the developmental process together with the ability of many differentiated cell types to respond to effector molecules (thus changing their state) are taken into account, many hundreds of combinations must necessarily be possible within the coding capacity of a single genome. Perhaps the most extreme example of the difficulties faced in trying to rationalize these problems concerns the flexibility of the response of lymphocytes to antigenic stimulation and the enormous range of gene products (in the form of antibody peptides) which can be individually induced.

To explain these observations on the basis of regulation at the RNA polymerase level alone would require that the enzyme be capable of existing in a large number of different states, each with its own promoter specificity. Assuming that only one species of eukaryotic RNA polymerase is involved in mRNA biosynthesis, it would be necessary to speculate upon the existence of complex equilibria between different enzyme forms mediated by unknown specificity factors characteristic of each cell type and state. It seems highly improbable that, even in the case of an enzyme as structurally complex as RNA polymerase, the capacity for such extensive modulation could exist. However, that is not to say that some discrimination could not be exerted at the polymerase level; a coarse control of large classes of mRNA populations might be feasible by invoking only a few enzyme forms, acting coordinately with more specific regulatory factors perhaps intrinsic to the gene sequences or associated proteins.

Despite the necessarily vague and speculative nature of RNA polymerase controls of this type, it is nevertheless possible to make certain predictions as to the kinds of situation one would expect to find if they were operative. For example, abundances of messenger RNAs would be strictly coordinated; if a number of types were abundant in one cell, it would be expected that all of these would vary with respect to different abundance levels in other cells dependent on the abundance of the polymerase form recognizing the class of promoters implicitly common to all of them. Secondly, the model requires that the form II RNA polymerase should in total be present at concentrations close to the optimal needed for adequate transcription of the gene complement; in the absence of other controls, excess enzyme would presumably lead to significant transcription of sequences not required by the particular cell type, i.e., "gene leakage" would result.

IV. SOME GUIDELINES FOR THE ASSESSMENT OF EXPERIMENTAL INFORMATION

In the foregoing section, an attempt has been made to assemble a set of coherent mechanisms for the regulation of RNA synthesis which might involve the RNA polymerase(s). The work of the last 10 years has led to our being able to formulate these models. But it should be emphasized that the published experiments which will be reviewed below were not designed to probe these regulatory mechanisms specifically, and inevitably many of them fail to satisfy completely the criteria prescribed by any one of the models. A number of potentially useful systems have been identified where changes in the rates of synthesis of distinct RNA species are evident. It might be useful at this time to lay down one or two guidelines, based on the strictures imposed by the control mechanisms described above, which will aid in the assessment of available data.

The experimental systems widely used to study RNA synthesis can be divided into three categories: (1) RNA synthesis in intact cells; (2) RNA synthesis in organelles and cell fractions; and (3) the resolution and purification of RNA polymerases either from whole cells or cell fractions. We have looked for unequivocal evidence of (1) *de novo* synthesis and/or degradation of specific RNA polymerases; (2) activation of existing (inert?) enzyme molecules; (3) changes in the rate of initiation or elongation of RNA chains; and (4) changes in the properties of an enzyme species which might be indicative of a change in template specificity.

Probably the most contentious issue which arises from this survey is what is meant by the term the "level of enzyme activity", and experiments which demonstrate changes in enzyme "level" dominate the literature. It is clear that, in principle, such measurements could provide useful information. However, a clear distinction must be drawn between two parameters which prescribe this phenomenon: the *total activity* of the enzyme molecules present in a system and the *absolute activity* of enzyme molecules present. The total activity of enzyme molecules can be defined in terms of RNA synthesized in vitro under *optimal* conditions of substrate (nucleoside triphosphates), divalent metal ion, ionic strength, and the DNA template; attention will be drawn to (frequent) instances where changes in the rate of RNA synthesis have been indicated but where these fundamental conditions have not been satisfied in the design of the experiment. UTP is commonly used as the labeled RNA precursor in in vitro experiments. Roeder and Rutter[24] showed that increasing the concentration from 5 to 120 μM gave rise to a sixfold increase in RNA synthesis, and Mondal et al.[69] have demonstrated that at least 150 μM UTP is required to avoid substrate limitation effects with the coconut endosperm RNA polymerases. Our own observations suggest that at least 40 μM pyrimidine nucleoside triphosphate and a minimum of 200 μM purine nucleoside triphosphate are required to support the maximum activity of the mammalian RNA polymerases. This is clearly an important point when experiments are designed to use "enzyme activities" as indicative of "enzyme levels" in different situations and one which has been neglected in a surprisingly large number of cases. Where the RNA synthetic capacity of whole cells or organelles is under investigation, a knowledge of the endogenous pool sizes of substrates and cofactors is critical so that the dilution of labeled precursors can be assessed accurately. Some attempt should also be made to screen any experimental system for the presence of contaminating activities (such as nucleases) which interfere with the study of RNA synthesis rates.

The absolute numbers of enzyme molecules present in a system may be defined using specific antisera raised to specific RNA polymerase species, bearing in mind the known sharing of some antigenic determinants between polymerases.[38,39] An alternative to immunoprecipitation is the purification of enzyme protein; however, the extreme lability of eukaryotic RNA polymerases and low yields (in the range of 2 to 15%) might lead to selective loss of less stable enzyme species and to intolerable error factors in quantitative comparisons.

Another area to which attention should be drawn is the distinction between potentially inert and physiologically active RNA polymerases. With the type of degraded and "nicked" DNA templates in common usage, it is unlikely that this distinction is possible at the moment. Using high concentrations (in excess of 50 $\mu g/m\ell$) actinomycin D to inhibit DNA-bound RNA polymerase, a pool of "free" enzyme can be identified using the synthetic deoxyribo-polymer poly d(A-T);[29,32] but it is not possible to construe whether the pool of "free" polymerase constitutes a physiologically active form of the enzyme because inactive (or inert) polymerase may transcribe the artificial templates used in this type of experiment. Furthermore, our lack of suitable DNA templates imposes severe limitations on our ability to define differential initiation specificity within a single class of RNA polymerase.

We have borne these general restrictions in mind when constructing our analysis of those published experiments which have laid the groundwork for future investigations of RNA synthesis control mechanisms.

V. SYSTEMS EXHIBITING TRANSCRIPTIONAL CONTROL

A number of situations have been examined in which changes in the state of cells and tissues appear to be accompanied by demonstrable alterations in the pattern of RNA synthesis. We will now consider the types of systems which have been investigated and the depth of biochemical understanding which has accrued in relation to fundamental mechanism.

A. Development and Differentiation

Developmental systems are attractive subjects for examining the regulation of gene expression for a number of reasons. Primarily, the processes of determination and terminal differentiation represent the most challenging and least understood areas of biology today; in addition, changes in the pattern of gene expression clearly occur and may be reflected in gross changes in the rates of RNA synthesis at various stages of ontogeny. Finally, the system is valuable because it usually requires little in the way of artificial instigation; virtually all other regulatory situations need to be induced in some specific way by the experimenter.

Perhaps the most thoroughly studied developmental program is that of the amphibia, and soon after methods became available for isolating the eukaryotic RNA polymerases, the presence of these enzymes in the germinal vesicles of *Rana* oocytes was detected.[70] The mature oocyte is essentially inactive in RNA synthesis, yet these cells contained some 400,000-fold more enzyme than an individual embryonic cell. All three classes of enzyme were present, with form II predominating. This observation was essentially confirmed by Roeder[71] who examined RNA polymerase levels both during oogenesis and early development in *Xenopus laevis*. Large amounts of all classes of polymerase accumulated through oogenesis, in no way reflecting the sequential expression of 5S, 40S, and HnRNA during the same period (Table 2). Thus, the turnover of the RNA polymerase itself coincides with other aspects of oogenesis during which large amounts of "maternal macromolecules" (including ribosomes and DNA polymerases) are assembled for utilization during the phase of rapid cell division following fertilization. The early phases of embryonic development are characterized by little change in the overall polymerase content of the embryo (but, of course, a rapid drop on a per cell basis), again without any correlation between the three enzyme types and the bursts of HnRNA, ribosomal, and transfer RNA synthesis which occur between blastula and gastrula stages (Table 3). Unlike *Rana, Xenopus* oocytes contain a large amount of form III RNA polymerase which gradually drops between the gastrula and swimming tadpole stages to the much smaller proportion characteristic of adult tissues.[63,71,72] Whether this phenomenon is in any way related to the very high number of 5S genes in *Xenopus* (some 25,000 per haploid genome) and the existence of distinct oocyte and somatic 5S RNAs remains to be resolved. These experiments on RNA polymerase levels merely reflect the enzyme activities assessed on exogenous templates and do not quantify the amounts of enzyme protein in the cells. In related work, Roeder[73] suggests that RNA polymerase II_A of *Xenopus* somatic tissues may be of cytoplasmic origin; this species is also present in relatively large amounts in the mature oocytes and tends to disappear during development,[71] perhaps reflecting the utilization of a soluble pool of enzyme. Interestingly, this latter observation has found support in studies of soybean germination. In this instance, ungerminated embryos contain predominantly soluble RNA polymerase II in the II_A form, with a heavy subunit of 200K daltons. Subsequent to germination, the enzyme is found mainly bound to chromatin and in the II_B form, with a large subunit of 170K daltons.[47] Also, *Drosophila* embryos contain polymerase II with a 215K heavy subunit which is replaced in cultured cells by one of 170K daltons.[74] This conversion could be observed in vitro in crossover experiments and was not prevented by the serine protease inhibitor phenyl-methyl-sulphonyl fluoride (PMSF).

Changes of this sort during development have not been observed in the other RNA polymerases. Form I exhibits microheterogeneity in *Xenopus,* but forms I_A and I_B are present in similar amounts during development and both occur in the anucleolar mutant which synthesizes no 40S rRNA and has no ribosomal genes. However, possible experimental interconversion of these two forms of this class of enzyme described above (Section IIC.1) somewhat clouds this particular issue.

Table 2
LEVELS OF RNA POLYMERASE ACTIVITIES DURING
XENOPUS LAEVIS OOGENESIS

		RNA polymerase activity					
		I		II		III	
Experiment	Stage	Units/10^4	%	Units/10^4	%	Units/10^4	%
1	Small oocyte (immature ovary)	22	31	27	37	24	32
2	Small oocyte (purified)	N.D.[a]	31	N.D.	32	N.D.	37
3	Medium oocyte	N.D.	37	N.D.	28	N.D.	35
4	Mature oocyte	11,200	33	12,400	36	10,600	31
5	Mature oocyte	15,800		14,100		11,800	
	Germinal vesicle	17,000		10,700		9,700	
6	Mature oocyte	10,800		21,600		7,400	
	Unfertilized egg	11,300		26,000		7,400	

Note: Various proportions of each RNA polymerase were calculated following DEAE-Sephadex® chromatography of the solubilized RNA polymerase preparations. Enzyme I activity includes I_A and I_B activities, and enzyme II activity includes both II_A and II_B activities. In experiment 1, the number of cells per ovary was estimated from the average amount of rDNA (rRNA genes) present in these ovaries. The data shown for experiments 3 and 4 represent, respectively, averages of three and six experiments, all performed under comparable conditions. In the other experiments, the data are from single representative experiments. In experiment 5, germinal vesicles were from the same batch of oocytes used for the mature oocyte determinations in the same experiment. In experiment 6, mature oocytes and unfertilized eggs were from the same female; the oocytes were removed from the excised ovary 1 day after ovulation of the eggs. For these experiments, three different DNA template preparations were used in the assay of the RNA polymerases: one for experiments 1 to 4, a second for experiment 5, and a third for experiment 6.

[a] N.D. — values not determined.

From Roeder, R. G., *J. Biol. Chem.*, 249, 249, 1974. With permission.

Hydration of encysted gastrulae of the brine shrimp *Artemia* has recently been used as a model system in which to observe the induction of RNA synthesis as development proceeds.[75] Levels of free and bound enzymes I and II were measured in isolated nuclei, using actinomycin D and poly d(A-T). The data indicate a drop in the level of unbound enzymes and a rise in the numbers attached to the template (confirmed by estimations of numbers of elongating RNA chains), concurrent with the rapid synthesis of new ribosomes and mRNAs. Some reservations must be expressed concerning the quantitation of enzyme levels in this work due to the use of rate-limiting concentrations of labeled RNA precursor (only 10 μM) when probing soluble enzyme activity; although nuclei potentially have an endogenous pool of nucleoside triphosphates which may prevent rate-limiting effects, account should be taken of the fact that this pool may itself vary between different metabolic situations and, thus, give rise to apparent changes in endogenous RNA polymerase activity due to altered specific activities of substrates.

Developmental systems of the above sorts suffer the disadvantage of increasing cell diversity which cannot easily be reconciled with examination of RNA polymerase levels

Table 3
LEVELS OF RNA POLYMERASE ACTIVITIES DURING EMBRYONIC DEVELOPMENT

RNA polymerase activity

Niewkoop-Faber stage		Cell number	Units/10⁴ embryos				Units/10⁴ cells			
			I	II$_A$	II$_B$	III	I	II$_A$	II$_B$	III
1	Unfertilised egg	1	10,500	7,700	17,200	9,500	10,500	7,700	17,200	9,500
2-6	Cleavage	8	10,900	9,500	15,600	11,800	1,700	1,200	1,900	1,500
11-14	Late gastrula	62,000	11,500	9,770	23,900	11,600	0.19	0.16	0.39	0.19
10-22	Late neurula	106,000	17,600	11,200	36,300	13,200	0.17	0.10	0.34	0.12
30-33	Heartbeat	255,000	50,800	16,300	70,700	18,200	0.20	0.06	0.28	0.07
38-40	Swimming tadpole	420,000	90,800	23,000	117,000	19,800	0.19	0.05	0.28	0.04
43-46	Swimming tadpole	900,000	131,000	18,000	113,000	20,000	0.15	0.02	0.13	0.02
	Cultured kidney cells						0.18	0.02	0.15	0.02

Note: Data were calculated from DEAE-Sephadex® chromatographic analyses of solubilized enzyme preparations. In all cases, the numbers of eggs and embryos were counted directly. The average number of cells per embryo at the cleavage stage was ascertained by microscopic examination. For later stage embryos and or cultured cells, cell numbers were determined by colorimetric estimation of DNA content in the homogenates, using a value of 6 pg of DNA per diploid cell. For full details, see Roeder.[71,73]

From Roeder, R. G., *J. Biol. Chem.*, 249, 249, 1974.

assessed on a "per embryo" basis; intercellular differences cannot be detected by these relatively crude approaches.[29] The problem has been circumvented to some extent by the examination of RNA polymerases in terminally differentiating erythrocytes. Van der Westhuyzen et al.[76] examined RNA polymerase levels in avian erythrocytes following anemia induced by phenyl-hydrazine. Only form II polymerase was detected; the level of the enzyme (measured by activity in nuclei after solubilization) rose three- to fourfold over the period of stimulated RNA and protein synthesis (2 to 4 days after induction) but was maintained at a high level long after these syntheses had returned to steady-state rates. Other workers[77,78] have found all three RNA polymerase species in avian erythrocytes. Longacre and Rutter[77] observed a decline in activities I and II (fractionated on DEAE-Sephadex®) over the differentiation period, with form I dropping off faster than form II. Tests with rat liver RNA polymerases ruled out the production of inhibitors during this period, but assays were performed at limiting substrate concentrations. Form III was low throughout. The drop in form I coincided with the decrease in rRNA biosynthesis, but residual amounts of I and II enzymes remained at times when RNA synthesis in vivo was no longer detectable. Kruger and Seifart[78] observed that forms I and III persisted in a soluble form (heparin-sensitive) after cessation of rRNA synthesis and that nuclei from mature erythrocytes contained only form II as a template-bound entity. The mature cells have no nucleoli.

The consensus from these experiments would seem to be that changes in rates of RNA synthesis during development are not reflected by overall amounts of RNA polymerase activities as measured on exogenous templates in vitro. However, there is evidence of changes in both the structure and functional states of certain enzymes during development, though the data on these aspects must be regarded as preliminary.

B. Tumor Cells

Some attempts have been made to compare RNA polymerase activities from cancerous and normal tissues. Of course, many of the cell lines routinely used to study RNA metabolism (such as HeLa and Ascites) are transformed, but these cannot be compared sensibly with any particular differentiated tissue. Chesterton et al.[79] looked at the types of enzymes in both cytosol and nuclear fractions of rat liver and a minimal deviation hepatoma cell line. This work was performed before the different properties of DEAE-cellulose and DEAE-Sephadex® were known (forms I and III cochromatograph on DEAE-cellulose[80] and, in the final analysis using phosphocellulose, forms I_B and III cochromatograph). Expressing their results as activity per milligram DNA, i.e., on a per cell basis, it was concluded that the tumor cells contained twice as much forms I_A and II but some nine times as much form I_B as the normal liver cells. As the latter component will be contaminated by form III, the actual species which is elevated in this situation is unknown and is of potential importance. More recent work on rat hepatoma[81] detected the same polymerase species as those seen by Chesterton et al.,[80] but these observations were confined to nuclear enzymes and no major differences in levels were observed. However, it was noticed that the tumor polymerases appeared to have very different ionic strength optima for in vitro activity when compared with the liver enzymes; form I was down from 40 to 10 mM ammonium sulfate and form II from 100 to 50 mM. If true, this would add a further complication to interpreting the earlier data, but it should be noted that a number of factors affect such optima including enzyme to DNA ratios, which do not necessarily reflect fundamental changes in the enzymes (personal observations). It is clearly important, however, to optimize assay conditions for each set of circumstances, and this has rarely been done in published work.

Capobianco et al.[82] fractionated RNA polymerases from four tumors of liver and

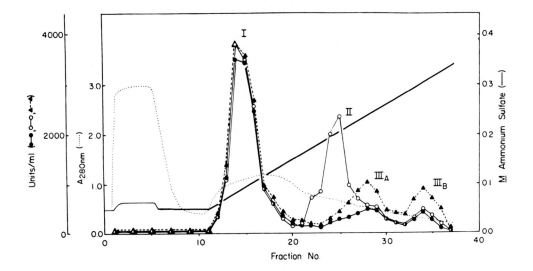

FIGURE 1. DEAE-Sephadex® chromatography of RNA polymerases from MOPC 315 tumors. This figure shows the classical resolution on DEAE-Sephadex® of the different classes of RNA polymerase derived from high-salt, sonication of 10 g MOPC 315 tumor cells.[37] Fractions eluted from the column by a salt gradient were assayed for RNA polymerase activity in the absence (○——○) or presence (●——●) of 0.5 μg/mℓ α-amanitin using calf thymus DNA as the template or with poly-d(A-T) as the template in the presence of 0.5 μg/mℓ α-amanitin (▲——▲); ———, ammonium sulfate concentration defining the salt gradient; ————, absorbance at 280 nm. (From Schwartz, L. B., Sklar, V. E. F., Jaehning, J. A., Weinmann, R., and Roeder, R. G., *J. Biol. Chem.*, 249, 5889, 1974. With permission.)

kidney on DEAE-Sephadex® and compared them with enzymes from normal tissues. Nuclei were used as the enzyme source. The tumors all exhibited two types of form I RNA polymerases and one form II, whereas normal tissues showed no microheterogeneity of form I on this chromedia. No form III was seen in any instance. The tumors were more active in RNA synthesis than their parent tissues, but no changes in enzyme levels (of the common forms) were apparent, perhaps because limiting substrate concentrations (15 μM) were used.

The most thorough investigations of tumor cells have been made by Schwartz et al.[37] and Schwartz and Roeder.[83,84] These workers isolated RNA polymerase from mouse myeloma MOPC 315 (Figure 1) and compared the types and amounts present with those of somatic tissues (Table 4). Polymerase levels were assessed primarily on the basis of enzyme activity, taking into account losses during the purification procedure as far as these could be estimated. The losses could be greater than calculated since no account was taken of the existence or fate of nuclease, etc. through the isolation steps. Conditions for optimal activity were established and high (nonlimiting) substrate concentrations were used. It was deduced that mouse myeloma cells contain a preponderance of form I polymerase (Figure 1), in agreement with the other work on tumor cells mentioned above. Levels of forms I, II, and III were estimated to be seven- to eightfold, twofold, and sixfold higher, respectively, in myeloma than in liver (expressed as units per milligram DNA). Form III$_B$ seemed to be a cytoplasmic species, and form III$_A$ nucleoplasmic in these tumor cells. Interestingly, liver cells from mice harboring MOPC tumors also had elevated RNA polymerase contents (forms, I, II, and III increased by factors of three-, 1.3-, and less than twofold, respectively). No new forms of enzyme were detected in the tumor cells, but Schwartz et al.[37] estimated, on the basis of calculations of enzyme content, that RNA polymerase I concentration might be rate-limiting in ribosomal gene expression: from known ribosomal gene con-

Table 4
LEVELS OF RNA POLYMERASE
ACTIVITIES IN DIFFERENT TISSUES

	I	II	III
	Units of RNA polymerase activity/ mg DNA		
MOPC 315 tumors	5500	2600	1100
BALB/c liver	764	1350	186
MOPC 315 BALB/c liver	2330	1780	292
BALB/c spleen	210	1138	137
MOPC 315 BALB/c spleen	1150	1380	310
Calf thymus	527	1040	46

Note: Data were calculated from DEAE-Sephadex® chromatographic analyses of enzymes solubilized from tissues and are presented as units of activity related to tissue DNA content. RNA polymerase III represents the summation of III_A and III_B activities. For further experimental details, the original paper should be consulted.[37]

From Schwartz, L. B., Sklar, V. E. F., Jaehning, J. A., Weinmann, R., and Roeder, R. G., *J. Biol. Chem.*, 249, 5889, 1974. With permission.

tent and polymerase packing ratios, it was deduced that 0.5 to 1.8×10^5 enzyme molecules would be needed to saturate the cistrons (assuming all were available for transcription). Liver cells contain only 2×10^4 polymerase I molecules, but MOPC cells could achieve saturation with their 1.5×10^5 enzyme molecules.

These data, taken overall, infer that some change in the form I polymerase may be a feature of tumor cells, but very much more information on this point is needed for any more meaningful conclusion. Whether this reflects a novel type of enzyme I or a change in the relative proportions of the well-known subspecies remains unclear. Interpretation of RNA polymerase patterns here is less meaningful than in most other situations because two stable states are being compared, rather than the temporal transition from one to another; tumor cells differ from normal ones in a great many ways, the simple observation of which tells us nothing about the process of carcinogenesis.

C. Tissue Regeneration

Perhaps one of the crudest methods of inducing dramatic metabolic changes in an organism has involved the partial removal of an organ (usually the liver) followed by careful monitoring of the subsequent recovery phase. Up to 90% of a mammalian liver can be removed and the loss made up by regeneration, providing that the body temperature of the animal is maintained by external sources. The new liver achieves essentially the same final size as the original, though it is amorphous and lacks distinct lobe structure. Following the operation, the cells of the residual stump hypertrophy to twice their original size over the initial 24 hr. This is accompanied by an enlargement of the nucleus, a decrease in the average number of nucleoli per cell, but an increase in their individual sizes and ribosomal gene content.[85] As the cells proceed towards DNA synthesis and division, there is a large increase in the synthesis of ribosomes, peaking at around 18 hr after hepatectomy.

Novello and Stirpe[86] investigated the endogenous RNA polymerases in rat liver nuclei from animals of various ages and following hepatectomy. The latter situation caused a doubling of endogenous form I activity and about a 50% increase in form II, peaking by about 18 hr. Yu,[87,88] using the actinomycin/poly d(A-T) technique, demonstrated that rat liver nuclei contain free as well as template-bound RNA polymerases of types I and II (about 70% of free enzyme was form I, though the presence of form III component was not tested for in the initial experiments). Some 17 hr after partial hepatectomy, both free and bound enzyme levels were elevated two- to threefold.[88] For this work, nuclei were isolated in hypertonic sucrose which increases the yields of nuclear RNA polymerases considerably by trapping enzymes which otherwise (in isotonic preparations) leak into the cytosol fraction.[35] Data of this kind, therefore, may be closely related to the total tissue RNA polymerase contents. Free enzyme was washed out of nuclei prepared in hypertonic media using an isotonic buffer and free and bound components were analyzed by DEAE-Sephadex chromatography. Hepatectomy resulted in apparent increases in the template-bound form I and in free form III$_A$. This work is broadly in agreement with the observation of Organtini et al.[89] using isotonically prepared nuclei 18 hr after hepatectomy; these authors also observed a doubling of endogenous nuclear activities (bound), free enzymes (active on poly d[A-T]) and in total activities chromatographed on DEAE-Sephadex®; in the latter experiments, form I was raised twofold and form II rather less. No form III was observed, presumably because of the ease with which it is lost from nuclei during isotonic preparation.[35]

Working with the same tissue, Schmid and Sekeris[90] looked specifically at the effects of form I RNA polymerase in isolated nucleoli 12 to 24 hr after partial hepatectomy. Endogenous and total enzyme activities (after solubilization) were elevated three- to fourfold. Free enzyme in nucleoli was measured simply by the addition of exogenous DNA. The authors went further and titrated enzymes isolated from normal and regenerating tissue against increasing amounts of DNA. They inferred from the results that enzyme from both sources was saturated by the same amount of DNA, a conclusion not entirely supported by the data presented (Figure 2) and that the increased activity was due to modification of preexisting enzyme rather than de novo synthesis of polymerase.

There are problems of interpretation with all of these studies. Conformity in expressing polymerase activity (per milligram protein, per milligram DNA etc.) has not always been maintained, an important factor in a situation where cell size doubles (and, therefore, the number of cells per gram of tissue falls significantly). As we have stressed above, the actinomycin concentration required to prevent a "read-off" contribution to the free pool of enzyme is at least 50 μg/mℓ, and all of the above experiments were carried out at much lower concentrations. The contribution of DNA-binding proteins to the point of DNA saturation of the polymerases was not considered by Schmid and Sekeris (see Figure 2), despite the fact that they observed an increase of 20 to 30% in solubilized nucleolar proteins following hepatectomy. These workers also saw an increase in ribonuclease activity, but neither here nor in most other instances have serious attempts been made to assess the role of factors of this type which may mask or inhibit polymerase activity; one of the simplest ways of probing for these factors is to look at the effects of protein fractions on the activity of a purified RNA polymerase preparation (as applied by Chesterton et al.[79]).

With all these reservations in mind, the consensus of opinion indicates an increase in the "activity levels" (on a per cell basis) of the RNA polymerases following hepatectomy, especially notable in the enzyme forms synthesizing stable RNAs. This increase seems to be reflected in both bound and free pools of the enzymes, though the relative proportions of these may change also. Insufficient data exist to support any particular mechanism for bringing these changes about.

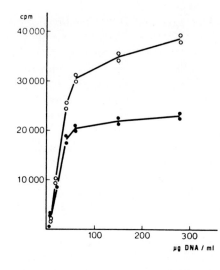

FIGURE 2. RNA synthesis by nucleolar RNA polymerase purified on Biogel A-1.5 derived from control and partially hepatectomized rats. Nucleolar RNA polymerase was solubilized from control rat liver nuclei or from nucleoli of partially hepatectomized rats and purified by fractionation on Bio-Gel® A-1.5. The RNA synthetic potential of these enzymes was then assessed by titrating each with increasing concentrations of DNA. •——•, c.p.m. labeled precursor incorporated into RNA by the control enzyme preparation; O——O, c.p.m. labeled precursor incorporated into RNA by enzyme preparation derived from partially hepatectomized animals. (From Schmid, W. and Sekeris, C. E., *Biochim. Biophys. Acta*, 402, 244, 1975. With permission.)

D. Chemical Effectors

A number of chemicals (carcinogens, mitogens, etc.) have been used to stimulate tissues and cells in ways which do not directly reflect situations normally occurring in vivo. Two particular instances will be considered.

Injection of rats with large doses of thioacetamide (50 mg/kg) has been used to induce the formation of hepatic tumors. Over short-term periods following single doses (up to 24 hr), the treatment results in a massive increase in the number of ribosomes accumulating in the liver cells. Andersen et al.[91] isolated nucleoli from treated animals and demonstrated five- to sevenfold increases in both endogenous and poly d(A-T)-dependent RNA polymerase I activity and interpreted the results as implying an increased number of initiation events. Rate-limiting substrate (15 μM) and low actinomycin D concentrations (20 μg/mℓ) were used: these reservations and the preliminary nature of the results preclude detailed analysis of a potentially interesting system at the present time.

One of the most thoroughly characterized sequence of events is that which follows treatment of resting mammalian lymphocytes with mitogenic plant lectins, especially phytohemaglutinin (PHA). In the continuous presence of this effector, peripheral lymphocytes cultured in vitro undergo a series of morphological and metabolic changes, including a large increase in cell volume (especially of the cytoplasm), the appearance of distinct nucleoli, increased synthesis of protein and RNA, and, ultimately (over about 72 hr), DNA replication leading to cell division.

These events have been studied in considerable detail in many laboratories, and this is one of the few systems in which accurate estimations of pool sizes and nucleotide transport processes have been taken into account when defining changes in the patterns of RNA synthesis in vivo.[92] It is the synthesis of ribosomal RNA which has been investigated most intensively, and a sequence of events has been characterized. Resting lymphocytes exhibit a "wastage" phenomenon; that is to say, a significant proportion of the small amounts of 45S pre-rRNA synthesized by the unstimulated cells is degraded without giving rise to mature 18S species in cytoplasmic ribosomes. Over the first few hours, PHA stimulation leads to a requirement for increased 45S biosynthesis by (1) causing the pool of inactive ribosomes (monomers) to engage in translation, depleting the free pool and (2) preventing wastage, such that virtually all 45S leads to functional rRNAs. There is then an increase in 45S transcription which may be insensitive to protein synthesis inhibitors; this is followed at later times (beyond 24 hr) by a greater increase which is sensitive to such inhibitors (and also a reappearance of wastage).

Several groups have examined the effects of these phenomena on the RNA polymerase activities. Cooke and Brown[93] found that over the first 20 hr, endogenous nuclear form I activity rose fivefold and form II some 1.6-fold. These changes were reflected almost exactly in the amounts of enzymes extracted from the nuclei. Interestingly, these authors also detected a change in the ionic strength optimum for both forms I and II RNA polymerases following PHA stimulation. A more detailed investigation of the total RNA polymerase content of lymphocytes over the time period of PHA stimulation (4 days) was carried out by Jaehning et al.[94] Polymerases were isolated at various time points and resolved on DEAE-Sephadex®; forms I, II, III$_A$, and III$_B$ were identified. All types of polymerases increased coordinately with time, the changes becoming particularly significant beyond the first 12 hr and ultimately leading to 17-fold higher forms I and III activities and eightfold higher form II (see Figure 4). Form II ultimately reaches a level (on a per cell basis) similar to that seen in the liver, whereas forms I and III become considerably more abundant than in that tissue (though none reach the levels seen in malignant plasmacytoma cells). Crossover type experiments designed to test for inhibitors were not carried out, but the authors concluded that the increased activity was most probably due to *de novo* synthesis of enzyme molecules rather than any form of allosteric activation. The observed changes explain to some extent the increases in RNA synthesis observed at later times but not the very early effect on rRNA transcription in particular. It is pertinent to note that an increase in the amount of RNase inhibitor during PHA stimulation has been observed,[95] again emphasizing the need to check out the possibility of such factors affecting polymerase assays. RNase levels are high in resting lymphocytes.

Early events in rRNA biosynthesis (in the first 8 hr) have recently been investigated by Dauphinais and Waithe.[96] Lysine-deprivation did not prevent the early rise in endogenous nuclear RNA polymerase I, though the increase occurred rather more slowly; nor did it affect the low activity of unstimulated lymphocytes. The authors demonstrated an effect of cycloheximide on endogenous form I activity over this early period and claimed (without providing data) that if PHA and cycloheximide were added simultaneously at the start, then even the early stimulations were not seen. Concentrations of radioactive substrates in these experiments were only 15 μM.

Recent work in one of our laboratories[185] has confirmed that measurements of soluble enzyme levels extracted from whole cells bear little relationship to endogenous, template-bound nuclear activities. Much of the increased RNA polymerase content apparent over the first 24 hr exists free in the cytoplasm.

The lymphocyte system offers exciting possibilities for the detailed investigation of

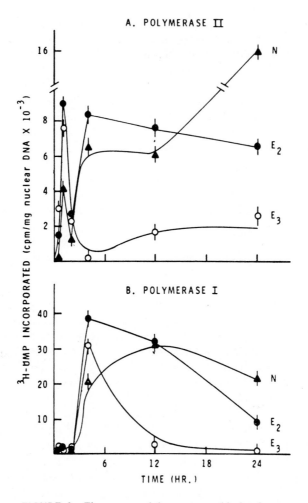

FIGURE 3. Time course of the response of isolated rat uterine nuclear RNA polymerases I and II following treatment of animals with hormones. Animals were injected with estradiol (E₂), estriol (E₃), and Nafoxidine (N) as described in detail by Hardin et al.[107] At the indicated times, uteri were removed, nuclei isolated, and endogenous RNA polymerase activities were determined. (A) RNA polymerase II activity. (B) RNA polymerase I activity. ●———●, E₂; ○———○, E₃; ▲———▲, N. (From Hardin, J. W., Clark, J. H., Glasser, S. R., and Peck, E. J., *Biochemistry*, 15, 1370, 1976. With permission.)

transcriptional control because the system is so well defined and the background work so thoroughly documented. Only the most recent and relevant publications are cited above. We still have no idea about how the early transcriptional events are regulated, and, though RNA polymerase levels apparently rise later on, the nature of the increased activities even at these times has not been defined satisfactorily.

E. Hormones

The molecular mechanisms by which hormones exert their effects on target tissues have received an enormous amount of attention in recent years. In many instances, alterations of the pattern of gene expression have been implicated; we will confine ourselves here with systems that have demonstrated effects on some aspect of RNA polymerase metabolism.

Indole acetic acid (auxin) is perhaps the most thoroughly studied of the plant hormones. Work on the stimulation of lentil root growth demonstrated an effect on RNA polymerases some 14 hr after treatment.[97] No change in nuclear RNA polymerase (endogenous) activities were seen over the first 2 hr during which time mRNA synthesis is apparently elevated, but at later times an increase of form I_B was observed on DEAE-Sephadex® chromatography. This correlated with the time of new ribosome synthesis in vivo. The authors titrated a fixed amount of lentil DNA with increasing amounts of RNA polymerases from control and auxin-stimulated tissues and found that enzymes derived from stimulated systems gave rise to further RNA synthesis when added to an incubation already saturated by control form I_B. This was interpreted to indicate an allosteric or covalent modification of RNA polymerase rather than de novo synthesis, but the enzymes were not highly purified and no account was taken of the effects of possible contaminating activities (such as nucleases, etc.). Guilfoyle et al.[98] looked at the effects of auxins on soybean seedlings after 12 hr and came to similar conclusions; elongating enzymes in nuclei (all apparently of form I type) were elevated five-to sevenfold, and there was an increase in solubilizable form I demonstrated by DEAE-Sephadex® chromatography. These authors also favored an increase in specific activity of preexisting molecules, but it should be noted that radioactive substrates were used at only 10 to 20 μM concentrations in these experiments.

Of the peptide hormones, the most detailed work at the transcriptional level has been carried out by Fuhrman and Gill[99,100] with adenocorticotropic hormone (ACTH) and guinea pig adrenals. Some 14 hr after hormone treatment, adrenal cells exhibit high rates of ribosomal and transfer RNA synthesis; nuclei isolated at this time and assayed for endogenous RNA polymerase activities showed twofold increases in forms I and III (assayed with low concentrations of α-amanitin), with 90% of the activity being of form I. End-group analysis of RNA on polyethyleneimine (PEI)-cellulose suggested no change in the number of chains being elongated by form I enzyme, but transcription in vitro continued for longer than in untreated controls and larger molecules were synthesized. No change was seen in RNase activity, but little account was taken of precursor pool sizes and labeled substrate was provided at only 15 μM. Elongation rates were around one to two nucleotides per second, considerably slower (by an order of magnitude) than those calculated in vivo. However, the authors concluded that a primary effect of ACTH treatment on polymerase I was a doubling of the elongation rates. The second paper examined mainly low molecular weight RNA synthesis by form III enzyme, mainly in terms of 5S and 4S RNAs (although the gel identifications were less than clear). The use of poly d(A-T) and actinomycin D (only 30 $\mu g/$ mℓ) showed that increases in free and template-bound enzymes were occurring; the increase in bound enzyme was mainly form I, whereas the free enzyme was form III. Poly d(A-T) competed with endogenous 4S and 5S RNA synthesis, indicating that reinitiation by polymerase III on the chromatin was occurring in the system. DEAE-Sephadex® analysis of the enzymes showed no change in the overall content of polymerase I following ACTH treatment but the appearance of the minor form I_A and a corresponding decrease in form I_B. Form III_A rose but form III_B, a cytoplasmic enzyme, did not change.

More popular for examination of gene-level effects have been the steroid hormones. Sajdel and Jacob[101] compared hydrocortisone-treated and adrenalectomized rats, isolating nucleoli and form I RNA polymerase fom liver 1.5 hr after hormone injection. Increases in excess of 900% in solubilized form I enzyme were observed on DEAE-Sephadex® between adrenalectomized and hormone-treated animals. Titrating against a fixed concentration of DNA again led the authors to infer allosteric change as the underlying mechanism. The effects were seen on endogenous nucleolar activity but not in solubilized forms II and III. Davies and Griffiths[102] isolated nuclei from castrated rat prostates and looked at the effects on polymerase activities of 5-α-dihydrotestosterone (5αDHT). In the presence of receptor proteins, stimulation of 100 to 150% of endogenous form I and of soluble form I on prostate nucleolar or nuclear chromatin was routinely observed. No effects were seen using liver chromatin or deproteinized DNA as templates, leading the authors to implicate nonhistone chromosomal proteins in the response. This is one of the few instances were direct effects on RNA polymerases have been demonstrated in vitro.

Several laboratories are currently engaged in elucidating the mechanism by which estradiol promotes the biosynthesis of ovalbumin in avian oviduct and the growth of uterine tissue in mammals. Some of these workers have looked at effects on the RNA polymerases of the target organs. Cox et al.[103] demonstrated an increase in endogenous polymerase activities of 300% (form I) and 50% (form II) over 24 hr in oviduct nuclei; these changes were reflected in the DEAE-Sephadex® profiles of isolated enzymes. Chromatin isolated after 24 hr was a twofold more effective template for exogenous form II polymerase, and little change in RNase content was detectable. After only 6 hr, Cox[104] determined increases in the number of RNA chains being elongated from 2×10^3 to 5×10^3 by form I, but the number of chains being synthesized by form II remained virtually constant at 10^4. Dierks-Ventling and Bieri-Bonniot[105] also observed increases in endogenous forms I and II in nuclei from stimulated chick oviduct and in nuclei from liver.[106] In the latter, solubilization of the enzymes demonstrated an increase in form I_B and a drop in I_A (resolved on CM-Sephadex®); form I_A sedimented faster through a glyercol gradient and appeared to be a significantly larger molecule than form I_B.

Work in mammalian systems (primarily rat) has shown a series of effects with an early stimulation of form II followed by more prolonged elevation of form I and II endogenous uterine nuclear activities over 24 hr[107] (Figure 4). However, Weil et al.[108] found 500% and 250% increases in endogenous form I and III, respectively, but no change in form II over the first 6 hr. No net changes in solubilized enzymes (analyzed on DEAE-Sephadex®) were noted for forms I, II, or III though III_A was reduced and III_B was elevated.

Work on steroid effects is, therefore, both preliminary and, in some instances, conflicting. Detailed analyses of free and bound enzyme levels remain to be performed, and no general concensus emerges from the above data except to say that endogenous nuclear activities do tend to increase though the mechanisms are not resolved. These systems represent some of the most widely investigated in the field of endocrinology and gene expression, but there are others which have received attention; generally, this has been of a preliminary nature and space does not permit the listing of all such instances. A very diverse range of molecules constitute the general class of effector substances which have been annotated as hormones, and, in view of this fact and the wide variety of responses which the compounds elicit, it seems scarcely surprising that there is no real agreement on the mechanism of action. In the RNA polymerase field, there are indications of form I stimulation (usually rather late after hormone treatment) of uncertain mechanism; the rather unsatisfactory data thus far available imply an activation of preexisting molecules in several instances. In terms of total activity, form II enzyme seems to respond to a much lesser extent, though there may be stimulation and quantitative changes in promoter selection which remain uninvestigated. Form III activity may also be elevated, though this enzyme has been less thoroughly studied to date, and there are no data on mechanisms.

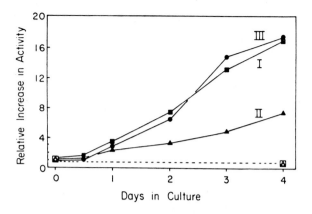

FIGURE 4. Relative increase in cellular RNA polymerase levels in PHA-stimulated lymphocytes. Enzyme levels were calculated from DEAE-Sephadex® chromatographic analyses of RNA polymerases solubilized from human lymphocytes at various times following the addition of PHA to the medium used to maintain the cells in culture. The data for each class of polymerase is plotted relative to its level present in the resting lymphocyte at day zero (closed symbols); data from control cells, cultured in the absence of PHA over the same period is also shown (open symbols). (From Jaehning, J. A., Stewart, C. C., and Roeder, R. G., *Cell,* 4, 51, 1975. With permission.)

F. The Stringent Response

When either prokaryotic or eukaryotic cells are deprived of amino acids or energy sources or when protein synthesis is directly inhibited, there follows a rapid shutdown of stable (ribosomal and transfer) RNA biosynthesis. This well-documented phenomenon has been the subject of intensive study since it offers the possibility of elucidating regulatory links between transcription and translation in simple experimental situations. The most detailed work has been carried out with bacteria where the accumulation of an unusual nucleotide (ppGpp) is thought to provide the connecting mechanism and to act at the RNA polymerase level.[6] The nature of the corresponding agent(s) in eukaryotic cells remains unknown, but it is worthwhile considering such information as is available concerning animal cells to decide whether the situation in such cells is truly analogous.

Barbiroli et al.[110,111] have investigated the effects of regimented starvation and refeeding cycles on the transcription apparatus of rat liver nuclei. Rats were starved overnight and either killed at 0900 or refed and killed at 1500 hr. Refeeding stimulated endogenous forms I and II polymerases about twofold over this period, accompanied by a slight increase in solubilizable form II. The authors described a marked change in the ionic strength optima for solubilized and for chromatin-associated form II polymerase after refeeding. Basic protein factors were isolated from starved or refed systems which affected the ionic strength optima, but it is very difficult to ascribe any fundamental mechanism to these observations: the assay systems were crude, and the possibilities of nucleases and other modifiers which might affect the observed activities were not assessed. Andersson and Von der Decker[112] starved rats of protein for up to 6 days, isolated RNA polymerases, and separated form I and II (from nuclei) on DEAE-Sephadex.® The difficulties in quantifying results from this kind of experiment were clearly discussed in their work which also checked for the appearance of inhibitors or activity effectors. Polymerases I and II were reduced by 75% and 50%, respectively (assessed as units per milligram DNA). On the other hand, Bailey et al.,[113] studying amino acid deprivation of rats, found a twofold stimulation of endogenous nucleolar polymerase I activity over 3 to 5 days; nucleolar volume also doubled, and the effects apparently coincided with an increased rate of ribosomal RNA synthesis. Deprivation of methionine alone sufficed to cause these effects. Assay conditions were rather unusual, since Mn^{++} was used as the cation together with limiting concentrations of labeled nucleoside triphosphate; no attempt was made to assess nucleotide pool sizes before or after deprivation, and the results are consequently difficult to interpret definitively.

Yu and Feigelson[114] observed that the administration of the translation (elongation) inhibitor cycloheximide at doses of up to 30 mg/kg caused a rapid cessation of protein synthesis in rat liver and also a coincident decrease in the endogenous nucleolar RNA polymerase I activity; the latter decayed with a time-life of 1.3 hr. Benecke et al.[115] showed that the levels of solubilizable RNA polymerases I, II, and III in rat liver did not vary over 24 hr following administration of rather lower doses of cycloheximide (4 mg/kg) which were nevertheless sufficient to obliterate protein synthesis. Problems have arisen with the use of cycloheximide because the doses necessary for the inhibition of protein synthesis and RNA synthesis in vivo may vary by up to an order of magnitude.[116] Subsequent work by Lampert and Feigelson[117] utilized lower cycloheximide doses and also looked for free and bound polymerase I using actinomycin D (only 20 μg/mℓ) and poly d(A-t). They concluded that whereas the endogenous (elongating) activity was reduced by prior cycloheximide administration in vivo, the soluble pool tended to rise in accord with the observations that total RNA polymerase content is unaffected by the inhibitor (Figure 5). These and similar observations have led to the idea that a "rapidly turning over protein" (RTOP) is required to maintain rRNA transcription, presumably acting at the level of initiation. Recently, the possibility of using sublethal doses of cycloheximide to look at the recovery phase has received preliminary attention, though the effects at the transcriptional level have still to be explored in vitro.[118]

If a RTOP does exist for the regulation of polymerase I activity, its synthesis might be controlled initially at the transcriptional level. Circumstantial evidence that this may be so comes from the work of Hadijiolov et al.[119] These workers looked at the effects of α-amanitin injected into mice on the synthesis and processing of preribosomal RNA in liver nuclei. Although this compound affects only RNA polymerases II and III in vitro, its administration in vivo leads, in many situations, to a rapid cessation of ribosome synthesis. Hadijiolov found that HnRNA transcription was quickly depressed, followed some 30 min later by cessation of 45S processing and between 30 and 150 min by inhibition of 45S transcription. Other RNA species (5S rRNA and tRNA) were also affected, and after 2.5 hr, nucleolar lesions appeared. However, this could be a case of feedback effects from processing on transcription; nucleolar RNA polymerase activity in vitro was not itself affected over the period of 45S inhibition in vivo. Further evidence stems from the observations of Penman et al.[120] that low concentrations of actinomycin D in vivo selectively inhibit ribosomal RNA synthesis. Lindell[121] looked at the effects of this agent on isolated rat liver nuclei and demonstrated that whereas form I polymerase was not sensitive over the concentration range effective in vivo (up to 0.05 μg/mℓ), a small and discrete proportion of form II polymerase was depressed by low actinomycin concentrations (see Figure 6). This was interpreted to imply that the gene coding for the RTOP might be the site of actinomycin sensitivity, though no further confirmation of this idea has yet been forthcoming. These ideas conflict with those of Widnell and Tata[23] who observed a selective effect on actinomycin on form I RNA polymerase in rat liver nuclei, albeit under different assay conditions.

Cultured mammalian cells are rather more amenable to studies of the stringent response. Chesterton et al.[122] examined the effects of valine starvation and the translation inhibitors cycloheximide and puromycin on ribosomal RNA synthesis in HeLa

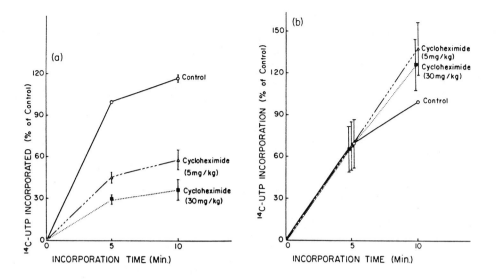

FIGURE 5. Effect of cycloheximide treatment on the chromosome-associated and "free" α-aman-itin-resistant RNA polymerase activity of rat liver nuclei. Following overnight starvation, rats received (1) 5 mg/kg cycloheximide in saline, (2) 30 mg/kg cycloheximide in saline, or (3) saline alone, each by intraperitoneal injection of a volume of 1 mℓ. Animals were sacrificed 3 hr after injection, and liver nuclei were isolated. (A) RNA synthesis on the endogenous template corresponding to the chromosome-associated RNA polymerase. (B) RNA synthesis by the "free" RNA polymerase assessed using the exogenous template poly-d(A-T). ○———○, control; △———△, 5 mg/Kg cycloheximide; ■———■, 30 mg/Kg cycloheximide. (From Lampert, A. and Feigelson, P., *Biochem. Biophys. Res. Commun.*, 58, 1030, 1974. With permission.)

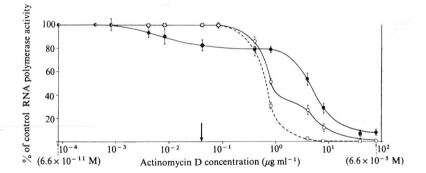

FIGURE 6. Effect of actinomycin D on transcription in isolated nuclei and nucleoli. Nuclei were isolated from rat liver and fractionated into nucleoli and nucleoplasm (see Lindell[121] for the complete details of these procedures). The extent of inhibition of nucleoplasmic polymerase II (●———●), nuclear polymerases I and III (○———○), and nucleolar polymerase I (□———□) is shown. The arrow indicates 0.04 μg/mℓ actinomycin D. (From Lindell, T. J., *Nature (London)*, 263, 347, 1976. With permission.)

cells. Valine starvation apparently exerted its effect primarily by inhibiting the processing of 45S RNA, whereas the inhibitors reduced the rate of synthesis of this molecule by 70 to 75%. No changes were observed in the total extractable amounts of polymerases I, II, or III, but using sarkosyl in isolated nuclei, the authors showed a reduction in endogenous RNA polymerase I molecules. There was no change in the template-bound form II enzyme. Sarkosyl strips proteins from the chromatin template and is thought to allow measurement of endogenous polymerase activity freed from feedback or steric constraints, an idea supported by the restoration of endogenous activity to near normal in the case of valine-starved nuclei. This kind of system would, nevertheless, benefit from a vigorous confirmation of the number of template-bound enzyme molecules since a covalently altered polymerase (exhibiting reduced elongation rates) might not be restored to control activity by sarkosyl in vitro. Similar sets of experiments with ascites cells[123,124] utilized amino acid starvation and the translation inhibitor pactomycin. Within 20 min following the administration of pactomycin or 60 min of starvation, there was a 50% decrease in the endogenous form I activity. There was no change in the endogenous form II or in the amounts of total extractable polymerases. RTOP was postulated, and the kinetics of 45S synthesis indicated a lowered elongation rate such that a complete molecule was taking 20, rather than 7, min to be synthesized. However, in vitro assays used only 10 μM ^{3}H-UTP, and the observed inhibition of 45S processing was not considered by the authors as relevant to the elongation rates. No measurements of nucleotide pool sizes were made in vivo or in vitro, and these reservations taken together must cast considerable doubts on the mechanisms proposed for the effects seen by the authors.

A series of recent publications has indicated that in ascites and mouse 3T3 cells, inhibition of rRNA transcription subsequent to depression of protein synthesis induced by amino acid or serum starvation may be related to a decrease in the intracellular concentrations of ATP and GTP.[125-127] Again, bound nucleolar RNA polymerase I activity was reduced with no loss in total cellular enzymes. No change in the RNase content was seen. The lowered endogenous activity was restored in nuclei isolated from cells which had been provided with an exogenous source of adenosine and guanosine although protein synthesis was not restored. Inhibition of protein synthesis by cycloheximide led to reduced nucleolar activities which could not be recovered by exogenous nucleosides. Addition of nucleosides was carried out after very long periods of starvation (18 hr), and there was no clear evidence that the nucleotide levels themselves directly regulated rRNA synthesis; nucleoli do not initiate rRNA synthesis in vitro irrespective of purine nucleoside triphosphate concentration, and there is no evidence that elongation of rRNA is more sensitive than other types to nucleotide levels. These are observations which scarcely support the proposed model. In 3T3 cells, azaserine (an inhibitor of purine nucleotide anabolism) suppressed the increase in ATP concentration normally observed after readdition of serum, but no data were provided on the effects on rRNA synthesis. Working with Friend leukemia cells, Dehlinger et al.[128] observed no effects on ATP and GTP pool sizes of functional histidine deprivation although tRNA and rRNA biosynthesis were depressed in the usual way. Perhaps the most important conclusion to be drawn from these observations is the need for careful measurement of nucleotide pools during regulatory processes if only for their potential effects on labeling kinetics.

The ease with which yeast cells can be grown in large amounts has encouraged their use as a model for many aspects of eukaryotic biochemistry. Included among these, the regulation of gene expression and the stringent response of yeast have been well characterized. Gross and Pogo[129] showed that starvation or cycloheximide treatment had no effects on the levels of extractable enzymes but reduced α-amanitin-resistant and -sensitive nuclear activities by 67% and 50%, respectively. Cycloheximide added after a period of starvation relaxed the inhibition of rRNA synthesis in vivo but not the depressed nuclear RNA polymerase activities. Later work[130,131] used a mutant temperature-sensitive with respect to protein synthesis together with starvation and translation inhibitors. Fluctuations (as opposed to labeling kinetics) of nucleotide pools were not extensively investigated although the authors discovered the importance of using uridine rather than uracil in vivo (due to the effects on nucleotide metabolism during stringency). As a result, the quantitative nature of in vivo changes was not clearly demonstrated. The RNA polymerases were not temperature-sensitive in themselves, but the endogenous nuclear activities were; shifting starved cells to the nonpermissive temperature again released rRNA inhibition as did cycloheximide, but again the release was not observed in isolated nuclei in vitro. The interpretation of these observations was that two factors were involved in rRNA synthesis: one switching on and the other switching off. Thus, starvation reduces the production of a positive factor, and complete shutdown of protein synthesis eliminates a negative factor also. No evidence is available concerning the nature of these factors or their sites of action, and their implied involvement is only a preliminary attempt to explain a rather complex series of events. Recent studies using methyl-labeling of RNA has indicated more accurately the degree of inhibition observed at the level of RNA metabolism in vivo,[132] and the yeast system continues to offer great promise in the elucidation of stringency in eukaryotic cells.

Virtually all of this work on the stringent response has implied that some separate gene product exists which is capable of influencing the level of ribosomal gene transcription in vitro using a fixed and invariant form I RNA polymerase. That is to say, either a type II regulation (alteration of polymerase-specific activity) or a direct effect on the ribosomal genes is indicated, with no information available to distinguish between these possibilities.

G. Mechanisms of RNA Polymerase Alteration

Notwithstanding the many ambiguities concerning the involvement of RNA polymerases in regulatory phenomena apparent from the above types of studies, many attempts have been made to look directly for modifiers of these enzymes in vitro.

1. Covalent Modification

The only covalent alteration of eukaryotic RNA polymerases reported so far involves phosphorylation of one or several of the peptide subunits. Varrone et al.[133] described a stimulation of rat liver polymerase of unspecified type in the presence of cytoplasmic proteins and cAMP; this effect was thought to involve template rather than polymerase modification and remains ill-defined. Martelo and Hirsch[134] investigated the effects of nuclear protein kinases I and II on rat liver RNA polymerases I and II, observing a stimulation of forms I (fivefold) and II (1.5-fold) with homologous DNA and kinase I only. Labeled phosphate was incorporated into material cochromatographing with the RNA polymerases, and both this and the increase in polymerase activity (also observed in isolated nuclei) could be stimulated further by cAMP. Unfortunately, the authors used only 2 μM ^{3}H-precursor in vitro and millimolar concentrations of cAMP, rather than the micromolar amounts usually seen in vivo. A more detailed study using calf ovary polymerases[135] and homologous protein kinases also indicated a stimulation of polymerase I (threefold) and II (ninefold) after preincubation at 37°C. The kinases were relatively unspecific: histones, casein, and *Escherichia coli* RNA polymerase were also phosphorylated. However, the effects were enhanced by only 5×10^{-9} M cAMP (Figure 7), and labeled phosphate again cochromatographed with the eukaryotic RNA polymerases. The authors considered that polymerase phosphorylation may be involved in the increased ovarian RNA synthesis which occurs subsequent to gonadotrophin stimulation. Most recently, a five- to sevenfold increase in the activity of the ascites RNA polymerase II in the presence of homologous protein kinase has been described which is not affected by cAMP[136] These effects are thought to involve initiation efficiency,[134] but in most instances little effort has been made to confirm that γ-^{32}P incorporation was into RNA rather than protein, a point which requires careful clarification.[137]

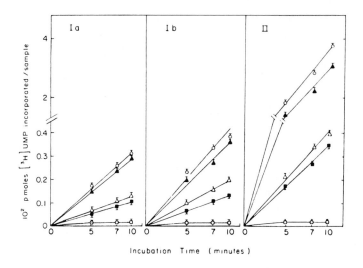

FIGURE 7.   Effect of cyclic AMP-dependent and -independent protein kinases on the activity of calf ovary RNA polymerases I_A, I_B, and II. RNA polymerases were solubilized from calf ovarian nuclei and resolved on DEAE-Sephadex®. Each enzyme was incubated with the relevant protein kinase at 30°C for 10 min prior to estimating its RNA synthetic potential (for experimental details, see Jungmann et al.[135]). The figure shows a time course of RNA synthesis by polymerases pretreated in the following ways: ■——■, RNA polymerase and 5×10^{-9} M cAMP; □——□, cAMP-dependent protein kinase and 5×10^{-9} M cAMP; ▲——▲, RNA polymerase and cAMP-independent protein kinase; △——△, RNA polymerase and cAMP-dependent protein kinase; ○——○, RNA polymerase, cAMP-dependent protein kinase and 5×10^{-9} M cAMP. (From Jungmann, R. A., Hiestrand, P. C., and Schweppe, J. S., *J. Biol. Chem.*, 249, 5444, 1974. With permission.)

Recent studies with the yeast RNA polymerases purified to homogeneity have confirmed that subunit phosphorylation occurs in vivo and can be mimicked in vitro. Buhler et al.[138] and Bell et al.[139] isolated enzymes from cells labldin vivo with ^{32}P and found a proportion of of the form I enzyme subunits (including the largest) and one or more of the forms II and III small subunits were phosphorylated. This labeling pattern was unaffected by the presence of cycloheximide in vivo.[139] Later work[140] demonstrated the existence of a protein kinase which phosphorylated in vitro the subunits found to be in this condition in vivo, although the specificity was not absolute and some extra peptides were also phosphorylated in vitro. No effects of either kinase or phosphatase treatments on enzyme activities in vitro could be detected, though rate-limiting (10 μM) labeled substrate concentrations were used.

2. Factors

The eukaryotic RNA polymerases have not fared equally with respect to the demonstration of factors affecting their activities in vitro. Polymerase II has been the subject of a considerable number of such reports, while there are only a few for form I which generally show only small effects on activity and, as yet, none specifically for form III. Factors tend to be specific for one of the main enzyme classes, but this rule is not absolute, and McNaughton et al.[141] isolated three unusual guanosine nucleotides (HSI, II, and III) from the water mold *Achyla* which apparently influence all three polymerase classes. These nucleotides were investigated as potential analogues of ppGpp in procaryotes but have not been structurally identified though their levels varied through the life cycle of the mold. HSI seemed the most specific, functioning at 1 to 10 $\mu g/ml$ and stimulating form III polymerase while inhibiting forms I and II. *E. coli* RNA polymerase was not affected, and ppGpp was not active on the eukaryotic enzymes. Whether there is a system linking translation with transcription in this primitive eukaryote which is mechanistically similar to that seen in bacteria remains to be resolved.

With regard to form I RNA polymerase, Higashinakagawa et al.[142] isolated a factor from nucleoli with the properties of a heat-stable, basic protein which stimulated the enzyme about 1.8-fold on native DNA. The protein did not affect polymerase II, but the presence of DNase was detected though not thought to be the positive agent due to its thermolability. The effects on the template were, nevertheless, not investigated. More recently, a nonhistone chromosomal protein from Novikoff Hepatoma nucleoli (C-14 protein) was found to stimulate polymerase I by about 30%; this peptide has a molecular weight of 70,000 daltons and also stimulated *E. coli* RNA polymerase, raising some questions as to any specific role in vivo.[143] Goldberg et al.[144] passed rat liver RNA polymerase I through a matrix of rRNA-Sepharose®, causing the release of two peptides (molecular weight 11,000 and 12,000, both basic and heat-stable) and leaving an enzyme with a greatly reduced affinity for DNA. Transcription of the artificial template poly-dC was not affected, and reconstitution with the factors restored synthesis on double-stranded DNA by a mechanism thought to involve the initiation reaction. The physiological relevance of these obervations remains obscure, since polymerase II was also affected and a molar ratio of 50:1 (factors to enzyme) was necessary for maximal stimulation. Manen and Russell[145] have suggested the possibility that orinithine decarboxylase may be the RTOP for polymerase I; affinity columns with bound polymerase retained this enzyme, which also stimulated transcription in isolated nuclei. This interesting possibility awaits more detailed investigation.

Hildebrandt and Sauer[146] observed an inverse correlation between polyphosphate levels and RNA polymerase I activity during the growth cycle of *Physarum*. Polyphosphate (2 μM) caused 50% inhibition of enzyme I in vitro but less than 10% inhibition of form II and associated more tightly with the former enzyme than the latter (measured by ^{32}P binding). Whether polyphosphates bind to the enzyme in vivo was not investigated.

Factors affecting the activity of RNA polymerase II in vitro have been reported from a number of different cells and tissues. Mostly these seem to be basic polypeptides increasing the ability of the enzyme to transcribe double-stranded DNA. Among the first systems to be characterized was coconut endosperm, from which two major types of RNA polymerases, CI and CII (equivalent to aimal forms II and I, respectively) have been isolated.[147] Three factors (A, B, and C) were also found. Later work[69,148] further characterizedthese enzymes and factors: B binds to enzyme CI causing an increase in initiation rate and trnscript size from double-stranded DNA; it also counteracts a sensitivity to rifamycin (unique among eukaryotic RNA polymerases) which is an inherent property of CI. Factor C stimulated enzyme CI only in the presence of factor B and was thought to be a termination factor. These observations defy extrapolation to other eukaryotic systems due to the unique nature of the enzyme forms which still awaits clarification; it certainly does not seem to be a general feature of plant tissues.

Another early discovery was the "S" factor from calf thymus cytoplasm.[149,150] This basic peptide proved to be a heat-stable stimulant of double-stranded DNA transcription by form II enzyme only (Figure 8). It acts after initiation, presumably on elongation rates, without altering the sizes of the final transcripts. The factor did not have any direct (irreversible) effect on the DNA and markedly lowered the ionic strength optimum for polymerase II in vitro. "S" factor has a molecular weight of

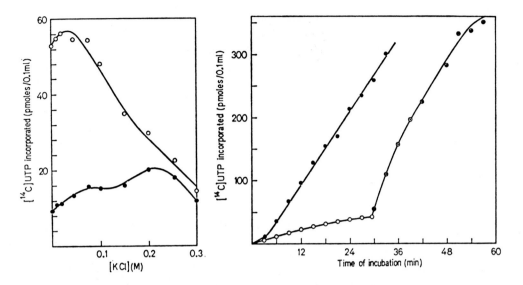

FIGURE 8.   The effect of "stimulating factor" on the transcription of calf thymus DNA by purified calf thymus RNA polymerase II. All the ingredients of a standard RNA polymerase in vitro assay were contained in 0.1 m*l* including RNA polymerase, nucleoside triphosphates, DNA, Mn[++], KCl, and stimulating factor (where relevant).[150] (A) Analyses the dependence of the RNA polymerase II reaction on the KCl concentration in the presence (O——O) and in the absence (●——●) of added factor. (B) Examines the kinetics of the RNA polymerase II reaction in the presence of factor (●——●), in the absence of factor (O——O), and the effect of factor addition after 30 min of RNA synthesis (☉——☉). (From Stein, H. and Hausen, P., *Eur. J. Biochem.*, 14, 270, 1970. With permission.)

27,500 daltons, associates directly with the enzyme, and is not the same as any of the small subunits of polymerase II.[151] Lukacs and Stein[152] recently reported another factor from calf thymus which is probably histone H1; they found that this protein stimulated transcription by form II enzyme tenfold at H1 to DNA ratios of 2:1, with a detectable but much lower stimulation of *E. coli* RNA polymerase also. Other histones inhibited RNA synthesis, but in this and earlier work, the use of limiting substrate concentrations again adds a complication to quantitative interpretation.

Analogous work with rat liver cytoplasm[153,154] revealed a 30,000-dalton peptide with properties almost identical to those of "S" factor. Five- to tenfold stimulation of form II was seen, and its effects were greatest on large DNA templates. In addition, a phosphorylated nonhistone protein fraction from rat liver has been shown to stimulate from II enzyme on homologous DNA only; addition of phosphatase obliterates the stimulation, though these observations remain otherwise poorly characterized.[155]

Sugden and Keller[156] isolated two basic protein fractions on CM-cellulose (SFA and SFB) capable of stimulating HeLa and KB cell polymerase II enzymes. Both were between 20,000 to 30,000 daltons and similar to "S" factor in most respects. However, they did lead to the synthesis of discrete size classes of RNA using adenovirus DNA templates, and their effects were countered by the initiation inhibitor rifampicin AF/0-15 suggesting a different, and perhaps more pecific, role compared with "S" proteins.

Lentfer and Lezius[157] isolated an "S"-type factor from mouse myeloma cells, and Ihara and Kawakami[158] have obtained a basic nuclear-protein fraction from myeloma cells which apparently promotes the formation of AF/0-13-resistant complexes between polymerase II and native calf thymus DNA. Polymerase II was stimulated fivefold in activity, but form I was also enhanced twofold; optimum results were obtained only when factor, polymerase, and DNA were preincubated together, although some effects were observed by preincubating either factor plus enzyme or factor plus DNA. The mechanism and significance of these results await clarification.

Lee and Dahmus[159] obtained fractions from ascites cells which could be resolved into heat-stable ("S"-like) and labile components capable of stimulating RNA polymerase II. Similar results were obtained by Sekimizu et al.,[160] though the mechanism of the factor investigated in detail which had a molecular weight of 38,000 daltons seemed to be rather more complex; initiation rates, elongation rates, and final transcript size may all have been elevated. DNases were apparently absent from these preparations. Ascites chromatin has also yielded transcription factors; Kostraba and Wang[161] obained an acidic, nonhistone chromosomal protein of molecular weight 10,000 to 11,000 which bound to DNA and, at high protein to DNA ratios (2:1 by weight), selectively inhibited initiation by polymerase II. This species was the most abundant acidic chromosomal protein, essentially the only type revealed by their extraction procedures. Later, however, using the same cells, Kostraba et al.[162] obtained a nonhistone chromosomal protein fraction which stimulated the initiation of RNA chains starting with ATP rather than GTP, and only on unique sequence homologous DNA. The factor bound to the template rather than the enzyme.

Other cells and tissues have also yielded polymerase factors, but these generally fit into the pattern of those described above. In no instance has a clear physiological role for any factor been established, and rarely is it possible to speculate on their significance at the present level of knowledge. Whether or not the levels or properties of these peptides vary under different physiological conditions remains unknown.

3. Polyamines

In the light of the general nature of the polymerase stimulation factors described above, it has been suggested[28] that the effects are a direct, yet rather unspecific, result of the presence of small, basic molecules which might reduce the inherent charge repulsion between the acidic RNA polymerases (especially form II) and DNA. It is, therefore, of interest to evaluate the effects of the very basic polyamines spermine and spermidine, small molecules often found associated with DNA in both prokaryotes and eukaryotes, on RNA polymerase activities. Moruzzi et al.[163] showed that in rat liver nuclei, exogenous spermidine stimulated transcription of the endogenous form I enzyme only at relatively high concentrations (10^{-3} to 10^{-2} M). Spermine did not stimulate under these conditions, and high concentrations of either polyamine were inhibitory. At higher salt concentrations, spermine showed biphasic stimulation at 10^{-6} M and again at 10^{-4} M; spermidine only increased polymerase activity in the 10^{-4} M range, i.e., primarily involving RNA polymerase II. Neither spermine nor spermidine apparently caused a measurable increase in protein displacement form the chromatin template, and the effects were slightly additive over increasing ionic strength (which itself probably does function by removing protein from the chromatin). The preparation of chromatin from these nuclei resulted in a system insensitive to 10^{-6} M spermine but capable of stimulation for 10^{-4} M spermine or spermidine with regard to both endogenous forms I and II polymerases, i.e., some specificity was apparently lost. However, transcription of chromatin by exogenous form II was stimulated biphasically by 10^{-6} and 10^{-4} M spermine, and the authors concluded that this polyamine at low concentrations might be important in the regulation of form II activity.

Janne et al.[164] looked at the effect of these polyamine on purified pig kidney RNA polymerases I and II using either calf thymus DNA or chromatin as template. Both spermine and spermidine stimulated the transcription of native DNA by form I polymerase (threefold) and form II (sevenfold), optimally at 2 mM or 5 to 10 mM, respectively (Figure 9). The effects were much reduced on single-stranded DNA and acted on the V_{max} rather than the K_m for UTP. End-group analyses of RNA molecules indi-

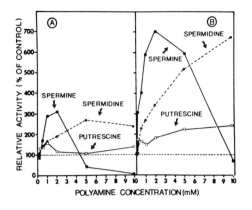

FIGURE 9.   The effect of polyamines on DNA transcription by pig kidney RNA polymerases. The ability of spermine, spermidine, and putrescine to stimulate in vitro transcription of DNA was assessed using (A) purified form I and (B) purified form II RNA polymerases. (From Janne, C. O., Bardin, W., and Jacob, S. T., *Biochemistry*, 14, 3589, 1975. With permission.)

cated that the stimulation was of elongation rate rather than initiation. With chromatin as template, a similar stimulation of exogenous form II was seen with spermine, but form I was inhibited, possibly by blocking initiation.

These results tend to confirm the notion that small basic molecules may have an intrinsic ability to enhance transcription by form II polymerase primarily by facilitating elongation along the electronegative DNA backbone. To what extent this property is used by the cell in a regulative manner remains a matter for speculation.

VI. GENERAL ASSESSMENT OF CURRENT KNOWLEDGE

Having related much of the available data concerning possible regulatory roles of RNA polymerases, it seems pertinent at this stage to make an assessment of the quality and quantity of this information and also to try to ascertain how it relates to the three types of theoretical controls outlined in Section IV.

Investigations of regulatory processes are among the most complex that biochemists undertake because the number of possible variables is so large. The review of experimental data in Section V, which is the basis of our current understanding of transcriptional control mechanisms in eukaryotes, is unashamedly critical although a good deal of invaluable information has obviously accrued. Criticism can usually be construed as being "wise after the event", and this is surely true in this case! The approach which has been adopted was designed to draw attention to fundamental aspects of experimental format which are obligatory if a definitive picture of RNA polymerase involvement in regulatory mechanisms is to be established. It is the complexity of the eukaryotic system which dictates this stringent approach to experimental protocol. A number of obvious problems are evident from the foregoing scrutiny of the literature, and it might be useful to spell them out and to indicate (where possible) experimental solutions.

1.   In the in vivo situation, changes in protein and RNA synthesis rates are virtually always based on labeled-precursor experiments, and, for accurate quantitative information, it is clearly essential that possible effects in the transport and pool

sizes of these precursors be worked out. Failure to do so may, at best, give rise to qualitatively accurate impressions; on the other hand, it may be totally misleading. For instance, Ho-Terry and Cohen[165] have recently demonstrated that the apparent stimulation of RNA synthesis in CV-1 cells following SV40 infection was a complete artifact resulting from effects on the specific radioactivity of the uridine pool.

2.   It is easy to underestimate the difficulty of obtaining quantitative extraction of RNA polymerases from any source. In Section II.A, the risks of using isolated cell fractions, rather than whole cells, as a source of enzymes was stressed. To emphasize this point, Figure 10 clearly demonstrates that the technique used to carry out the initial cell fractionation for the preparation of nuclei dictates the distribution of various RNA polymerases between nucleus and the extranuclear ("cytosol") fractions:[35] the use of a "hypertonic" sucrose medium for the homogenization of tissues results in the retention of a large proportion of the activity within the nucleus, whereas RNA polymerase activity is lost to the cytosol when homogenization is carried out in "isotonic" sucrose media. Neither of the two basic techniques for solubilizing the RNA polymerase activity can be guaranteed to give quantitative results: in the case of the high-salt, sonication technique,[24] there is evidence of enzyme loss[34,166] and interconversion within a single class of polymerase;[34] in our experience, the low-salt extraction procedure gives rise to at least a twofold increase in polymerase yield over the alternative technique if conducted under conditions of optimum ionic strength and time of extraction, conditions which are somewhat empirical (see Reference 30). A problem here is the risk of proteolysis[42] (see below for a further discussion of proteolytic artifacts).

3.   In estimating the extent of solubilization of polymerase activity from organelles, perhaps the greatest difficulty is to establish the 100% figure. There are a number of reasons for this. There is no way in which a comparison can be drawn between rates of RNA synthesis by bound (nuclear) RNA polymerases and the activity of the solubilized enzymes using "nicked" DNA templates. In vitro RNA synthesis in isolated nuclei is primarily the result of the elongation of RNA chains initiated in vivo. Using β-^{32}P-nucleoside triphosphates, Gilboa et al.[167] have confirmed this, and their data suggest that what initiation does occur in this in vitro system is restricted to the form III RNA polymerase. The time course of the elongation reaction tends to be relatively short. One major implication of this situation is that comparisons of RNA synthetic potential between nuclei from different physiological states or between nuclear and solubilized RNA polymerase activity requires the comparison of initial reaction rates: attention has not been drawn to this important criterion in preceding sections because it is nearly always impossible to assess whether or not this protocol has been followed. Finally, the initial extracts of organelles or tissues are invariably contaminated by nucleases which obscure their true synthetic potential, and most, if not all, purification steps lead to some losses.

4.   In laying down preliminary guidelines (Section IV), it was stressed that for quantitative comparisons of enzyme activities it is necessary to use saturating concentrations or substrates, and, in the case of organelles, it is crucial to obtain an estimate of potential endogenous pool sizes. Nothing would be gained from laboring this point further save to say that there is abundant evidence that these parameters are frequently ignored. Similarly, it is worth pointing out that those workers who have looked for changes in optimum activity conditions (with respect to ionic strength and interference by RNase and DNase) for polymerases from cells in different physiological states have usually found them: this consti-

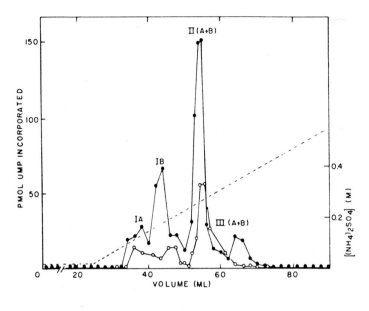

A

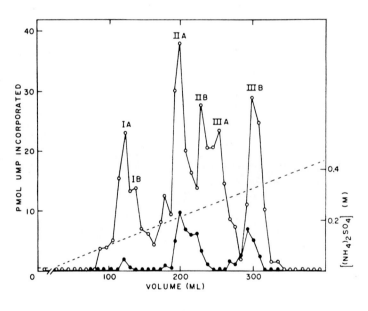

B

FIGURE 10.   The variation in the distribution of RNA polymerase activities between the nucleus and the cytosol depending on the initial sucrose concentration in the homogenizing medium used to prepare nuclei from rat liver. Nuclei were resolved from the cytosol of rat liver by differential centrifugation following homogenization of 14 g of tissue in a medium containing either 0.25 *M* sucrose ("isotonic") or 2.2 to 2.3 *M* sucrose ("hypertonic"). RNA polymerase activity was solubilized from nuclei by high-salt sonication. This extract and the cytosol fraction were analyzed for polymerase activity by gradient elution from DEAE-Sephadex® (as shown). DEAE-Sephadex® profiles are shown derived from (A) nuclear solubilized polymerase activity and (B) the cytosol. O——O, "isotonic" preparation; ●——●, "hypertonic" preparation. (From Lin, Y. C., Rose, K. M., and Jacob, S. T., *Biochem. Biophys. Res. Commun.*, 72, 114, 1976. With permission.)

tutes another very important reservation regarding the majority of investigations which have failed to explore these possibilities.

5.   All of the experiments discussed in Section V described RNA polymerase "levels" on the basis of total activity. This was generally expressed as units per milligram DNA, i.e., on a per cell basis, though some of the data were not even clear on this point. To differentiate clearly between the numbers of enzyme molecules and their activity, we wish to reemphasise the potential of the immunoprecipitation techniques.[38,39,56,168,169] The most detailed study so far using this technology has been by Guialis et al.[170] using fused cells derived from normal and α-amanitin-resistant Chinese hamster ovary (CHO) cell lines. In the presence of α-amanitin, the fused cells rapidly lost their α-amanitin-sensitive polymerase activity; this seemed to involve selective enzyme degradation, since (1) binding capacity for labeled α-amanitin decreased rapidly and (2) total RNA polymerase II content of the cells was maintained, as determined by competition (displacement) studies using I^{125}-labeled calf thymus RNA polymerase II and antisera which showed no apparent species specificity in this instance. This is undoubtedly the most convincing demonstration to date that cells have a sensitive mechanism for modulating their RNA polymerase content; synthesis of resistant enzyme was clearly stimulated at a rate adequate to maintain the total level during the decay of inactivated polymerase, which occurred with a halflife of about 5 hr. We feel that this kind of approach has great value in studies on RNA polymerase levels during regulatory sequences and, indeed, may become the most definitive approach in the near future.

6.   In attempting to ascribe mechanisms to polymerase-mediated alterations of transcription, several groups have detected changes in subunit sizes or composition of the eukaryotic enzymes. It is necessary to sound a note of caution here; in addition to the general difficulty of ascertaining functional requirements of individual subunits,[29] the problems of proteolytic conversion during extraction (perhaps arising through changes in protease activities during regulatory sequences) warrant continued attention. Coupar et al.[41] have shown that the low-salt extraction method for isolating rat liver polymerase I results in the proteolytic degradation of the heavy subunit (from 195K to 175K daltons). A similar situation may be responsible for the microheterogeneity of form II RNA polymerase. Careful use of the serine protease inhibitor PMSF results in the isolation of a single enzyme II from yeast; a protease can be extracted which selectively reduces the size of the heavy subunit to create the diversity usually observed.[46] Of course, if changes in the subunit size do have a regulatory function, there would clearly have to be an enzyme to bring about the change, and the demonstration of proteolytic effects may be interpreted as a fruitful area of research rather than just an in vitro artifact.

VII. CONTROL AT THE RNA POLYMERASE LEVEL

In Section III, three mechanisms were proposed for control at the level of the RNA polymerase: type 1, gross alteration in the amounts of active enzymes; type 2, a change in the catalytic "efficiency" of active polymerase; and type 3, modulation of RNA polymerase specificity. How far do the data support these ideas?

The first observation which can be made is that transcriptional control is not *always* linked to RNA polymerase "levels" in terms of amounts of enzyme activity measurable in vitro. The mature amphibian egg has large amounts of all three polymerase species but makes little or no RNA. This makes very unlikely either a type 2 or 3 regulation but does not rule out type 1 entirely since we do not know *a priori* whether these polymerases are functionally capable of initiating RNA synthesis in vivo; they could represent physiologically inactive pools. However, nuclear transplantation experiments between eggs of different species (*Xenopus laevis* and *Discoglossus pictus*) have shown that the subsequent patterns of RNA synthesis depends on the source of nuclei.[171] Cell fusion experiments in which hen erythrocyte nuclei enter cells active in RNA synthesis, e.g., HeLa, have shown that the erythrocyte nuclei do not begin to synthesize RNA immediately (despite the presence of HeLa polymerases) but take some 4 days to become active.[172] Also, the expression of *Xenopus* oocyte 5S ribosomal genes has been detected in cultured cells subsequent to translocation of the cistrons to the nucleolus.[173] All of these observations mitigate against regulation at the RNA polymerase level, indicating variable availability of genes. That is not to say that polymerases play no part in early development but only that they are not a limiting factor in quantitative terms.

The consensus of opinion with respect to neoplastic tissues seems to be that levels of RNA polymerases, especially form I, are elevated: this is a type 1 regulatory system giving rise to an increase in enzyme protein. However, type 2 regulation, enhancement of preexisting enzyme activity, has not been rigorously excluded. There is no information on the temporal nature of this change.

Effector molecules such as mitogens and hormones apparently have rather complex results on their target cells; it may be that early responses involve the activation or alteration of existing enzyme molecules (type 2), whereas establishment of the new cell state is accompanied at later times by changes in the amounts of the enzymes (type 1 effects). Unfortunately, the evidence purporting to demonstrate type 2 regulation is sketchy at best in these systems and requires extensive investigation before any single instance can be unequivocally identified. What is clear, however, is that there are several instances where endogenous nuclear RNA polymerase levels reflect the in vivo situation whereas total amounts of solubilized enzymes do not; this probably indicates either a type 2 control or the analogous situation in which the efficiency of the gene (promoter?) itself is regulated, and no experimental approach has yet successfully distinguished between these possible mechanisms.

In some ways, the regenerating liver is analogous to the PHA stimulation of lymphocytes (a cell population with a low mitotic index stimulated to hectic division) and in other ways relates to development (since there are clear morphological constraints of the ultimate extent of proliferation). Published data tend to support a type 2 control mechanism at the level of the RNA polymerase, at least of stable RNA synthesis, and in this respect the lymphocyte analogy might prove to be the closer.

Virtually all the work concerning the stringent response indicates that here also regulation of stable RNA synthesis is exerted via a type 2 mechanism (if at the polymerase level at all). There is good evidence that some aspects of stringency in eukaryotes may involve processing controls in the case of 45S pre-rRNA, and as yet there are no data identifying mechanisms involving polymerase I directly or other factors modifying the accessibility or conformation of the ribosomal RNA coding sequence.

To summarize: (1) not all transcriptional regulation can possibly depend on the amounts of RNA polymerase present; (2) type 2 regulation (the modulation of activity) may be the most widespread, at least over the first few hours of cell state changes; (3) type 1 alterations tend to occur at later stages and probably involve *de novo* synthesis or degradation of enzyme (rather than activation of totally inert pools of enzyme); and (4) type 2 regulation has not been clearly distinguished from effects at other levels (such as posttranscriptional processing) in gene expression and not even from factors affecting the DNA coding sequence directly.

We have said nothing of type 3 regulation which is concerned with the modulation of enzyme specificity. The simple reason is that there are no data having a direct bearing on this issue at the present time. We have seen that in amphibian eggs there is a large excess of form II polymerase, confirming the notion that HnRNA synthesis cannot be controlled in all instances by a type 3 mechanism alone. However, polymerase excesses of this sort may not be a general feature of eukaryotic cells. A more usual circumstance may be that reflected in differentiated tissues such as liver. Our own observations suggest that form II enzyme in liver nuclei is mainly template-bound, an idea supported by estimates of the numbers of active genes compared with numbers of polymerase molecules. Thus, if there are only about 10^3 cistrons being transcribed in a liver cell (a conservative estimate) and only about 2×10^4 polymerase II molecules (assuming all HnRNA synthesis is by this enzyme),[24] an average packing ratio of only 20 enzymes per gene would result. Since there are probably many more genes than this active in liver, the data imply that somatic cells may not have much more form II polymerase than they are actually using at any point in time. Electron micrographs of putative HnRNA transcription units confirm that each has many polymerases associated with it.[174] One prediction of the modulation model, the occurrence of limiting amounts of the relevant enzyme, may therefore be met in some, or even perhaps in the majority, of the instances in differentiated organisms. The recent observations of Kleene and Humphreys[175] that the HnRNA population of sea urchin cells does not vary in sequence content between blastula and pluteus stages in any detectable way (and is complementary to as much as 34% of the unique-sequence DNA) also indicate that transcriptional controls important at later times may not feature in the early development of an organism. Of course, somatic cells do exhibit some free (cytoplasmic) form II enzyme, but it is notable that this may be a different form from that bound to the chromatin; annotated as polymerase II_A in *Xenopus*,[73] it presumably contains the heavier subunit, and we have no information on whether it is physiologically active in vivo. The possibility exists that this enzyme may represent an ''inert'' pool of the sort postulated for type 1 regulation, though we have no evidence on this point.

Studies on the complexity of mRNA populations in eukaryotes are also in accord with the existence of type 3 regulation, at least in some instances; thus far, only a few cell types have been analyzed in this way. In agreement with the above observations on HnRNA transcription, Hough-Evans et al.[176] have shown that during early development of the sea urchin, the complexity of the mRNA population is much grater than in somatic cells and that similar sequences are produced in the oocyte and in early development; the more precise controls apparent in differentiated tissues are not seen at these times. However, Hereford and Rosbash[177,178] have shown three abundance classes of mRNAs in yeast and also that shifting a temperature-sensitive mutant to nonpermissive temperatures results in a drop in the components of one of these abundance classes. Furthermore, messenger RNA studies in mouse tissues have shown that although cDNAs complementary to kidney, brain, and liver mRNA populations cross-react up to 70 to 85% with different populations, more detailed analysis reveals the complementarity to be in the intermediate and low abundance (high complexity) classes; sequences present in great abundance in one tissue are low as a group in another. In regenerating rat liver, some 10 to 15% of the mRNA population (in terms of sequence complexity) is unique to the growing tissue 12 hr after the operation, though the abundance class(es) involved were not defined.[179] These observations are compatible with the predictions of, but in no way demonstrate, a type 3 regulation of mRNA synthesis mediated by RNA polymerase II specificity. Interestingly, three abundance classes of mRNA have recently been demonstrated in *E. coli*,[180] an organism in which there is considerably more evidence implicating RNA polymerase specificity as a modulator at least of the major RNA classes and perhaps of different mRNAs also.[6] Direct experimental approaches to this problem in eukaryotes face major obstacles, both with regard to suitable in vitro assay systems and because modulating factors may combine reversibly and weakly with the polymerase and be readily lost on isolation if prokaryotic precedent is to be maintained here.

Finally, it seems worthwhile having a look at some of the most recent direct evidence of the nature of transcription and the implications of electron microscope observations in any consideration of regulatory processes. Franke et al.[181] examined ribosomal genes from several organisms, and it is apparent from these studies that the mechanical operations enacted on these cistrons may be rather more complex than at first thought. In particular, Franke observed "prelude pieces" indicating that the initiation of the 45S precursor may actually start some way upstream of the known transcript. Combining electron microscopy and autoradiography following in vivo labeling, Angelier et al.[182] arrived at the conclusion that different cistrons within the same ribosomal gene population (again amphibian) were elongating RNA at different rates. McKnight and Miller[183] examined the switch-on of ribosomal genes during *Drosophila* development and showed the existence of some "Christmas tree" formations which consisted only of early region transcripts; it seemed that different genes were switched on independently, since others were simultaneously fully activated. In all cases, maximum polymerase packing densities were observed, but in the ribosomal cistrons of *Triturus* during oogenesis, different densities were seen of different genes, leading the authors to speculate on the possibility of differing initiation rates within the population.[184]

All of these data, on a single gene type, merely serve to emphasize the probable complexity of regulatory processes in vivo. It is perhaps facile to look for a single mechanism even for a single gene, a point emphasized by the interaction of positive and negative elements influencing operon activity in prokaryotes and well established in several specific instances.

VIII. FUTURE POSSIBILITIES

It seems to us that the most promising way forward in this field requires a thorough characterization of the early events of a suitable regulatory sequence with regard to the fate of the RNA polymerases. The PHA stimulation of lymphocytes seems well suited to such a study, with the advantages that nucleotide pool effects have largely been determined and the sequence of events in vivo has been documented in detail with regard to RNA synthesis and processing. There are also advantages in dealing with populations of single cells. None of this is to decry a need for pursuing the course of events in other cells and tissues also. We need to know in particular (1) whether early effects on endogenous nuclear RNA synthesis are dependent or independent of protein synthesis; (2) whether amounts of polymerase protein varies (by immunoassay); and (3) whether the effects are on the genes or on the polymerases directly. The answers to these questions will largely dictate future plans, but if the enzymes do turn out to be directly involved, then even more urgent will become the need to establish in vitro systems whereby fidelity of transcription (especially initiation) can be adequately demonstrated. The microheterogeneity of each polymerase may prove important in this respect, since it now seems as if the two subforms of each type may reflect "bound" and "free" forms or perhaps (in some cases) active and inactive pool, respectively. Thus forms I_A, II_B, and III_A may be chromatin-bound whereas I_B, II_A, and III_B may be soluble enzymes. II_A and III_B each have one subunit larger than their chromatin-bound counterparts, whereas I_B lacks a peptide present in I_A. These observations may provide clues to the mechanisms of polymerase alteration and regulation. Covalent modification of RNA polymerases may also prove a fruitful area of research, since the recent detailed observations on phosphorylated subunits should permit a ready measure of changes in these parameters under different growth (or other) conditions. It remains to be seen whether phosphorylation can be interpreted more precisely with RNA polymerases than has thus far been possible with histones or nonhistone chromosomal proteins and whether other modifications seen on histones (such as acetylation, methylation, etc.) occur on polymerases also.

The nature of RNA polymerase alteration remains largely speculative with no clear consensus arising from published work. Many observations imply (but do not prove) a regulatory event at or near initiation, whereas others indicate that elongation rates may be controlled (as in the cases of most of the "factors" thus far discovered). This is another aspect which awaits the development of suitable assay systems for convincing resolution in any particular instance.

We share the view of Travers[21] that the complexity of the RNA polymerase molecules and their sheer size (some ten times larger than the smallest enzymes known to be able to transcribe DNA in mitochondria) imply regulatory functions for these enzymes. It is interesting that many regulatory events lead to enzymes with altered ionic strength optima, one of the criteria by which changed promoter specificities are assayed using the prokaryotic enzyme. It seems likely that when many of the technical problems in this difficult field are overcome, significant regulatory roles for the eukaryotic RNA polymerase will ultimately be defined.

IX. RECENT PROGRESS

Since the body of this manuscript was laid down in the late part of 1977, several notable technical advances have had a profound impact on our understanding of the organization and expression of the eukaryotic genome. The advent of rapid nucleic acid sequencing techniques[186,187] has already given rise to complete base sequences of viral genomes[188] and suggests that base sequence analysis is going to be to eukaryotic systems what genetics has been to bacterial systems. The synthesis of complete DNA copies (cDNA) of messenger RNA sequences using the avian myoblastosis reverse transcriptase, the cloning of these copies in bacterial plasmids and subsequent sequencing has resulted in complete base sequences being resolved for many abundant mRNAs (see, e.g., Reference 189). This technology has provided unique probes to search within restriction enzyme fragments of total cellular DNA and libraries of cloned genomes[190] for those which contain structural genes. Detailed analysis of the organization of many structural gene coding sequences has now established that the protein coding sequences can contain one or more interruptions ("intervening sequences"). These intervening sequences are transcribed and the appearance of a mature messenger RNA involves a number of splicing events to yield a contiguous protein coding sequence (reviewed by Abelson[191]). The formidable growth of this type of information on a large number of structural genes has led to a radical reappraisal of our concept of the transcription unit. It is no longer rational (as we suspected, see Section II.E) to make any generalisation which suggests that protein coding sequence is located in the 3′-terminal regions of transcription units. In the most thoroughly studied eukaryotic genes, the chick ovalbumin[192] and conalbumin genes[193] are interrupted 7 and at least 17 times, respectively; protein coding sequences are distributed over the full length of the transcription units and the evidence suggests that a region of the transcription unit very close to the RNA synthesis initiation point is capped[18] and, therefore, retained in the mature messenger RNAs. A splicing activity (which removes intervening sequence from a yeast tRNA precursor) has been isolated and partially characterised[194,195] and very recently a role for the so-called "small RNAs" (snRNAs) has been predicted in the orientation of the splice junctions.[196]

From the point of view of the emphasis of this review, the genomic cloning techniques and subsequent sequencing data has not only provided this new picture of the organization of the transcription unit, but has also provided experimental tools (which were previously lacking) which will permit an absolute definition of correct initiation of RNA synthesis. Already, these tools have been put to good use. The most distinguished piece of work in this respect has resulted in the demonstration by Roeder and his colleagues of "selective and accurate initiation of transcription at the Adenovirus-2 Major Late Promoter in a soluble system dependent on purified RNA polymerase II and DNA".[197]

Current evidence suggests that the Late Adenovirus-2 genes are transcribed as a gigantic polycistronic message (approx. 30,000 bases).[198] The maturation of individual late mRNAs requires the splicing of 3 short sequences from the 5′-end to a protein coding sequence from within the primary gene transcript.[14] Ziff and Evans[199] identified and sequenced the late transcription initiation point at 16.45 map units in the Adenovirus-2 genome. Using a restriction enzyme fragment containing this presumptive promoter and purified RNA polymerase II, Weil et al.[197] were able to reconstitute an in vitro transcription system which initiated RNA synthesis accurately. They corroborated what others had recently found that the purified RNA polymerase lacked certain initiation "determinants" (see Reference 197). In this case, accurate initiation was only achieved when the transcription system was supplemented with a crude cellular extract ('S-100').

The resolution of the relevant components from these crude extracts which appear to be required to direct accurate initiation in reconstituted transcription systems is inevitably a vigorous area of current research. It is ironic that the astonishing structural complexity which has long been recognized in the purified eukaryotic RNA polymerases (see Table 1) still may not contain crucial initiation factors. These findings may account for the apparent (though controversial) success of one or two early experiments which were claimed to demonstrate selective sequence transcription using crude rather than purified RNA polymerase preparations.[61,63,200] While detailed dissection of the components which make up competent transcriptional machinery proceeds apace, the microinjection of cloned eukaryotic structural genes into Xenopus oocytes[201,202] and the use of crude extracts derived from oocytes which contains RNA polymerase activity[203] are both providing essential information on the DNA sequences surrounding eukaryotic genes which are required for faithful transcription. We can anticipate a formidable increase in our understanding of the catalytic and DNA sequence requirements for eukaryotic gene expression within the next few years.

It seems fair to say that the information explosion on structural aspects of eukaryotic transcription units over the last few years has not yet revolutionized our understanding of regulatory mechanisms, though there is every reason to anticipate major improvements in this field as a consequence of gene manipulatory methods in the near future. Some new observations have been made however and are worthy of brief consideration.

Recently Gillam et al.[204] have investigated spermatogenesis in trout testes and have shown that a general decline in RNA synthetic activity between spermatogonium and spermatid was paralleled by a loss of polymerase activities; ^{3}H-α-amanitin-binding studies were carried out and confirmed that at least in the case of polymerase II, this decline of activity was commensurate with an actual loss of enzymes from the cells. Another developmental system increasingly attracting the attention of biochemists has been the myogenesis of myoblasts isolated from mammalian or avian embryos and cultured in vitro; in a cell line derived from rats, it has been shown that the 5 to 10 fold decrease in ribosomal RNA synthesis which occurs at or about the time of fusion is regulated exclusively at the transcriptional level[205] and in another study levels of soluble RNA polymerases I and II rose 1 to 8 and 1 to 5 fold, respectively, during the same period.[206] Whether shut-down of transcription, a feature of all these investigations, will turn out to be as interesting as the more widely studied 'on' switches remains to be seen.

There has been some further progress in the area of the eukaryotic stringent response, though the problems here are far from resolved and the mechanisms underlying the phenomenon remain elusive and controversial. Coupar et al.[207] showed that in starved rats the elongation rates of template-bound polymerase I molecules were lowered substantially, but the number of enzymes bound (presumably all to ribosomal genes) were unchanged in liver nuclei. On the other hand, numbers of template-bound polymerase II molecules were reduced by more than 50% but elongation rates were unchanged. Lindell et al.[208] injected rats with low concentrations of actinomycin D and showed that template-bound polymerase I and II activities in liver were much reduced 1 hr later, as was a fraction of rapidly-labeled nuclear proteins (down by 30%); this was interpreted to support the notion of a rapidly-turning-over protein factor regulating ribosomal RNA synthesis, but Iapalucci-Espinoza and Franze-Fernandez[209] performed similar experiments with ascites cells and came to a different conclusion. They found that pactamycin, a translation inhibitor, reduced 45S RNA transcription more slowly than actinomycin D and thus have cast doubt on the similarity of actinomycin D effects and protein synthesis inhibitors in this regard. So there is still no consensus as to the way in which protein and ribosomal RNA synthesis are coordinated in eukaryotic cells.

Guialis et al.[210] have made further use of a hybrid CHO cell line derived from normal and α-amanitin-resistant strains to show coordinate synthesis of 3 of the polymerase II subunits, including the largest of 214,000 daltons, and that several of the smaller polypeptides (34,000, 23,000 and 16,500 daltons) are not coordinately regulated in the same way. This type of approach continues to offer great promise for gaining information on RNA polymerase II metabolism.

There has been little definitive progress in sorting out the mechanisms of transcriptional regulation. Kuehn et al.[211] have isolated a 70,000-dalton protein from *Physarum* nuclei which, when phosphorylated, stimulated the transcription of ribosomal genes some fivefold. This may well relate to previous observations of phosporylated components of polymerase I in yeast.[138,139] Crampton and Woodland[212,213] have also obtained four factors from *Xenopus* oocyte extracts which appear to stimulate RNA synthesis in nuclei isolated from embryos, though this system requires more thorough characterization before the importance of these proteins can be at all clear.

In a series of papers, Ueno et al.[214] and Sekimizu et al.[215,216] have shown that antisera raised to 'S' factor selectively inhibits RNA polymerase II activity in isolated nuclei and does not affect the purified soluble enzyme (which has lost the 'S'-protein). Immunofluorescence studies also demonstrated the intranuclear location of 'S' protein during interphase and its evolutionary conservation (the antiserum reacted in nuclei from many different species). All of these experiments go some considerable way towards confirming the status of 'S' proteins as a true part of the transcriptional apparatus in vivo, but we are still without any definitive evidence concerning factors that may be important for the specific regulation of particular genes.

ACKNOWLEDGMENTS

The authors wish to express their appreciation to the Science Research Council, the Medical Research Council, and the Wellcome Trust for grants which have supported their research in this area over the past several years.

REFERENCES

1. Lewin, B., *Gene Expression-1*, John Wiley & Sons, London, 1974.
2. Zubay, G., Schwartz, D., and Beckwith, J., Mechanism of activation of catabolite sensitive genes: a positive control system, *Proc. Natl. Acad. Sci. U.S.A.*, 66, 104, 1970.
3. Chen, B., de Crombrugghe, B., Anderson, W. B., Gottesman, M. E., Pastan, I., and Perlman, R. L., On the mechanism of action of lac repressor, *Nature (London), New Biol.*, 233, 67, 1971.
4. Golomb, M. and Chamberlin, M., Characterisation of T_7-specific Ribonucleic acid polymerase, *J. Biol. Chem.*, 249, 2858, 1974.
5. Duffy, J. J. and Geiduschek, E. P., Purification of a positive regulatory subunit from phage SPOI-modified RNA polymerase, *Nature (London)*, 270, 28, 1977.
6. Travers, A., RNA polymerase specificity and the control of growth, *Nature (London)*, 263, 641, 1976.
7. Kornberg, R. D., Structure of chromatin, *Annu. Rev. Biochem.*, 46, 931, 1977.
8. Lewin, B., Units of transcription and translation, *Cell*, 4, 77, 1975.
9. Davidson, E. H. and Britten, R. J., Organisation, transcription and regulation in the animal genome, *Q. Rev. Biol.*, 48, 565, 1973.
10. Perry, R. P., Processing of RNA, *Annu. Rev. Biochem.*, 45, 605, 1976.
11. Lewin, B., Units of transcription and translation, *Cell*, 4, 11, 1975.
12. Molloy, G. R., Jelinek, W., Salditt, M., and Darnell, J. E., Arrangement of specific oligonucleotides within poly(A)-terminated hnRNA molecules, *Cell*, 1, 43, 1974.
13. Jelinek, W., Molloy, G. R., Fernandez-Munoz, R., Salditt, M., and Darnell, J. E., Secondary structure in heterogeneous nuclear RNA, *J. Mol. Biol.*, 82, 361, 1974.
14. Klessig, D. F., Two adenovirus mRNAs have a common 5'-terminal leader sequence encoded at least 10kb upstream from their main coding regions, *Cell*, 12, 9, 1977.
15. Jeffreys, A. J. and Flavell, R. A., The rabbit β-globin gene contains a large insert in the coding sequence, *Cell*, 12, 1097, 1977.
16. Bastos, R. N. and Aviv, H., Globin RNA precursor molecules, *Cell*, 11, 641, 1977.
17. Brawerman, G., Characteristics and significance of the polyadenylate sequence in mammalian messenger RNA, *Prog. Nucleic Acid Res. Mol. Biol.*, 17, 118, 1976.
18. Schibler, U. and Perry, R. P., Characterisation of the 5'-termini of HnRNA in mouse L cells, *Cell*, 9, 121, 1976.
19. Lodish, H. F., Translational control of protein synthesis, *Annu. Rev. Biochem.*, 45, 39, 1976.
20. Cooper, H. L., Ribosomal nucleic acid wastage in resting and growing lymphocytes, *J. Biol. Chem.*, 244, 5590, 1969.
21. Travers, A., Transcription control mechanisms, *Int. Rev. Biochem.*, 7, 233, 1978.
22. Weiss, S., Enzymatic incorporation of ribonucleoside triphosphates into the interpolynucleotide linkages of ribonucleic acid, *Proc. Natl. Acad. Sci. U.S.A.*, 46, 1020, 1960.
23. Widnell, C. C. and Tata, J. R., Studies on the stimulation by ammonium sulphate of the DNA-dependent RNA polymerase of isolated rat liver nuclei, *Biochim. Biophys. Acta*, 123, 478, 1966.
24. Roeder, R. G. and Rutter, W. J., Specific nucleolar and nucleoplasmic RNA polymerases, *Proc. Natl. Acad. Sci. U.S.A.*, 65, 675, 1970.
25. Kedinger, C., Nuret, P., and Chambon, P., Structural evidence for two α-amanitin sensitive RNA polymerases in calf thymus, *FEBS Lett.*, 15, 169, 1971.
26. Jacob, S. T., Mammalian RNA polymerases, *Prog. Nucleic Acid Res. Mol. Biol.*, 13, 93, 1973.
27. Chambon, P., Animal RNA polymerases, in *The Enzymes*, Vol. 10, 3rd ed., Boyer, P. D., Ed., Academic Press, New York, 1974, 261.
28. Chambon, P., Eucaryotic nuclear RNA polymerases, *Annu. Rev. Biochem.*, 44, 613, 1975.
29. Beebee, T. J. C. and Butterworth, P. H. W., Eucaryotic deoxyribonucleic acid-dependent RNA polymerases, *Biochem. Soc. Symp.*, 42, 75, 1977.
30. Coupar, B. E. H. and Chesterton, C. J., Purification of forms AI and AII DAN-dependent RNA polymerases from rat liver nucleoli using low-ionic-strength extraction conditions, *Eur. J. Biochem.*, 59, 25, 1975.
31. Flint, S. J., de Pomerai, D. I., Chesterton, C. J., and Butterworth, P. H. W., Template specificity of eucaryotic DNA-dependent RNA polymerases, *Eur. J. Biochem.*, 42, 567, 1974.
32. Yu, F.- L. and Feigelson, P., Cortisone stimulation of nucleolar RNA polymerase activity, *Proc. Natl. Acad. Sci. U.S.A.*, 68, 2177, 1972.
33. Grummt, I. and Lindigkeit, R., Pre-ribosomal RNA synthesis in isolated rat-liver nucleoli, *Eur. J. Biochem.*, 36, 244, 1973.
34. Kellas, B. L., Austoker, J. L., Beebee, T. J. C., and Butterworth, P. H. W., Forms AI and AII DNA-dependent RNA polymerases as components of two defined pools of polymerase activity in mammalian cells, *Eur. J. Biochem.*, 72, 583, 1977.

35. **Lin, Y. C., Rose, K. M., and Jacob, S. T.,** Evidence for the nucleolar origin of RNA polymerases identified in the cytosol, *Biochem. Biophys. Res. Commun.*, 72, 114, 1976.
36. **Seifart, K. H., Benecke, B. J., and Juhasz, P. P.,** Multiple RNA polymerase species from rat liver, *Arch. Biochem. Biophys.*, 151, 519, 1972.
37. **Schwartz, L. B., Sklar, V. E. F., Jaehning, J. A., Weinmann, R., and Roeder, R. G.,** Isolation and partial characterisation of the multiple forms of deoxyribonucleic acid-dependent ribonucleic acid polymerases in the mouse myeloma, MOPC 315, *J. Biol. Chem.*, 249, 5889, 1974.
38. **Buhler, J.-M., Iborra, F., Sentenac, A., and Fromageot, P.,** Structural studies on yeast RNA polymerases, *J. Biol. Chem.*, 251, 1712, 1976.
39. **Kedinger, C., Gissinger, F., and Chambon, P.,** Animal DNA-dependent RNA polymerases, *Eur. J. Biochem.*, 44, 421, 1974.
40. **Sklar, V. E. F. and Roeder, R. G.,** Purification and subunit structure of deoxyribonucleic acid-dependent ribonucleic acid polymerase III from the mouse plasmacytoma, MOPC 315, *J. Biol. Chem.*, 251, 1064, 1976.
41. **Coupar, B. E. H., Chesterton, C. J., and Butterworth, P. H. W.,** The subunit structure of the form AII DNA-dependent RNA polymerase from rat liver, *FEBS Lett.*, 77, 273, 1977.
42. **Gissinger, F. and Chambon, P.,** Animal DNA-dependent RNA polymerases, *Eur. J. Biochem.*, 28, 277, 1972.
43. **Matsui, T., Onishi, T., and Muramatsu, M.,** Nucleolar DNA-dependent RNA polymerases from rat liver, *Eur. J. Biochem.*, 71, 361, 1976.
44. **Weaver, R. F., Blatti, S. P., and Rutter, W. J.,** Molecular structures of DNA-dependent RNA polymerase (II) from calf thymus and rat liver, *Proc. Natl. Acad. Sci. U.S.A.*, 68, 2994, 1971.
45. **Dezelee, S., Wyers, F., Sentenac, A., and Fromageot, P.,** Two forms of RNA polymerase B in yeast, *Eur. J. Biochem.*, 65, 543, 1976.
46. **Guilfoyle, T. J. and Key, J. L.,** The subunit structure of soluble and chromatin-bound RNA polymerase II from soybean, *Biochem. Biophys. Res. Commun.*, 74, 308, 1977.
47. **Sklar, V. E. F., Schwartz, L. B., and Roeder, R. G.,** Distinct molecular structures of nuclear class I, II and III DNA-dependent RNA polymerases, *Proc. Natl. Acad. Sci. U.S.A.*, 72, 348, 1975.
48. **Zylber, E. A. and Penman, S.,** Products of RNA polymerases in HeLa cell nuclei, *Proc. Natl. Acad. Sci. U.S.A.*, 68, 2861, 1971.
49. **Reeder, R. H. and Roeder, R. G.,** Ribosomal RNA synthesis in isolated nuclei, *J. Mol. Biol.*, 67, 433, 1972.
50. **Weinmann, R. and Roeder, R. G.,** Role of DNA-dependent RNA polymerase III in the transcription of tRNA and 5 *S* RNA genes, *Proc. Natl. Acad. Sci. U.S.A.*, 71, 1790, 1974.
51. **Beebee, T. J. C. and Butterworth, P. H. W.,** Transcription fidelity and structural integrity of isolated nucleoli, *Eur. J. Biochem.*, 77, 341, 1977.
52. **Ballal, N. R., Choi, Y. C., Mouche, R., and Busch, H.,** Fidelity of synthesis of pre-ribosomal RNA in isolated nucleoli and nucleolar chromatin, *Proc. Natl. Acad. Sci. U.S.A.*, 74, 2446, 1977.
53. **Ingles, C. J., Guialas, A., Lam, J., and Siminovitch, L.,** α-amanitin resistance of RNA polymerase II in mutant Chinese hamster ovary cell lines, *J. Biol. Chem.*, 251, 2729, 1976.
54. **Amati, F., Blasi, F., di Porzio, U., Riccio, A., and Trabeni, C.,** Hamster α-amanitin-resistant RNA polymerase II able to transcribe polyoma virus genome in somatic cell hybrids, *Proc. Natl. Acad. Sci. U.S.A.*, 72, 753, 1975.
55. **Gariglio, P. and Mousset, S.,** Characterisation of a soluble Simian virus 40 transcription complex, *Eur. J. Biochem.*, 76, 583, 1977.
56. **Jamrich, M., Greenleaf, A. L., and Bautz, E. K. F.,** Localisation of RNA polymerase in polytene chromosomes of *Drosophila melanogaster*, *Proc. Natl. Acad. Sci. U.S.A.*, 74, 2079, 1977.
57. **Marzluff, W. F., White, E. L., Benjamin, R., and Huang, R. C. C.,** Low molecular weight RNA species from chromatin, *Biochemistry*, 14, 3715, 1975.
58. **Price, R. and Penman, S.,** A distinct RNA polymerase activity synthesising 5.5 *S*, 5 *S* and 4 *S* RNA in nuclei from adenovirus-2 infected HeLa cells, *J. Mol. Biol.*, 70, 435, 1972.
59. **Weinmann, R., Raskas, H. J., and Roeder, R. G.,** Role of DNA-dependent RNA polymerase II and III in transcription of the adenovirus genome late in productive infection, *Proc. Natl. Acad. Sci. U.S.A.*, 71, 3426, 1974.
60. **Van Keulen, H., Planta, R. J., and Retel, J.,** Structure and transcription specificity of yeast RNA polymerase A, *Biochim. Biophys. Acta*, 395, 179, 1975.
61. **Van Keulen, H. and Retel, J.,** Transcription specificity of yeast RNA polymerase A, *Eur. J. Biochem.*, 79, 579, 1977.
62. **Beebee, T. J. C. and Butterworth, P. H. W.,** Template specificities of *Xenopus laevis* RNA polymerases, *Eur. J. Biochem.*, 45, 395, 1974.
63. **Beebee, T. J. C. and Butterworth, P. H. W.,** Transcription specificity of *Xenopus laevis* RNA polymerase A, *FEBS Lett.*, 47, 304, 1974.

64. **Parker, C. S. and Roeder, R. G.,** Selective and accurate transcription of the *Xenopus laevis* 5S RNA genes in isolated chromatin by purified RNA polymerase III, *Proc. Natl. Acad. Sci. U.S.A.,* 74, 44, 1977.

65. **Yamamoto, M., Jonas, D., and Seifart, K. H.,** Transcription of ribosomal 5S RNA by RNA polymerase C in isolated chromatin from HeLa cells, *Eur. J. Biochem.,* 80, 243, 1977.

66. **Galau, G. A., Klein, W. H., Davis, M. M., Wold, B. J., Britten, R. J., and Davidson, E. H.,** Structural gene sets active in embryos and adult tissues of sea urchin, *Cell,* 7, 487, 1976.

67. **Bishop, J. O., Morton, J. G., Rosbash, M., and Richardson, M.,** Three abundance classes in HeLa Cell messenger RNA, *Nature (London),* 250, 199, 1974.

68. **Hastie, N. D. and Bishop, J. O.,** The expression of three abundance classes of messenger RNA in mouse tissues, *Cell,* 9, 761, 1976.

69. **Mondal, H., Mandal, R., and Biswas, B.,** RNA polymerase from eucaryote cells, *Eur. J. Biochem.,* 25, 463, 1972.

70. **Wasserman, P. M., Hollinger, T. G., and Smith, L. D.,** RNA polymerases in the germinal vesicle contents of *Rana pipiens* oocytes, *Nature (London) New Biol.,* 240, 208, 1972.

71. **Roeder, R. G.,** Multiple forms of deoxyribonucleic acid-dependent ribonucleic acid polymerase in *Xenopus laevis, J. Biol. Chem.,* 249, 249, 1974.

72. **Wilhelm, J., Dina, D., and Crippa, M.,** A special form of deoxyribonucleic acid-dependent ribonucleic acid polymerase from oocytes of *Xenopus laevis, Biochemistry,* 13, 1200, 1974.

73. **Roeder, R. G.,** Multiple forms of deoxyribonucleic acid-dependent ribonucleic acid polymerase in *Xenopus laevis, J. Biol. Chem.,* 249, 241, 1974.

74. **Greenleaf, A. L., Haars, R., and Bautz, E. K. F.,** In vitro proteolysis of a large subunit of *Drosophila melanogaster* RNA polymerase B, *FEBS Lett.,* 71, 205, 1976.

75. **Hentschel, C. C. and Tata, J. R.,** Differential activation of free and template-engaged RNA polymerase I and II during the resumption of development of dormant *Artemia gastrulae, Dev. Biol.,* 57, 293, 1977.

76. **Van der Westhuyzen, D. R., Boyd, M. C. D., Fitschen, W., and von Holt, C.,** DNA-dependent RNA polymerase in maturing avian erythrocytes, *FEBS Lett.,* 30, 195, 1973.

77. **Longacre, S. S. and Rutter, W. J.,** Nucleotide polymerases in the developing avian erythrocyte, *J. Biol. Chem.,* 252, 273, 1977.

78. **Kruger, C. and Seifart, K. H.,** RNA polymerases during differentiation of avian erythrocytes, *Exp. Cell Res.,* 106, 446, 1977.

79. **Chesteron, C. J., Humphrey, S. M., and Butterworth, P. H. W.,** Comparison of the multiple deoxyribonucleic acid-dependent ribonucleic acid polymerase forms of a whole rat liver and a minimal-deviation rat hepatoma cell line, *Biochem. J.,* 126, 675, 1972.

80. **Austoker, J. L., Beebee, T. J. C., Chesterton, C. J., and Butterworth, P. H. W.,** DNA-dependent RNA polymerase activity of Chinese hamster kidney cells sensitive to high concentrations of α-amanitin, *Cell,* 3, 227, 1974.

81. **Rose, K. M., Ruch, P. A., Morris, H. P., and Jacob, S. T.,** RNA polymerases from a rat hepatoma, *Biochim. Biophys. Acta,* 432, 60, 1976.

82. **Capobianco, G., Farina, G., Pelella, E., and Musiella, V.,** Sensitivity to α-amanitin of multiple DNA-dependent RNA polymerases from experimental tumors, *Biochem. Biophys. Res. Commun.,* 77, 306, 1977.

83. **Schwartz, L. B. and Roeder, R. G.,** Purification and subunit structure of deoxyribonucleic acid-dependent ribonucleic acid polymerase I from the mouse myeloma MOPC 315, *J. Biol. Chem.,* 249, 5898, 1974.

84. **Schwartz, L. B. and Roeder, R. G.,** Purification and subunit structure of deoxyribonucleic acid-dependent ribonucleic acid polymerase II from the mouse plasmcytoma MOPC 315, *J. Biol. Chem.,* 250, 3221, 1975.

85. **Takatsuka, Y., Kohno, M., Higashi, K., Hirano, H., and Sakamoto, Y.,** Redistribution of chromatin containing ribosomal cistrons during liver regeneration, *Exp. Cell Res.,* 103, 191, 1976.

86. **Novello, F. and Stirpe, F.,** Simultaneous assay of RNA polymerase I and II in nuclei isolated from resting and growing rat liver with the use of α-amanitin, *FEBS Lett.,* 8, 57, 1970.

87. **Yu, F.-L.,** Two functional states of the RNA polymerase in the rat hepatic nuclear and nucleolar fractions, *Nature (London),* 251, 344, 1974.

88. **Yu, F.-L.,** Increased levels of rat hepatic nuclear free and engaged RNA polymerase activities during liver regeneration, *Biochem. Biophys. Res. Commun.,* 64, 1107, 1975.

89. **Organtini, J. E., Joseph, C. R., and Farbar, J. L.,** Increases in the activity of the solubilised rat liver nuclear RNA polymerases following partial hepatectomy, *Arch. Biochem. Biophys.,* 170, 485, 1975.

90. **Schmid, W. and Sekeris, C. E.,** Nucleolar RNA synthesis in the liver of partially hepatectomised and cortisol-treated rats, *Biochim. Biophys. Acta,* 402, 244, 1975.

91. **Andersen, M. W., Ballal, N. R., and Busch, H.,** Nucleoli of thioacetamide-treated liver as a model for studying regulation of pre-ribosomal RNA synthesis, *Biochem. Biophys. Res. Commun.,* 78, 129, 1977.

92. **Cooper, H. L.,** *Biochemistry of Cell Division,* Baserga, R., Ed., Charles C Thomas, Springfield, Illinois, 1969, 91.

93. **Cooke, A. S. and Brown, M.,** Stimulation of the activities of solubilised pig lymphocyte RNA polymerases by phytohaemagglutinin, *Biochem. Biophys. Res. Commun.,* 51, 1042, 1973.

94. **Jaehning, J. A., Stewart, C. C., and Roeder, R. G.,** DNA-dependent RNA polymerase levels during the response of human periperal lymphocytes to phytohaemagglutinin, *Cell,* 4, 51, 1975.

95. **Kraft, N. and Shortman, K.,** A suggested control function for the animal ribonuclease-ribonuclease inhibitor system based on studies of isolated cells and phytohaemagglutinin-transformed lymphocytes, *Biochim. Biophys. Acta,* 217, 164, 1970.

96. **Dauphinais, C. and Waithe, W. I.,** Phytohaemagglutinin stimulation of human lymphocytes during amino acid deprivation, *Eur. J. Biochem.,* 78, 189, 1977.

97. **Teissere, M., Peron, P., and Ricard, J.,** Hormonal control of chromatin availability and of the activity of RNA polerases in higher plants, *FEBS Lett.,* 30, 65, 1973.

98. **Guilfoyle, T. J., Lin, C. Y., Chen, Y. M., Nagao, R. T., and Key, J. L.,** Enhancement of soybean RNA polymerase I by Auxin, *Proc. Natl. Acad. Sci. U.S.A.,* 72, 69, 1975.

99. **Fuhrman, S. A. and Gill, G. N.,** Adrenocorticotropic hormone stimulation of adrenal RNA polymerase I and III activities, *Biochemistry,* 14, 2925, 1975.

100. **Fuhrman, S. A. and Gill, G. N.,** Adrenocorticotropic hormone regulation of adrenal RNA polymerases, *Biochemistry,* 15, 5520, 1976.

101. **Sajdel, E. and Jacob, S.,** Mechanism of early effect of hydrocortisone on the transcriptional process, *Biochem. Biophys. Res. Commun.,* 45, 707, 1971.

102. **Davies, P. and Griffiths, K.,** Stimulation in vitro of prostatic ribonucleic acid polymerase by 5α-dihydrotestosterone-receptor complexes, *Biochem. Biophys. Res. Commun.,* 53, 373, 1973.

103. **Cox, R. F., Haines, M. E., and Carey, N. H.,** Modification of the template capacity of chick oviduct chromatin for form B RNA polymerase by estradiol, *Eur. J. Biochem.,* 32, 513, 1973.

104. **Cox, R. F.,** Quantitation of elongation rates of form A and B RNA polymerases in chick oviduct nuclei and effects of estradiol, *Cell,* 7, 455, 1976.

105. **Dierks-Ventling, C. and Bieri-Bonniot, F.,** Stimulation of RNA polymerase I and II activities by 17-β-estradiol receptor on chick liver chromatin, *Nucleic Acid Res.,* 4, 381, 1977.

106. **Bieri-Bonniot, F. and Dierks-Ventling, C.,** Multiple forms of DNA-dependent RNA polymerase I from immature chick liver, *Eur. J. Biochem.,* 73, 507, 1977.

107. **Hardin, J. W., Clark, J. H., Glasser, S. R., and Peck, E. J.,** RNA polymerase activity and uterine growth, *Biochemistry,* 15, 1370, 1976.

108. **Weil, P. A., Sidikaro, J., Stancel, G. M., and Blatti, S. P.,** Hormonal control of transcription in the rat uterus, *J. Biol. Chem.,* 252, 1092, 1977.

109. **Smuckler, E. and Tata, J. R.,** Changes in hepatic nuclear DNA-dependent RNA polymerase caused by growth hormone and triiodothyronine, *Nature (London),* 234, 37, 1971.

110. **Barbiroli, B., Tadolini, B., Moruzzi, M. S., and Monti, M. G.,** Modification of the template capacity of liver chromatin for form B ribonucleic acid polymerase by food intake in rats under controlled feeding schedules, *Biochem. J.,* 146, 687, 1975.

111. **Barbiroli, B., Monti, M. G., Moruzzi, M. S., and Mezzetti, G.,** Functional modification of liver form B RNA polymerase activity by a protein fraction from rats accustomed to controlled feeding schedules, *Biochim. Biophys. Acta,* 479, 69, 1977.

112. **Andersson, G. M. and Von der Decker, A.,** Deoxyribonucleic acid-dependent ribonucleic acid polymerase activity in rat liver after protein restriction, *Biochem. J.,* 148, 49, 1975.

113. **Bailey, R. P., Vrooman, M. J., Sawai, Y., Tsukada, K., Short, J., and Lieberman, I.,** Amino acids and control of nucleolar size, the activity of RNA polymerase I and DNA synthesis in liver, *Proc. Natl. Acad. Sci. U.S.A.,* 73, 3201, 1976.

114. **Yu, F.-L. and Feigelson, P.,** The rapid turnover of RNA polymerase of rat liver nucleolus and of its messenger RNA, *Proc. Natl. Acad. Sci. U.S.A.,* 69, 2833, 1972.

115. **Benecke, B. J., Ferencz, A., and Seifart, K. H.,** Resistance of hepatic RNA polymerases to compounds effecting RNA and protein synthesis in vivo, *FEBS Lett.,* 31, 53, 1973.

116. **Farber, J. L. and Farmar, R.,** Differential effects of cycloheximide on protein and RNA synthesis as a function of dose, *Biochem. Biophys. Res. Commun.,* 51, 626, 1973.

117. **Lampert, A. and Feigelson, P.,** A short-lived polypeptide component of one of two discrete functional pools of hepatic, nuclear, α-amanitin resistant RNA polymerases, *Biochem. Biophys. Res. Commun.,* 58, 1030, 1974.

118. **Ch'ih, J. J., Pike, L. M., and Devlin, T. M.,** Regulation of mammalian protein synthesis in vivo, *Biochem. J.,* 168, 57, 1977.

119. Hadijiolov, A. A., Dabeva, M. D., and Mackedonski, V. V., The action of α-amanitin in vivo on the synthesis and maturation of mouse liver ribonucleic acids, *Biochem. J.*, 138, 321, 1974.

120. Penman, S., Vesco, C., and Penman, M., Localisation and kinetics of formation of nuclear heterodisperse RNA, cytoplasmic heterodisperse RNA and polysome-associated messenger RNA in Hela cells, *J. Mol. Biol.*, 34, 49, 1968.

121. Lindell, T. J., Evidence for an extranucleolar mechanism of actinomycin D action, *Nature (London)*, 263, 347, 1976.

122. Chesterton, C. J., Coupar, B. E. H., Butterworth, P. H. W., Buss, J., and Green, M. H., Studies on the control of ribosomal RNA synthesis in Hela cells, *Eur. J. Biochem.*, 57, 79, 1975.

123. Cereglini, S. and Franze-Fernandez, M. T., Ehrlich Ascites cell DNA-dependent RNA polymerases, *FEBS Lett.*, 41, 161, 1974.

124. Franze-Fernandez, M. T. and Fontanive-Sanguesa, A. V., Control of rRNA synthesis, *FEBS Lett.*, 54, 26, 1975.

125. Grummt, F., Smith, V. A., and Grummt, I., Amino acid starvation affects the initiation frequency of nucleolar RNA polymerase, *Cell*, 7, 439, 1976.

126. Grummt, I. and Grummt, F., Control of nucleolar RNA synthesis by the intracellular pool sizes of ATP and GTP, *Cell*, 7, 447, 1976.

127. Grummt, F., Paul, D., and Grummt, I., Regulation of ATP pools, rRNA and DNA synthesis in 3T3 cells in response to serum or hypoxanthine, *Eur. J. Biochem.*, 76, 7, 1977.

128. Dehlinger, P. J., Hamilton, T. A., and Litt, M., Amino acid control of stable RNA synthesis in Friend leukemia cells in relation to intracellular purine nucleoside triphosphate levels, *Eur. J. Biochem.*, 77, 495, 1977.

129. Gross, K. J. and Pogo, A. O., Control of ribonucleic acid synthesis in eucaryotes, *J. Biol. Chem.*, 249, 568, 1974.

130. Gross, K. J. and Pogo, A. O., Conrol of ribonucleic acid synthesis in eucaryotes, *Biochemistry*, 15, 2070, 1976.

131. Gross, K. J. and Pogo, A. O., Control of ribonucleic acid synthesis in eucaryotes, *Biochemistry*, 15, 2082, 1976.

132. Schulman, R. W., Sripati, C. E., and Warner, J. R., Non-coordinated transcription in the absence of protein synthesis in yeast, *J. Biol. Chem.*, 252, 1344, 1977.

133. Varrone, V., Ambesi-Impiombata, F., and Macchia, V., Stimulation by cyclic-3',5'-adenosine monophosphate of RNA synthesis in a mammalian cell-free system, *FEBS Lett.*, 21, 99, 1972.

134. Martelo, O. J. and Hirsch, J., Effect of nuclear protein kinases on mammalian RNA synthesis, *Biochem. Biophys. Res. Commun.*, 58, 1008, 1974.

135. Jungmann, R. A., Hiestrand, P. C., and Schweppe, J. S., Adenosine-3',5'-monophosphate-dependent protein kinase and the stimulation of ovarian nuclear ribonucleic acid polymerase activities, *J. Biol. Chem.*, 249, 5444, 1974.

136. Dahmus, M. E., Stimulation of Ascites tumor RNA polymerase II by protein kinase, *Biochemistry*, 15, 1821, 1976.

137. Beebee, T. J. C., Incorporation of γ ^{32}P-ATP by eucaryotic RNA polymerase A, *FEBS Lett.*, 35, 133, 1973.

138. Buhler, J. M., Iborra, F., Sentenac, A., and Fromageot, P., The presence of phosphorylated subunits in yeast RNA polymerases A and B, *FEBS Lett.*, 71, 37, 1976.

139. Bell, G. I., Valenzuela, P., and Rutter, W. J., Phosphorylation of yeast RNA polymerases, *Nature (London)*, 261, 429, 1976.

140. Bell, G. I., Valenzuela, P., and Rutter, W. J., Phosphorylation of yeast DNA-dependent RNA polymerases in vivo and in vitro, *J. Biol. Chem.*, 252, 3082, 1977.

141. McNaughton, D. R., Klassen, G. R., and LeJohn, H. B., Phosphorylated guanosine derivatives of eucaryotes: regulation of DNA-dependent RNA polymerase I, II and III in fungal development, *Biochem. Biophys. Res. Commun.*, 66, 468, 1975.

142. Higashinakagawa, T., Onishi, T., and Muramatsu, M., A factor stimulating the transcription by nucleolar RNA polymerase I in the nucleolus of rat liver, *Biochem. Biophys. Res. Commun.*, 48, 937, 1972.

143. James, G. T., Yeoman, L. C., Matsui, S., Goldberg, A. H., and Busch, H., Isolation and characterisation of non-histone chromosomal protein C-14 which stimulates RNA synthesis, *Biochemistry*, 16, 2384, 1977.

144. Goldberg, M. I., Perriard, J. C., and Rutter, W. J., A protein cofactor that stimulates the activity of DNA-dependent RNA polymerase I on double-stranded DNA, *Biochemistry*, 16, 1648, 1977.

145. Manen, C. A. and Russell, D. H., Ornithine decarboxylase may function as an initiation factor for RNA polymerase I, *Science*, 195, 505, 1977.

146. Hildebrandt, A. and Sauer, H. W., Transcription of ribosomal RNA in the life cycle of *Physarum* may be regulated by a specific nucleolar initiation inhibitor, *Biochem. Biophys. Res. Commun.*, 74, 466, 1977.

147. **Mondal, H., Mandal, R., and Biswas, B.,** Factors and rifampicin influencing RNA polymerase isolation from chromatin of eucaryotic cells, *Biochem. Biophys. Res. Commun., 40,* 1194, 1970.

148. **Mondal, H., Ganguly, A., Das, A., Mandall, R. K., and Biswas, B. B.,** Ribonucleic acid polymerase from eucaryotic cells, *Eur. J. Biochem., 28,* 143, 1972.

149. **Stein, H. and Hausen, P.,** Factors influencing the activity of mammalian RNA polymerase, *Cold Spring Harbor Symp. Quant. Biol., 35,* 709, 1970.

150. **Stein, H. and Hausen, P.,** A factor from calf thymus stimulating DNA-dependent RNA polymerase isolated from this tissue, *Eur. J. Biochem., 14,* 270, 1970.

151. **Brand, J., Spindler, E., and Stein, H.,** The role of basic proteins in the DNA-dependent RNA polymerase reaction, *FEBS Lett., 80,* 173, 1977.

152. **Lukacs, N. and Stein, H.,** Evidence that there are two basically different types of protein present in calf thymus which stimulate the DNA-dependent RNA polymerase reaction, *FEBS Lett., 69,* 295, 1976.

153. **Seifart, K. H.,** A factor stimulating the transcription on the double-stranded DNA by purified RNA polymerase from rat liver nuclei, *Cold Spring Harbor Symp. Quant. Biol., 35,* 719, 1970.

154. **Seifart, K. H., Juhasz, P. P., and Benecke, B. J.,** A protein factor from rat liver tissue enhancing the transcription of native templates by homologous RNA polymerase B, *Eur. J. Biochem., 33,* 181, 1973.

155. **Shea, M. and Kleinsmith, L. J.,** Template-specific stimulation of RNA synthesis by phosphorylated non-histone chromatin proteins, *Biochem. Biophys. Res. Commun., 50,* 473, 1973.

156. **Sugden, B. and Keller, W.,** Mammalian deoxyribonucleic acid-dependent ribonucleic acid polymerases, *J. Biol. Chem., 248,* 3777, 1973.

157. **Lentfer, D. and Lezius, A. G.,** Mouse myeloma RNA polymerase B template specificities and the role of a transcription-stimulating factor, *Eur. J. Biochem., 30,* 278, 1972.

158. **Ihara, S. and Kawakami, M.,** Stimulatory effect of a factor extracted from mouse myeloma nuclei on preinitiation process of RNA synthesis, *Arch. Biochem. Biophys., 183,* 123, 1977.

159. **Lee, S. C. and Dahmus, M. E.,** Stimulation of eucaryotic DNA-dependent RNA polymerase by protein factors, *Proc. Natl. Acad. Sci. U.S.A., 70,* 1383, 1973.

160. **Sekimizu, K., Kobayashi, N., Mizuno, D., and Natori, S.,** Purification of a factor from Ascites tumor cells specifically stimulating RNA polymerase II, *Biochemistry, 15,* 5064, 1976.

161. **Kostraba, N. C. and Wang, T. Y.,** Inhibition of transcription in vitro by a non-histone protein isolated from Ehrlich Ascites tumor chromatin, *J. Biol. Chem., 250,* 8938, 1975.

162. **Kostraba, N. C., Montagna, R. A., and Wang, T. Y.,** Mode of action of non-histone proteins in the stimulation of transcription from DNA, *Biochem. Biophys. Res. Commun., 72,* 334, 1976.

163. **Moruzzi, G., Barbiroli, B., Moruzzi, M. S., and Tadolini, B.,** The effects of spermine on transcription on mammalian chromatin by mammalian deoxyribonucleic acid-dependent ribonucleic acid polymerase, *Biochem. J., 146,* 697, 1975.

164. **Janne, C. O., Bardin, W., and Jacob, S. T.,** DNA-dependent RNA polymerases I and II from kidney, *Biochemistry, 14,* 3589, 1975.

165. **Ho-Terry, L. and Cohen, A.,** Effects of SV40 infection of (^{3}H)-uridine incorporation, *Biochim. Biophys. Acta, 479,* 24, 1977.

166. **Yu, F.-Y.,** An improved method for the quantitative isolation of rat liver nuclear RNA polymerases, *Biochim. Biophys. Acta, 395,* 329, 1975.

167. **Gilboa, E., Soreq, H., and Aviv, H.,** Initiation of RNA synthesis in isolated nuclei, *Eur. J. Biochem., 77,* 392, 1977.

168. **Hildebrandt, A., Sebastian, J., and Halvorson, H. O.,** Yeast nuclear RNA polymerase I and II are immunologically related, *Nature (London) New Biol., 246,* 73, 1973.

169. **Hodo, H. G. and Blatti, S. P.,** Purification using polyethylenimine precipitation and low molecular weight subunit analysis of calf thymus and wheat-germ DNA-dependent RNA polymerase II, *Biochemistry, 16,* 2334, 1977.

170. **Guialis, A., Beatty, B. G., Ingles, C. J., and Crerar, M. M.,** Regulation of RNA polymerase II activity in α-amanitin-resistant CHO hybrid cells, *Cell, 10,* 53, 1977.

171. **Woodland, H. R. and Gurdon, J. B.,** RNA synthesis in an amphibian nuclear transplant hybrid, *Dev. Biol., 20,* 89, 1969.

172. **Harris, H., Sidebottom, E., Grace, D. M., and Bramwell, M.,** The expression of genetic information: a study with hybrid animal cells, *J. Cell Sci., 4,* 499, 1969.

173. **Ford, P. J. and Mathieson, T.,** Control of 5 S RNA synthesis in *Xenopus laevis, Nature (London), 261,* 433, 1976.

174. **Foe, V. E., Wilkinson, L. E., and Laird, C. D.,** Comparative organisation of active transcription units in *Oncopeltus fasciatus, Cell, 9,* 131, 1976.

175. **Kleene, K. C. and Humphreys, T.,** Similarity of HnRNA sequences in blastula and pluteus stage sea urchin embryos, *Cell, 12,* 143, 1977.

176. **Hough-Evans, B., Wold, B. J., Ernst, S. G., Britten, R. J., and Davidson, E. H.,** Appearance and persistence of maternal RNA sequences in sea urchin development, *Dev. Biol.,* 60, 258, 1977.

177. **Hereford, L. M. and Rosbash, M.,** Number and distribution of polyadenylated RNA sequences in yeast, *Cell,* 10, 453, 1977.

178. **Hereford, L. M. and Rosbash, M.,** Regulation of a set of abundant mRNA sequences, *Cell,* 10, 463, 1977.

179. **Colbert, D. A., Tedeschi, M. V., Atryzek, V., and Fausto, N.,** Diversity of polyadenylated messenger RNA sequences in normal and 12 hr regenerating liver, *Dev. Biol.,* 59, 111, 1977.

180. **Hahn, W. E., Pettijohn, D. E., and Van Nes, J.,** One strand equivalent of the *Escherichia coli* genome is transcribed: complexity and abundance classes of mRNA, *Science,* 197, 582, 1977.

181. **Franke, W. W., Scheer, U., Spring, H., Trendelenburg, M. F., and Krohne, G.,** Morphology of transcriptional units of rDNA, *Exp. Cell Res.,* 100, 233, 1976.

182. **Angelier, N., Hemon, D., and Bouteille, M.,** Electron microscopic autoradiography of isolated nucleolar transcription units, *Exp. Cell Res.,* 100, 389, 1976.

183. **McKnight, S. L. and Miller, O. L.,** Ultrastructural patterns of RNA synthesis during early embryogenesis of *Drosophila melanogaster, Cell,* 8, 305, 1976.

184. **Scheer, U., Trendelenburg, M. F., and Franke, W. W.,** Regulation of transcription of genes of ribosomal RNA during amphibian oogenesis, *J. Cell Biol.,* 69, 465, 1976.

185. **Tillyer, C. R. and Butterworth, P. H. W.,** unpublished data.

186. **Maxam, A. M. and Gilbert, W.,** A new method for sequencing DNA, *Proc. Natl. Acad. Sci. U.S.A.,* 74, 560, 1977.

187. **Sanger, F., Nicklen, S., and Coulson, A. R.,** DNA-sequencing with chain-terminating inhibitors, *Proc. Natl. Acad. Sci. U.S.A.,* 74, 5463, 1977.

188. **Reddy, V. B., Thimmappaya, B., Dhar, R., Subramanian, B., Zain, S., Pan, J., Ghash, P. K., Celma, M. L., and Weissman, S. M.,** The genome of Simian Virus 40, *Science,* 200, 494, 1978.

189. **Efstratiadis, A., Kafatos, F. C., and Maniatis, T.,** The primary structure of rabbit β-globin mRNA as determined from cloned DNA, *Cell,* 10, 571, 1977.

190. **Hohn, B. and Murray, K.,** Packaging recombinant DNA molecules into bacteriophage particles *in vitro, Proc. Natl. Acad. Sci. U.S.A.,* 74, 3259, 1977.

191. **Abelson, J.,** RNA processing and the intervening sequence problem, *Ann. Rev. Biochem.,* 48, 1035, 1979.

192. **Gannon, F., O'Hare, K., Perrin, F., LePennec, J. P., Benoist, C., Cochet, M., Breathnach, R., Royal, A., Garapin, A., Cami, B., and Chambon, P.,** Organisation and sequence studies at the 5′ end of a cloned complete ovalbumin gene, *Nature (London),* 278, 428, 1979.

193. **Cochet, M., Gannon, F., Hen, R., Maroteaux, L., Perrin, F., and Chambon, P.,** Organisation and sequence studies of the 17-piece chicken conalbumin gene, *Nature (London),* 282, 567, 1979.

194. **Peebles, C. L., Ogden, R. C., Knapp, G., and Abelson, J.,** Splicing of yeast tRNA precursors; a two-stage reaction, *Cell,* 18, 27, 1979.

195. **Knapp, G., Ogden, R. C., Peebles, C. L., and Abelson, J.,** Splicing of yeast tRNA precursors: structure of the reaction intermediate, *Cell,* 18, 37, 1979.

196. **Lerner, M. R., Boyle, J. A., Mount, S. M., Wolin, S. L., and Steitz, J. A.,** Are snRNPs involved in splicing? *Nature (London),* 283, 220, 1980.

197. **Weil, P. A., Luse, D. S., Segall, J., and Roeder, R. G.,** Selective and accurate initiation of transcription at the Ad2 Major Late Promoter in a soluble system dependent on purified RNA polymerase II and DNA, *Cell,* 18, 469, 1979.

198. **Goldberg, S., Weber, J., and Darnell, J. E., Jr.,** The definition of a large viral transcription unit late in Ad2 infection of HeLa cells: mapping by effects of ultraviolet irradiation, *Cell,* 10, 617, 1977.

199. **Ziff, E. B. and Evans, R. M.,** Coincidence of the promoter and capped 5′ terminus of RNA from the Adenovirus 2 Major Late transcription unit, *Cell,* 15, 1463, 1978.

200. **Wu, G.-J. and Zubay, G.,** Prlonged transcription in a cell-free system involving nuclei and cytoplasm, *Proc. Natl. Acad. Sci. U.S.A.,* 71, 1803, 1974.

201. **Mertz, J. E. and Gurdon, J. B.,** Purified DNAs are transcribed after microinjection into X. oocytes, *Proc. Natl. Acad. Sci. U.S.A.,* 74, 1502, 1977.

202. **Kressmann, A., Hofstetter, H., de Capua, E., Grosschedl, R., and Birnsteil, M. L.,** A tRNA gene of *Xenopus laevis* contains at least two sites promoting transcription, *Nucleic Acid Res.,* 7, 1749, 1979.

203. **Birkenmeier, E. H., Brown, D. D., and Jordan, E.,** A nuclear extract of *Xenopus laevis* oocytes that accurately transcribes 5S RNA genes, *Cell,* 15, 1077, 1978.

204. **Gillam, S., Aline, R., Wylie, V., Ingles, C. J., and Smith, M.,** RNA synthesis and RNA polymerase activities during spermatogenesis in trout, *Biochim. Biophys. Acta,* 565, 275, 1979.

205. **Krauter, K. S., Soeiro, R., and Nadal-Ginard, B.,** Regulation of ribosomal RNA synthesis at the transcriptional level during rat myoblast differentiation, *J. Mol. Biol.,* 134, 727, 1979.

206. **Van der Westhuyzen, D. R.**, Alteration in RNA polymerase activities during fusion of myoblasts in culture, *Dev. Biol.*, 68, 280, 1979.
207. **Coupar, B. E. H., Davies, J. A., and Chesterton, C. J.**, Quantification of hepatic transcribing RNA polymerase molecules, polyribonucleotide elongation rates and messenger RNA complexity in fed and fasted rats, *Eur. J. Biochem.*, 84, 611, 1978.
208. **Lindell, T. J., O'Malley, A. F., and Puglisi, B.**, Inhibition of nucleoplasmic transcription and translation of rapidly-labelled nuclear proteins by low concentration of actinomycin D, *Biochemistry*, 17, 1154, 1978.
209. **Iapalucci-Espinoza, S., and Franze-Fernandex, M. T.**, Effects of actinomycin D and pactamycin on ribosomal RNA synthesis in ascites cells, *FEBS Lett.*, 107, 281, 1979.
210. **Guialis, A., Morrison, K. E., and Ingles, C. J.**, Co-ordinate synthesis of RNA polymerase II subunits in a hybrid CHO cell line, *J. Biol. Chem.*, 254, 4171, 1979.
211. **Kuehn, G. D., Affolter, V. J., Seebeck, T., Gubler, U., and Braun, R.**, Regulation of ribosomal RNA transcription in *Physarum* nuclei by a phosphoprotein *in vitro*, *Proc. Natl. Acad. Sci. U.S.A.*, 76, 2541, 1979.
212. **Crampton, J. M. and Woodland, H. R.**, A cell-free assay system for the analysis of changes in RNA synthesis during the development of *Xenopus laevis*, *Developmental Biology*, 70, 453, 1979.
213. **Crampton, J. M. and Woodland, H. R.**, Isolation from *Xenopus laevis* embryonic cells of a factor which stimulates ribosomal RNA synthesis by isolated nuclei, *Developmental Biology*, 70, 467, 1979.
214. **Ueno, K., Sekimizu, K., Mizuno, D., and Natori, S.**, Antisera to S-II protein inhibits RNA polymerase II activity in isolated nuclei, *Nature (London)*, 277, 145, 1979.
215. **Sekimizu, K., Nakanishi, Y., Mizuno, D., and Natori, S.**, Preparation and purification of antisera to ascites factor S-II and its effects on RNA polymerase II, *Biochemistry*, 18, 1582, 1979.
216. **Sekimizu, K., Mizuno, D., and Natori, S.**, Intracellular distribution of S-II protein as determined by immunofluorescence, *Exp. Cell Res.*, 124, 63, 1979.

Chapter 2

ROLE OF HISTONES IN CELL DIFFERENTIATION

R. Tsanev

TABLE OF CONTENTS

I. INTRODUCTION

The difficult and complex problem of the role of histones in cell differentiation has been discussed for 30 years since the suggestion of Stedman and Stedman.[1] In spite of the enormous progress in molecular biology, the answer to this problem is still obscure. Nevertheless, our advancing knowledge of the chemistry and structure of histones and chromatin has stimulated new ideas which may be useful for those who study cell differentiation.

The discussion of this problem cannot be successful unless we make clear two essential points. The first concerns the concept of cell differentation which is often used in a different sense, and the second point refers to the occurrence and properties of histones which may be relevant for their functional role.

II. THE PROBLEM OF CELL DIFFERENTIATION

The analysis of the great number of facts and hypotheses in this field is made difficult by the different meanings given to the term cell differentiation. Many discussions and disagreements concerning the molecular mechanism and the characteristics of this process arise from the very broad sense in which this term is used. It has been originally proposed to describe the appearance of different specialized cells in the course of embryonic development of multicellular organisms. Later, however, it was used in a much wider context as "a process whereby any cell whether of a unicellular or a multicellular organism, is able to respond to the demands made on it by selecting between the alternative potentialities of its gene complement".[2] The same broad meaning of the term is also expressed in the biochemical definition of cell differentiation: "Two cells are differentiated with respect to each other if, while they harbor the same genome, the pattern of protein which they synthesize is different".[3]

Such a concept of cell differentiation includes a variety of biological phenomena which have different characteristics and are controlled by different mechanisms. Even in its original meaning, the process of cell differentiation comprises a chain of events which do not share the same molecular basis.

Table 1
MAIN CHARACTERISTICS OF CELLULAR
REPROGRAMMING

Characteristics

Cellular reprogramming	1. Altered protein pattern
	2. No changes in DNA
A. Functional changes	1. Reversible
(labile form of cell	2. Monophasic
differentiation)	3. Short latent period
	4. Inducer permanently needed
	5. Cell-cycle independent
B. Cellular types	1. Normally irreversible
(stable form of cell	2. Multiphasic
differentiation)	3. Long latent period
	4. Inducer temporarily needed
	5. Cell-cycle dependent

The broad meaning of the term cell differentiation includes practically all cases of changing gene activity (cellular reprogramming) and does not help to understand its molecular mechanisms and particularly the role of histones. A better approach to the problem would be to classify different biological phenomena of cellular reprogramming according to their biological characteristics.

The analysis of various cases of cellular reprogramming, i.e., processes of altering protein pattern without changing DNA sequences, shows that a first level of classification may be to distinguish between two major groups markedly different in their biological characteristics.[4] The first group includes processes changing the *functional state* of a cell which are reversible and cell-cycle independent, while the second group is represented by processes changing the *cellular type* which are normally irreversible and cell-cycle dependent. All biological characteristics of these two types of cellular reprogramming are so different that it would be impossible to explain their control by one and the same molecular mechanism (Table 1).

The reversibility and the cell-cycle independence of the functional changes suggest that such processes may be controlled by a mechanism of reversible binding of regulatory molecules to DNA similar to the phenomena of repression-derepression in prokaryotic cells. On the contrary, the irreversible and cell-cycle dependent changes leading to a cellular type may be easily explained by some structural changes in the chromatin requiring an irreversible and cell-cycle dependent binding of macromolecules. While the terms repression and derepression may be preserved for mechanisms regulating the first kind of changes, we have found it reasonable to use another terminology — blocking and deblocking —[5] to specify a second kind of molecular mechanism controlling the irreversible commitment of the cell to become a particular cellular type. The need of two different control mechanisms in the process of cell differentiation has been felt by other authors, too, who have spoken of modulations and true differentiation, masking of genes, permanent repression, lightly and firmly repressed genes, labile and stable forms of cell differentiation, etc.

The theoretical conclusion that two basically different molecular mechanisms are needed for the transcription of a gene in eukaryotic cells[4,5] is experimentally supported by some recent data on the transcription of the globin gene in Friend leukemia cells. Fractionation of their chromatin into "active" and "inactive" portions by the use of DNAse II[6] has shown that both in dimethylsulfoxide (DMSO)-stimulated cells (with active globin genes) and in nonstimulated cells (with silent globin genes) the globin genes are present in the so-called "active" chromatin fraction.[7,7a] These data show that independently of whether this gene works or not, it is localized in a structurally different portion of the genome where it can be activated by a second mechanism. The same holds true for the ribosomal genes which were found to be preferentially degraded by DNase I both in G2 when rRNA synthesis is maximal and in mitosis when no rRNA is synthesized.[7b] A third example supporting this view was obtained in the case of the albumin gene which remained sensitive to DNase I even after estrogen action was blocked with the anti-estrogen tamoxifen.[7c]

Thus it can be concluded that various cellular types differ in their potentially active genomic regions (deblocked portion of the genome), i.e., in their DNA sequences which are made available for transcription due to some structural changes in the chromatin but are not transcribed unless a second mechanism is switched on. Structural changes in chromatin were experimentally found to take place in the heat shock loci of Drosophila after their activation.[7d]

If we consider the problem of histone involvement in cell differentiation from this point of view, it is clear that their role may be discussed with respect to both mechanisms. It is most likely, however, that they are involved in the second one, which irreversibly determines the cellular type. This mechanism seems to be based on the structural organization of chromatin, the essential features of which are determined by histones (see Section V). We shall first briefly discuss the present data on histones which may be relevant to their function. In most cases, reviews and some more recent data will be quoted.

III. OCCURRENCE OF HISTONES AND CELL DIFFERENTIATION

A. Histones in Different Species
1. Histones in Lower Eukaryotes[8,9]

The isolation and characterization of the proteins associated with DNA in prokaryotic and in primitive eukaryotic organisms is of fundamental importance for elucidating the evolutionary history of histones. Since the chromatin in lower eukaryotes can be condensed into chromosomes, it may be expected that at this stage of the evolution basic nuclear proteins forming regular complexes with DNA should have already appeared.

Studies on the basic DNA-associated proteins of lower organisms is difficult to perform and to interpret due to several reasons: (1) technical difficulties in isolating useful quantitites of clean nuclear material; (2) contamination of the nuclear material with basic ribosomal proteins;[10] (3) acid proteases which can degrade histones during their isolation;[11] and (4) varying results obtained with different extraction procedures.

All these difficulties show that reports on both the presence and the absence of histones in lower organisms may be due to artifacts. For this reason, only a few recent papers are more informative.

Prokaryotes — It is generally agreed that no histone-like proteins are associated with DNA of bacterial cells, although recently the presence of DNA-associated proteins in *Escherichia coli* was reported.[8] A low molecular weight DNA-binding protein, HU, was found in this species, which in some of its properties resembled the H2b eukaryotic histone.[11a,b] It is interesting that this protein was able to introduce negative superhelical turns in the DNA molecule condensing it by a ratio similar to that created by the four histones.[11c] In the thermophilic organism *Thermoplasma acidophilum,* a highly basic DNA-associated protein was isolated which was similar to calf thymus H3 in amino acid composition, to H4 in electrophoretic mobility, and to *Neurospora crassa* histones in the high content of glutamine and asparagine.[12] Another group of prokaryotes — the blue-green algae — also lack histones.[8] Some DNA-associated proteins isolated from *Anacystis nidulans* showed an amino acid composition very different from that

Table 2
MAJOR HISTONE SPECIES

Histone type	Localization	New nomenclature[36]	Earlier designations	Molecular weight (daltons)[55]
Lysine-rich	Extra-nucleosomal	H1	F1, I, KAP	21,000
		H5	F2c, V, KAS	16,000
Slightly lysine-rich	Nucleosomal	H2a	F2a2, IIb1, ALK	14,000
		H2b	F2b, IIb2, KSA	13,774
Arginine-rich	Nucleosomal	H3	F3, III, ARK	15,324
		H4	F2a1, IV, GRK	11,282
Sperm-specific		Basic histone-like proteins		Variable
		Protamines		
		Cysteine-protamines		

of histones,[13] but two other blue-green algae contained a protein which had immunological identity with the histone-like protein HU of *E. coli*.[13a]

Mesokaryotes — In the group of the *dinoflagellates,* which are considered as an intermediate group between pro- and eukaryotes, acid-soluble proteins were isolated[8,14,15] which also differed from the known histones. Their amount in *Gyrodinium cohnii* was much smaller than in a higher eukaryote, but a protein of this species was found to migrate as H4 from corn root chromatin.[15] In the binucleate dinoflagellate *Peridinium balticum,* the acid nuclear extracts gave four bands that comigrated with four of the five mammalian histones.[16]

Algae — In the colonial green alga *Volvox,* acid-soluble proteins were found with amino acid composition similar to that of histones from *N. crassa.* Their electrophoretic pattern, however, differed considerably from that of calf thymus histones.[17] Three lysine-rich histone-like fractions were isolated from *Chlorella.*[8] It was shown by the immunofluorescence test that the nuclei of the green algae *Chlamidomonas reinhardi, Haematococcus pluvialis* and *Dunaliella salina* contained proteins which reacted with antisera against the calf thymus histones H2a, H3, and H4.[17a]

Fungi — Some earlier data showing the absence of histones in fungi[8] were not confirmed by more recent results. In the primitive species *Phycomyces blakesleeanus,* relatively large quantities of DNA-associated basic proteins were found which were related to the typical histone species H1, H2a, H2b, and H4[18] (see Table 2). Two acid-soluble, slightly lysine-rich proteins were isolated from the chromatin of *Cordyceps militaris* and *Achlia bisexualis.*[8] More recent data have shown that *N. crassa* chromatin contains a full complement of five histones[19] with two fractions similar to the arginine-rich histones H3 and H4 of higher eukaryotes and two histones similar to the plant histones H2a and H2b. The presence of the five major histones was also demonstrated in the chromatin of *Aspergillus nidulans.*[20] H3 and H4 histones of this fungus were nearly identical to those of calf thymus with respect to net charge and molecular weight. In yeasts, four types of histones were detected in *Saccharomyces ceravisiae* resembling H3, H2a, H2b, and H4 of animal cells,[21,22] although earlier studies gave unclear results, or H3 was reported to be missing. In all studies, the lysine-rich histone H1 was found to be absent in yeasts, but three proteins that electrophoresed similarly were detected instead.[22] More recent data demonstrate the presence of H1-type histones in yeast.[22a-c]

Slime molds — The presence of basic proteins in the chromatin of slime molds was clearly shown. Their electrophoretic mobilities were similar to those of calf thymus.[8,9,23] An interesting case is *Dictyostelium discoideum* where two fractions were found to migrate in urea-polyacrylamide gels like animal H2a and H2b, while two other fractions migrated like plant histones H2a and H2b. The suggestion was made[9] that *D. discoideum* may represent a species where, in evolution, the slightly lysine-rich histones were diverging into an animal and a plant pattern.

Protozoa — A good evidence for the presence of histones was obtained also in protozoa. In four species (*Tetrahymena pyriformis, Paramecium aurelia, Euglena gracilis,* and *Stylonychia mytilus*), five major histone fractions were identified corresponding to the main types of mammalian histones.[8a,9,23a,23b] More recently, it was shown that H4 of these protozoa strongly resembles H4 of calf thymus with respect to relative electrophoretc mobility, molecular weight, amino acid composition, and even the presence of multiple acetylated forms in the macronucleus.[24,25] However, a partial aminoacid sequence of *Tetrahymena* histone H4 revealed that it differed significantly from that of calf or pea H4.[25a]

Comparison of different strains of *Tetrahymena* revealed that both H3 and H4 were constant, but H3 migrated faster than H3 of calf thymus showing that this histone was not so rigidly conserved as H4.[26] H1 of *Tetrahymena* was also shown to be similar in many respects to that of other species,[27] but was found to be absent in the micronucleus,[27a] where an unusual histone HX was found. The latter shows an evolutionary conservatism like H3 and H4 and can intereact with H4.[27a] This histone has been subsequently redefined as *Tetrahymena* H2a.[23a] The genes of *S. mytilus* coding for the five histones have been recently characterized.[27b]

Subunit structure — Very strong evidence that histones are present in lower eukaryotes are the recent results from nuclease digestion of their chromatin which show the presence of a subunit structure[22,27c-32] with the same length of DNA in the core particle (140 bp) as in higher eukaryotes[22,27c,28-32,32a-d] (see Section VII. A and B). A somewhat lower value was reported for *D. dictyostelium*.[32d] Electron microscopic pictures of the chromatin of *D. dictyostelium* and of the macromolecular chromatin of *S. mytilus* showed the presence of typical nucleosomes.[32e,f]

These important results demonstrate that the standard chromatin particle containing 140 bp of DNA has already arisen in the primitive eukaryotes. Since the formation of this structure requires, as a rule, all four nucleosomal histones (see Section VII.E), its presence is a strong argument that histones very similar to those of higher eukaryotes are present in the group of such primitive eukaryotic organisms as *Ascomycetes* and slime molds.

Thus, there are several species from the group of the fungi, slime molds, and protozoa where the presence of histones has been demonstrated beyond doubt. It seems very likely that this conclusion will be extended to other species from the lower eukaryotes. It cannot be excluded that a simpler subunit organization of chromatin may be discovered in some evolutionarily more primitive species.

Conclusions —

1.   In prokaryotic cells, histones are absent but some DNA-binding proteins have been found which can induce compact structures of DNA.
2.   In mesokaryotes basic acid-soluble proteins are associated with DNA but it is not yet clear what is their relationship to histones.
3.   In a number of lower eukaryotes the presence of a full complement of histones has been well documented which makes it most probable that typical histones exist in all lower eukaryotes.

2. Histones in Animals[33-35]

a. General Occurrence

There is no disagreement that histones in all animal species studied are represented by five major fractions. Depending on their lysine and arginine content, they are designated as lysine-rich histones H1, slightly lysine-rich histones H2a and H2b, and arginine-rich histones H3 and H4.[36] A lysine-rich histone H5 was found in the nucleated erythrocytes of birds, reptiles, amphibia, and fish,[33] (Table 2).

Comparative studies have shown that the electrophoretic mobility of the arginine-rich histones H3 and H4 in polyacrylamide gels is remarkably constant in all animals, indicating a great conservatism of their structure. This has been confirmed by studies on the primary structure of these histones (see Section V.A).

It has also been clearly shown that the two slightly lysine-rich animal histones H2a and H2b are more variable, which was first detected by their variable electrophoretic mobility in urea-polyacrylamide gels. In all animal species, however, they migrate in the zone between the two histones H3 and H4. Studies on the amino acid sequences of H2a and H2b have confirmed the greater variability of these histones (see Section V.A).

A new technique of gel electrophoresis in the presence of Triton® X100 has led to a discovery which may turn out to be of essential significance for the problem of cell differentiation. This technique has shown that all histone species in animals, with the exception of H4, are represented by several variants (isohistones) — two for H2a, three for H2b, and three for H3.[38-40c] Three molecular species of H2a were found in rat chloroleukemic cells.[41] The histone variants differ by several amino acid substitutions, mainly in their hydrophobic regions. The presence of two forms of H3 in calf thymus — one minor component (20% with only one cysteine residue and a major component with two cysteine residues — has already been shown.[42] It is important that the histone variants were found to be nonallelic and present in all tissues in different relative amounts.[39]

The biggest variability among histones exhibit the lysine-rich histones. In all animal species studied, H1 was represented by up to five subfractions which showed differences in their electrophoretic mobility, amino acid composition, and exhibited some species specificity. The partial amino acid sequence of some of these histones confirmed this variability (see Section V.A).

The similarities and differences between histones of different animal species were also revealed by immunochemical cross-reactivity. The index of dissimilarity between calf and *Drosophila* histones when assayed by this criterion showed no difference in amino acid composition for H4 and H2b, 4% and 6% difference for H3 and H2a, respectively, and 27% difference for H1.[43] By direct amino acid analysis, the histones of these two species were found to vary in the order H4, H3, H2a, H2b, and H1 from most to least conserved.[44] This order of evolutionary stability of the histones is indicated by all present studies.

An exception from this limited variability in animal histones are the special sperm-specific histones which will be discussed separately (see Section IV.C).

b. Conclusions

1. The arginine-rich histone pair H3 and H4 is the same in all animal species, H4 having the most conservative structure.
2. The slightly lysine-rich histone pair H2a and H2b shows relatively bigger species differences.
3. Nonallelic variants (isohistones) of H2a, H2b, and H3 exist.

4.   The lysine-rich histones are the most variable group showing some species-specific heterogeneity.

3. Histones in Plants
a. General Occurrence

The presence of a full complement of histones in plants is well established. The electrophoretic mobility of two plant histones significantly differs from that of animal histones.[45-49] There is a strong evidence that these two plant histones are functionally and structurally equivalent to the animal histones H2a and H2b. The partial sequence of H2b from pea confirmed this conclusion. This histone was very similar to calf thymus H2b in its middle and C terminal hydrophobic regions, while the N terminal basic region was different.[50] The same variations were suggested for H2a, as judged by its amino acid composition.[50] Three variants of H2a have been isolated from *Triticum*.[50a] On the other hand, plant chromatin was also found to have the same subunit structure and the same standard DNA length of the core particles (140 bp) as animal chromatin.[51,52]

The arginine-rich histones of plants were studied in more detail and were shown to be almost identical to the corresponding animal histones. The primary structure of these histones shows only two conservative replacements in H4 from pea bud when compared with calf thymus H4,[53] while H3 had relatively more substitutions.[34,54-56] The N terminal amino acid sequence of H3 of a lower plant (cycad) was found identical to that of H3 from animal origin except for a single replacement of Tyr-41 by Phe.[55] In all studies, the lysine-rich histones H1 of plants exhibited a lower electrophoretic mobility than the animal H1. An immunological comparison indicated an aminoacid difference of less than 2% between rye and calf histone H3 and of 10 to 20% for histones H2a and H2b, while rye H1 gave no immnological crossreaction with calf H1.[56a]

The comparison of a variety of different higher plants has shown that, like in animals, no species differences can be established in the arginine-rich histones H3 and H4, relatively more species differences show in the slightly lysine-rich pair H2a and H2b, while pronounced differences can be detected in the group of the lysine-rich histones H1.[45,47,48]

b. Conclusions

1.   Like animals, all plants possess a full complement of histones.
2.   The arginine-rich histones H3 and H4 are the same in all plants and correspond to the animal histones, even in their primary structure.
3.   The slightly lysine-rich plant histones H2a and H2b, although different from the corresponding animal histones, are closely related to them in structure and show variability in their N terminal region mostly.
4.   Microheterogeneity of plant H2a and H2b seems also to exist as indicated by partial sequences.[50,50a]
5.   As in animal cells, the lysine-rich histones of plants are subjected to more variations and show some species-specific heterogeneity.

B. Evolution of Histones and Cell Differentiation
1. History of Histones

The data on the occurrence of histones in different species do not permit to fix precisely the exact philogenetic origin of histones. It is reasonable to accept that these proteins have emerged at the epoch of the divergence of the organisms into prokaryotes and eukaryotes. The lack of reliable data on the intermediate group of the mesokaryotes makes it difficult to say definitely whether they have appeared before or after the formation of the nuclear membrane. However, the presence of condensed chromosomes in dinoflagellates shows that some DNA-associated proteins should be already present in these organisms, and it seems possible that they might be histone precursors.

It was speculated that histone precursors may have originated from ribosomal proteins at an epoch when the appearance of the nuclear membrane was associated with the migration into the nucleus of precursor ribosomal proteins.[10] This may have been an evolutionary step which has allowed such proteins to associate with DNA. This attractive hypothesis, however, was based only on some similarities between ribosomal proteins and basic chromosomal proteins of fungi.[10] The suggestion was also made that histones may have evolved from the DNA-associated proteins of some thermophilic prokaryotes where their first role may have been to protect DNA from thermal denaturation,[12] but later the condensing effect on DNA has led to another structural role.

The occurrence of internal regularities and homologies between the major histone classes has suggested that the four histones H2a, H2b, H3, and H4 have evolved from one or two common precursors.[56,57,57a] This is also strongly indicated by the specific clustering of their genes.[58]

Much more data are needed on the proteins and structural organization of the chromatin in lower eukaryotes in order to establish the evolution of the histone complex. The greater variability in the acid-soluble chromatin proteins of these organisms, however, indicates that the most advantageous histone structure has not yet been reached in these species.

The highly conservative structure of the histones in higher eukaryotes is a strong indication that some selected histone structures were of great evolutionary advantage to the organisms and their evolution. This is especially true for the arginine-rich pair H3 and H4 where almost no alternatives have been permitted, while the slightly lysine-rich pair H2a and H2b has had more freedom for evolutionary changes expressed as species differences and as a microheterogeneity within the same species. The biggest species differences in these histones occur in the primitive eukaryotes where they seem to have diverged into plant and animal histones as indicated by the histone pattern of the slime mold *D. discoideum*.

It can be speculated that there have been three periods in the evolutionary history of histones: (1) a period of *histone progenitor,* where many mutations have occurred leading to the histones or histone-like proteins of some lower eukaryotes; (2) a period of evolutionarily still *unstable histones* in some lower eukaryotes, where the possibility has existed to create the most advantageous structure; and (3) a period of relatively *frozen structure,* where the great advantage acquired has created a strong selection pressure against the survival of histone mutations.

2. Cell Differentiation and Emergence of Histones

If we compare this histone history to the history of cell differentiation, it can be seen that before the appearance of histones, the process of cellular reprogramming in prokaryotic cells has all the features of functional changes (labile form of cell differentiation). After the appearance of histones, a second type of cellular reprogramming has evolved leading to the emergence of different cellular types in multicellular organisms (stable form of cell differentiation).

In the intermediate forms of lower eukaryotes there are examples of changes which alter profoundly the morphology of the cell but, nevertheless, have most of the characteristics of functional changes. Such is, for example, the case of the unicellular *Neglaeria,* where the striking transitions between the flagellate and the ameboid forms is dependent on the permanent presence of the inducer, is reversible, and was also shown to be cell-cycle independent.

It is suggestive, however, that in the lower eukaryotes, primitive forms of stable cell differentiation have also started to appear. They are expressed as an intracellular differentiation of the nucleus into macro- and micronucleus in protozoa, as an intracolonial differentiation into two major cell types — somatic and reproductive — in the aggregates of colonial organisms, and as more complex developmental changes in some other lower eukaryotes. Thus, the appearance of histones in lower eukaryotes coincides with the emergence in these organisms of some primitive forms of stable cellular differentiation.

It is possible to consider the appearance of histones as a starting point for the development of a new molecular mechanism leading to the stable form of cell differentiation found in all eukaryotes. A serious problem in this line of thought is the small number of different histones and their remarkable evolutionary stability, which is in contrast to the rapid evolution and cell diversity in eukaryotic organisms. The limited number of evolutionarily conserved histone species has been the main reason for ascribing to these proteins a structural role only. Such a conclusion, however, seems too premature, a second alternative being that a relationship between the evolution of a stable form of cell differentiation and histones does exist, but it is not so simple as originally proposed.

IV. TISSUE SPECIFICITY OF HISTONES

The possible involvement of histones in cell differentiation raises also the important question of their tissue specificity. All data show that this problem should be treated separately for the group of the lysine-rich histones H1 and the group of the four nucleosomal histones. The male gametes have a different pattern of basic DNA-associated proteins which also needs a special treatment.

A. The Nucleosomal Histones

Both earlier and more recent studies have failed to reveal any tissue specificity of histones H4, H3, H2a, and H2b.[33] Many data showing quantitative changes in the ratios between different histones in different tissues are most probably artifacts due to incomplete isolation or degradation of some histone species. This conclusion seems justified in the light of the new data on the organization of chromatin in repeating units where all four histones are present in equimolar ratios (see Section VII).

The finding of histone variants (see Section III.A.2) opens the possibility that various tissues, although having the same major histones, may differ in their variants. Comparative data from several tissues show that they contain the same variants but in different quantitative ratios.[39] Although many more studies are needed on the tissue specificity of histone variants, it seems that the strict conservation of such variants in evolution is an indication of their functional significance. In this connection, an interesting finding is the changing ratio of the $H2a_1$ to $H2a_2$ variants in Friend leukemia cells. In normal mouse spleen and liver, this ratio was 3:1 while a decreased ratio of 2:1 was found in Friend cell lines established in vitro. The ability of these cell lines to be induced to synthesize hemoglobin was paralleled by an increased amount of variant $H2a_2$.[59]

Conclusions —

1. The four major nucleosomal histones H2a, H2b, H3, and H4 are the same in all tissues and, thus, should be considered as tissue nonspecific.

2.   Some tissue differences seem to exist with respect to the relative proportions of the histone variants of H2a, H2b, and H3. It is also possible that some other minor histone components may increase the tissue specificity of nucleosomal histones.

3.   The amino acid substitutions which occur mostly in the hydrophobic regions of the histone variants may strongly affect the histone-histone interactions and, thus, alter the properties of the chromatin, making it functionally heterogeneous and inducing tissue specificity.

B. The Lysine-Rich Histones[59a]

It is largely accepted that the expressed microheterogeneity of the lysine-rich histones is not only species- but also tissue-specific. The analysis of the literature data shows that this tissue specificity is mainly quantitative, being expressed as differences in the relative content of different subfractions rather than as the presence or absence of some H1 species. Although some qualitative differences have been reported, it seems that they were due to an incomplete resolution of different subfractions. A better separation technique has shown that a number of different tissues from mammalian and avian origin have the same full complement of lysine-rich histones although in different relative quantities.[60] A cochromatography of differentially labeled and mixed lysine-rich histones from mouse liver, spleen, uterus, and mammary gland also showed the occurrence of identical subfractions in these different tissues.[61] On the other hand, some of the differences observed, namely the lack of one special subfraction, seem to reflect a difference between proliferating and resting tissues rather than a tissue-specific difference.[62] Some of the subfractions of H1 may be also due to metabolic modifications.[63] A slight difference between H1 subfractions of rat thymus and rat liver was observed immunologically.[63a]

Taking into account that tissue-specific differences may arise as artifacts due to incomplete separation of subfractions[60] or to their proteolytic degradation,[64,65] it is difficult to say whether tissue-specific differences in the lysine-rich histones really exist. The meaning of some quantitative tissue differences is not clear, and the available data are not sufficient to see whether they are exceptional for a given tissue or are related to cell proliferation. The fact that there are a number of different tissues with identical pattern of H1 subfractions speaks against a direct role of these histones in cell differentiation.

The only case of a tissue-specific histone of this group is the well-studied histone H5 which appears during the process of final differentiation of the nucleate erythrocytes. More recent data show that the process of phosphorylation and subsequent dephosphorylation of H5 seem to be responsible for the chromatin condensation leading to its total inactivation.[66] This is a special case of terminal differentiation controlled by a specific histone. In mammalian species, however, the same type of erythroid differentiation is accomplished by another mechanism which completely eliminates the nucleus without the appearance of a specific histone.[67]

C. Histones in Male Gametes

The nature of the basic nuclear proteins of the male gametes is of special interest for two reasons. On the one hand, the emergence of such cells in ontogenesis is a special case of final differentiation, and on the other hand, earlier cytochemical data have already shown that some peculiar changes take place in the nuclear basic proteins during spermatogenesis. These changes led to the widely held view that, in spermatozoa, somatic histones are replaced by sperm-specific histones.

More recent biochemical data have confirmed the general conclusion that in all species studied the spermatozoa contain some unusual basic nuclear proteins (sperm-histones) which in molecular weight and in amino acid composition differ from the typical somatic histones.

There are several questions which are of first importance for our discussion. What are the characteristics of these proteins; how are they related to histones; what is their function; and to what extent are somatic histones eliminated by sperm-specific histones?

In *plants,* the microsporocytes of lily and tulip were found to contain a unique histone (meiotic histone) which was absent in somatic cells. It was synthesized during the premeiotic stage and persisted in mature pollen grains, but at the same time, the full somatic histone complement was present.[68]

Comparative studies of 14 species of *molluscs* have shown that their spermatozoa contain unusual histone-like proteins which vary considerably in the type and relative amounts of different components.[69] In some species, the main components are rich in arginine and are similar to the fish protamines but have a larger size. Most of the species contain a complex protein mixture including proteins identical or similar to somatic histones together with proteins intermediate in size and composition between protamines and histones.

The sperm-histones of *echinoderms* were found to contain all major five histones.[70-72] This is confirmed by nuclease digestion of sea urchin sperm chromatin which reveals a subunit structure similar to that of embryo chromatin.[73] In gel electrophoresis, the sperm-histones H3 and H4 have the same mobilities as the corresponding somatic histones. Sequence analysis has shown, indeed, that they are identical with calf thymus histones, except for the substitution by cysteine of one serine residue in calf H3 and one threonine residue in calf H4.[55,74]

Unlike the arginine-rich histones, the lysine-rich histones and the fractions H2a and H2b of echinoderms were found to be different from the corresponding somatic histones of mammalian origin.[70,72] Very interesting structural features of the sperm H2b were revealed when the complete amino acid sequence of the two variants of this histone became known.[75,76] A comparison with calf thymus H2b has shown that the N terminal region of the sperm H2b is extended by about 20 amino acid residues which may be accommodated into a repeating pentapeptide.[76]

Thus, the echinoderm sperm-histones $H2b_1$ and $H2b_2$ combine in their primary structure two different features: the characteristics of typical somatic histones in one part of their molecule and the characteristics of protamines expressed as a repeating basic pentapeptide at the N terminal region. In this connection it is interesting to recall the suggestion that a typical protamine found in fish (clupeine) may have evolved from an ancestral arginine-rich pentapeptide by repeated gene duplication and point mutations.[77] The primary structure of the sperm H2b histones of echinoderms lends support to such an idea and shows, in addition, that the protamines have most probably evolved from somatic histones.[69] Thus, it seems that echinoderms and some molluscs represent a step in the evolution when the ancestral protamine sequence has emerged within the chain of the somatic histones.

In *insects,* the spermatids and spermatozoa of house cricket were reported to contain the same five major histones as somatic tissues plus some additional histone-like basic proteins different from the typical protamines and from the sperm-specific histones of other species.[78,79] In this species, meiosis and much of the spermatid differentiation proceed with only the typical somatic histones present. Only at the very late stage of spermatogenesis do the unusual histone-like proteins appear which are later replaced by a complex mixture of protamine-like proteins.[80,81] The replacement of the somatic histones in cricket sperm by the new protamine-like proteins is not complete, as shown by the presence of the former in most of the electrophoregrams.[78,79,81]

A classical example of characteristic changes taking place in the histone pattern during spermatogenesis is the replacement of somatic histones by protamines in *fish*. The typical arginine-rich and small molecular weight protamines have been isolated from more than 50 species belonging to different families. Some of the protamines have been well characterized, and the primary structure of several species is known.[82] Their typical features are the low molecular weight (below 10,000) and the extremely high content of arginine which, in some species, reaches 90%. They do not contain cysteine, and only in some cases is a very low content of lysine found.[82] In trout, six different protamine genes were described.[82a]

The replacement of somatic histones by protamines has been well studied in the trout where this process takes place during the very late stage of spermatogenesis[83] although the group of protamine mRNAs are synthesized and stored in the cytoplasm at the earlier stage of the primary spermatocyte.[83a] It is widely accepted that in this case a complete histone replacement takes place, and the trout spermatozoa do not contain histones. While this seems true for 80 to 90% of the DNA, the possibility cannot be ruled out that some DNA sequences of the order of 10% have still retained their somatic histones, as in the case of other species. Electrophoregrams of acid-soluble chromatin proteins from spermatozoa of carp, goldfish, and toadfish show the presence of typical somatic histones.[84] It has not been possible to study the structure of trout sperm chromatin by the method of nuclease digestion since it was found to be completely resistant to this enzyme.[85]

The basic proteins associated with *amphibian* sperm display also a great variability. In the anurans, a mixture of sperm and late spermatid nuclei was shown to retain the somatic type histones together with the appearance of new fast migrating components,[86] which exhibited a great diversity among different species.[86a] The presence of rapidly migrating protamine-like proteins was shown also in unfractionated testis cells of the newt.[87] All typical somatic histones were found in the spermatozoa of frogs.[84]

In *reptilia* the testis-specific histones from lizards and snakes showed a remarkably similar pattern in contrast to its diversity in anurans,[86a] but it remains unclear whether their mature spermatozoids contain somatic histones.

In *birds,* the situation seems to be similar to that in fish. Eight main fractions were obtained by ion-exchange chromatography of acid-soluble extracts from fowl sperm. These proteins had the typical (for fish) protamines high content of arginine.[88] Proteolytic degradation of the spermatozoal basic proteins of the rooster was recently reported.[89]

In all *mammalian* species studied, sperm-specific proteins have also been isolated. In all cases, they differed in amino acid composition but shared many common features — a molecular weight intermediate between that of somatic histones and protamines and a high content of arginine. However, unlike fish protamines, they have a relatively high content of cysteine involved in -S-S- cross-linking,[90-98] resulting in their association with DNA in a highly polymerized form.[93] The mammalian sperm-specific proteins are supposed to be phylogenetically related to the protamines of teleost and avian sperm and were called cysteine-protamines.[69,98] It was pointed out that single-point mutations in the six arginine codons could lead to the replacement of arginine by cysteine and by some other amino acids which are frequent in mammalian protamines.[98]

In some species, the cysteine-protamines were reported to migrate as a single band in gel electrophoresis,[90-92,92a] while in others, as human spermatozoids, they consisted of several fractions.[94,96,96a] Transitory proteins unique to testis cells only and disappearing in spermatozoids were also isolated in some cases[92,92a,95,99,100] showing that the process of condensation of DNA during spermiogenesis is more complex than a simple replacement of somatic histones by one basic sperm-specific protein.[100a,b]

It has been often reported that the cysteine-protamines are the only acid-extractable proteins in mammalian spermatozoa.[92a,97,98,101] However, it seems very likely that not all of the somatic histones are replaced by protamines. In several studies, it can be clearly seen that in addition to sperm-specific proteins, somatic histones are present in the electrophoretic pattern of the acid extracts from spermatozoa of mouse, rat,[92,95,102] and humans.[94,96] The possibility that their presence may be due to contamination with other cells or late spermatids, which still contain all somatic histones, seems unlikely since they were found also in semen samples practically free of other cells[96] or with a contamination less than 2%.[102] The presence of small amounts of somatic histones in human spermatozoids has been confirmed by the immunofluorescence test.[102a,b]

The failure to detect any somatic histones in mammalian spermatozoa may be due to proteolytic degradation. It was shown that prolonged incubation of bull sperm chromatin in the presence of urea and mercaptoethanol at pH 8 resulted in extensive proteolysis of nuclear basic proteins.[103] A slight proteolysis of bull sperm protamines was detected also after only 20 min incubation in 8 M urea/dithiothrietol at pH 9.[98] Thus, it seems more probable that in mammalian spermatozoa somatic histones are also present, maybe in strongly reduced quantity, but remain undetected due to difficulties in their extraction and to proteolytic degradation.

Conclusions

1. In the male gametes of all species, some special basic proteins (sperm-histones) appear which significantly differ in structure from the somatic histones.
2. Sperm-histones offer an intriguing paradox: in contrast to the rigidly conservative structure of somatic histones, they display a highly variable structure which differs even within closely related species.
3. A common feature of all sperm-histones is their extremely high content of basic amino acids (in most cases arginine) which in eutherian mammals is accompanied by an unusual increase in cysteine.
4. Sperm-histones were derived in evolution from histones, most probably from a lysine-rich histone, by means of gene duplication and mutations. The following evolutionary scheme seems probable: ancestor somatic slightly lysine-rich histone → slightly lysine-rich histone extended by arginine-rich sequences → protamine-like proteins → protamines → cysteine-protamines.
5. The sperm-histones are synthesized before meiosis, most probably during the last mitotic division, and enter chromatin during meiosis and sperm maturation.
6. The appearance of sperm-histones in chromatin is associated with a process of replacement of somatic histones. The extent of replacement varies in different species between the two extreme cases of a "complete" replacement in some fish families and a "complete" conservation in some amphibians. Due to technical problems of extraction and proteolysis, the question of whether in some species *all* somatic histones are replaced by protamines remains open.
7. The role of sperm-histones seems to be a complex one related to high degree of DNA packing, total gene inactivation, and increased resistance to damage.

D. Histones During Embryonic Development

The very early stages of embryogenesis are characterized by the reappearance of the somatic histone pattern. The exact mechanism of this process is not known, and some controversial data have been reported concerning the time of the appearance of different somatic histones. Earlier data have led to the conclusion that there are no histones in female gametes and in cleaving zygotes of sea urchin, typical histones appearing in blastula or during gastrulation.[104]

More recent data, however, have shown the presence of stored histones in the eggs of sea urchin[105] and of *Xenopus,*[105a] the synthesis of histone mRNA in early blastula,[106] a cyclic synthesis of acid-soluble nuclear proteins beginning from the first cleavage almost in parallel with DNA replication,[107] and the presence of all histones in 1 to 16 cells stage of sea urchin.[108-109a] The finding of a repeating unit in the chromatin of sea urchin blastule[73] is a confirmation of the analytical data showing that a full complement of histones is present in the sea urchin embryo at least at the blastula stage.

There are no disagreements concerning the later stages of development. Most studies show that in different species — sea urchin,[104,110,111] *Xenopus laevis,*[65,112] *Drosophila,*[113] etc. — no qualitative changes in the histone pattern could be detected usually after blastulation. Developmental changes in the relative content of different histone species which are often reported are most probably due to technical reasons. No changes in the histone pattern were observed during wheat germination in spite of the increasing template activity of the chromatin.[114]

The most interesting observation concerning nucleosomal histones is the finding of stage-specific changes in the histone variants during the embryonic development of sea urchin.[109,113a-113e] It was found that different forms of H2a and H2b were synthesized at different stages of development and were preserved so that the multiplicity of nucleosomal histones increased concomitantly with the beginning of cell differentiation.[109,113a] These data show that although the main nucleosomal histones may not change during embryonic development, regular changes in the histone variants may be expected.

The same holds true for the group of the lysine-rich histones. In sea urchin, the microheterogeneity of H1 was reported to increase from one single fraction in morula to several different species in gastrula.[108,115,116] Although some authors reported the absence of H1 in the first stages of development, this histone was later found at the first cleavages (1 to 16 cells stage) in the sea urchin[109] and in the early blastula (16 to 32 cells stage) of the trout.[117] Differences in the relative synthesis of two H1 variants were observed in the three different cell types following the 4th cleavage of the sea urchin, which may have an implication for the emergence of diverging chromatin structures at a time when determination is in progress.[117a] The presence of newly synthesized H1 subfractions before gastrulation and their qualitative changes around gastrulation were found also in *Xenopus.*[117b]

Since maternal histone messenger RNA (mRNA) is stored in the egg and is additionally transcribed from the embryonic genome, it is not clear which histone species are represented in the stored maternal mRNA population and which are synthesized during different stages of embryonic development.[118] It is of interest that a programmed switch of the synthesis of lysine-rich histone species takes place at gastrulation, probably controlled at the level of transcription[118] and/or at the level of translation of stored maternal histone mRNAs.[116,119]

Conclusions

1. The replacement of sperm-histones by somatic histones takes place early in embryogenesis, most probably during the first cleavages, but it is probable that in this respect species differences may exist.

2. Maternal stored histones in the egg cytoplasm, translation of stored maternal histone mRNA, and transcription of new histone genes most likely participate in the reorganization of the gamete chromatin into somatic chromatin. A regularly programmed switch of the synthesis of different histone variants seems to exist both in the group of the H1 histones and in the group of the nucelosomal histones, so that qualitative developmental variations emerge in the pattern of histone variants.

3.   The five major histone species do not show qualitative variations during embryonic development, and the quantitative variations reported are likely to be due to technical reasons.

E. Histones in Tumors

Since malignant transformation is considered to be a disease of cell differentiation, data on histones in tumors may be relevant for understanding the role of these proteins.

No differences between the pattern of nucleosomal histones from normal and malignant tissues have been reported. The tryptic peptides of H2b from Walker tumor were identical to those of normal tissue.[120] Analysis of the C terminal sequences of H4 from bovine lymphosarcoma, Novikoff hepatoma, and fetal calf thymus showed complete identity.[121]

Some changes in histone variants have been observed in malignant cells. There were marked differences in the relative content of the two H2a histone subfractions isolated from different Friend leukemia cells (see Section III.A.2).

As may be expected, some variations were observed in the subfractions of H1. Quantitative differences in these subfractions were reported in tumors.[61] H1 histones derived from rat liver and rat hepatoma yielded different chromatographic profiles, H1 of the tumor being more heterogeneous, while regenerating liver did not differ from normal liver.[122] In three different rabbit mammary tumors, eight H1 subfractions were reported which were the same in all three tumors but different from a dog mammary tumor.[123] It is very likely that this multiplicity of H1 subfractions was due to phosphorylation. Differences in the microheterogeneity of tumor H1 were found to be due to phosphorylation correlated with the rate of tumor growth.[123a] Differences between H1 of normal and malignant tissues were indicated also by their immunological specificity.[124]

A subfraction of H1 which was originally found in resting cells only[62] was also reported to be decreased in malignant cells,[124] the decrease being correlated with the growth rate of hepatomas.[125] However, a decreased amount of this subfraction was reported also in regenerating rat liver[126] and in regenerating pancreas[127] but not in hyperplastic and neoplastic thyroid tissue.[128] A correlation between decreased cell proliferation and increased amount of this fraction was shown in the postnatal development of pancreas.[129] We did not find a decrease in this fraction in regenerating liver, but in primary hepatomas it was decreased and completely absent in their metastases.[130] It seems possible that the disappearance of this fraction is related to some step in the malignant transformation[125] connected with the control of cell proliferation.

The comparative data on histones in tumors, although scarce, show that no qualitative changes in the major histone species occur in tumors, but some changes in the histone variants, especially in H1, are likely to occur.

V. MAIN STRUCTURAL PROPERTIES OF HISTONES[33-35,56,131-133]

A. Primary Structure

Four features of the amino acid composition and sequence of the histone polypeptide chain are of special interest. First, histones are very rich in basic lysyl and arginyl residues, contain little aromatic amino acids and no tryptophan. Cysteine is present only in H3 and in H4 of echinoderms.

Secondly, a quite exceptional characteristic of the primary structure of histones is its remarkable stability in evolution. All comparative studies show that H4 is the most conservative protein known. As compared to other proteins, its evolutionary rate is at

Table 3
EVOLUTIONARY RATE OF
SOME PROTEINS[133a-133c]

Protein	Point mutations per 100 amino acid residues per 10^9 years
Fibrinopeptide A	400
Ribonuclease	250—300
Hemoglobin β	100—130
Cytochrome C	40
Insulin A and B	30
Histone H4	1

least one order of magnitude lower (Table 3). With the possible exception of some lower eukaryotes,[25a] its primary structure has remained identical in all species with only two conservative mutations preserved during the time separating plants from mammals.[53] The most striking replacement was found in H4 from echinoderms where a threonine residue was replaced by cysteine.[110,134] H3 is the next rigidly conserved histone, which shows a slightly higher number of mutations. When the whole sequence of this histone from mammalian, bird, fish, and plant origin was compared, only four substitutions, three of them conservative, were found between evolutionarily most distant species.[34,55,56,135-137] The N terminal portion of H3 seems to be strictly conserved, since its amino acid sequence was the same in evolutionarily quite distant species with only one replacement of Phe for Tyr in a primitive plant.[55]

In all species studied, H2a and H2b showed relatively much larger variations in their primary structure. A comparison of H2b from calf,[50] trout,[138] sea urchin,[74-76] pea,[50] chicken, crocodile, *Xenopus*,[40a] the mollusc *Patella granatina*,[138a] and man[138b] shows that most of the substitutions in these histones have occurred in the N terminal basic fragment which is the main DNA-binding site (see Section V.D). Relatively well conserved are the sequences in the middle and C terminal hydrophobic regions of the molecule which are involved in protein-protein interactions. The same is the situation with H2a as shown by comparative studies of this histone from calf, rat, chicken, trout, and sea urchin origin.[139-140b] Bearing in mind that in the nucleosome assembly H2a-H2b dimers bind to H3-H4 tetramers (see Section VI.E) the significant fact arises that the histone-histone binding sites show a remarkable evolutionary conservation.[140c] This may explain why nucleosomes can be reconstituted using mixtures of even philogenetically so distant species as plants and animals.[140d]

The most variable group was found to be the lysine-rich species H1 whose changes in the primary structure were comparable to those of some other proteins. It is interesting, however, that H1 seems also to contain a region which is relatively conservative and other portions which are more variable. Analysis of the primary structure of different fragments of H1 subfractions from mammalian thymus has shown that almost all amino acid substitutions have occurred in the N terminal part of the molecule in a fixed region between position 14 and 40.[141,142] It is difficult to say whether this is due to some functional role or to the lack of selection pressure since this variable fragment is situated in a portion of the molecule which has a random coil conformation (see Section V.B) and does not seem to be involved in some specific interactions.

This difference in the evolutionary stability of the three groups of histones — arginine-rich, slightly lysine-rich, and lysine-rich — can be correlated with their different localization in the chromatin: the most conservative arginine pair forms the center of the nucleosomal protein core, the relatively well-conserved but more variable slightly lysine-rich pair seems to occupy a more external position, while the less conserved H1 has an extranucleosomal localization (see Section VII). This correlates with the general observation that the most conservative part of a globular protein is the inner part which is not in contact with the solvent, while most variable are the external sites.[143]

The evolutionary conservatism of histones is a highly significant fact showing that most of the mutations affecting the primary structure of these proteins have been lethal, especially those which affect sites involved in protein-protein interactions and also in protein-DNA interactions in the case of arginine-rich histones.

A third important feature of histone primary structure is the uneven distribution of the basic amino acids along the polypeptide chain. In all histones, more such residues are concentrated toward the two ends of the molecule than in its central region. Thus, the terminal regions of the histone molecules are highly basic having a charge density which, for the nucleosomal histones, is 5 to 20 times higher than in other regions.[56] With the exception of H2b, the charge density of all histones is higher at one of the ends — the N terminal of H2a, H3, and H4 and the C terminal for H1.[56] This specific distribution of the basic amino acids is correlated with the main sites for interaction with DNA (see Section V.D).

Another important characteristic of histones which is often supposed to be correlated with their function are the various posttranslational modifications of the different amino acid residues, mainly O-phosphorylation of serine, N^6-acetylation, and N^6-methylation of lysine, and poly-ADP-ribosylation (see Section VI) leading to introduction, neutralization, or retention of charge. These frequent changes of charge in the histone molecule were found paradoxical when compared with the evolutionary rigidly conserved positions of charged residues along the polypeptide chain.[56] It is important that even within the same cell never does a histone species have all of its molecules modified in the same way. This is an additional indication of the functional role of these modifications.

B. Conformation of Histones[35,131]

Knowledge of histone conformation is of first importance for understanding their interaction with DNA and between themselves. In aqueous solutions, the polypeptide chain of histones has a secondary structure which strongly depends on the ionic conditions. No ordered structures are formed at very low ionic strength, low pH, or in the presence of urea, while increasing the ionic strength results in the appearance of regions organized in α-structures. The use of nuclear magnetic resonance (NMR) spectroscopy and the knowledge of the primary structure have permitted approximate localization of these regions in different histone species. Such studies have shown that the ordered structures are localized in the central regions and in the C terminal half of the polypeptide chain which are rich in hydrophobic amino acids. Thus, in the slightly lysine-rich histones H2a and H2b, a larger segment of the N terminal end and a smaller part of the C terminal end do not form ordered structures while α-helix formation takes place in the central regions.[144] In H4, two segments in the center and in the N terminal half of the molecule form secondary structures while the first 37 N terminal residues remain in a random-coil conformation.[145] The lysine-rich histone H1 has also a heterogeneous polypeptide chain showing three distinct structural domains: a random-coil fragment ("nose") comprising 35 to 40 residues from the N terminal end; a globular portion ("head") in the center; and a random-coil C terminal and ("tail").[146]

The precise conformation of histones in chromatin is not known, but probably they do not form β-structures. Studies on isolated core proteins of the nucleosomes and on histone complexes show that ordered secondary and tertiary structures are present in the chromatin subunits, most likely with the same localization as in isolated histones.[144,147,148]

C. Histone-Histone Interactions[35,131]

Earlier studies have shown the pronounced tendency of histones to form aggregates.[33] Only recently has it been shown that under suitable ionic conditions the interactions between histones represent a process of self-assembly, leading to the formation of specific complexes — dimers, tetramers, and octamers — which are an important step in the structural organization of chromatin (see Section VII.E).

The uneven distribution of the basic amino acid residues along the polypeptide chain is the molecular basis of the formation of these specific histone complexes. In salt-containing aqueous solutions, the nonbasic regions of the histone molecules become structured and come into contact to form a hydrophobic protein core, while the highly basic ends remain in a random coil for interactions with DNA.[148] This interaction seems to be more important for binding internucleosomal (spacer) DNA (see Section VI.A) rather than nucleosomal DNA. Experiments with the elimination of the N-terminal ends of the nucleosomal histones show that such trimmed histones are capable of binding and folding DNA into nucleosomes,[148a] while they fail to give the specific digestion pattern in which spacer DNA is involved.[148b]

Thus, two principally different regions in the histone molecule can be distinguished — basic DNA-binding sites and hydrophobic sites involved in protein-protein interactions. The conservation in evolution of the highly hydrophobic regions in the histone molecule with a frozen primary structure shows the importance of these histone regions for specific histone-histone interactions (as also indicated by the complementarity observed in histone structures[148c]) and probably also for interactions with other proteins.

The process of histone self-assembly in solution most probably proceeds through the formation of dimers, which then associate into tetramers and into octamers. At moderate ionic strength, the histone dimers were shown to be the most stable structure.[149] The dimers H3.H4 and H2a.H2b have been found in solution.[150-152] The dissociation of heterotypic tetramers into dimers has been also observed,[153] and an equilibrium was found between H3.H4 dimers and tetramers.[154] Heterotypic histone tetramers have been isolated at pH 7.4,[153] while at pH 9 an octamer was obtained.[155] The existence of heterotypic tetramers in solution has been questioned by some new data showing that in $2M$ NaCl and at neutral pH the histones form an octamer which can dissociate into a H3-H4 tetramer and two H2a-H2b dimers.[155a]

D. Histone-DNA Interactions[33,35]

The data from the primary structure of histones and their conformation in salt-containing aqueous solutions show that the highly heterogeneous polypeptide chains of these proteins cannot bind uniformly to DNA. Recent studies on the peptides which remain bound to DNA after tryptic digestion of chromatin have permitted confirmation of this conclusion and more precise identification of the sites of contact between nucleosomal histones and DNA. It was shown that the chief sites of interaction are at the N terminal region, but all these histones have secondary interaction sites at their C terminal part, while H2b and H2a interact also with some lysine residues at their central portions.[156]

Many earlier studies have confirmed the ionic character of the histone-DNA interaction in vitro but did not contribute very much to understanding the interactions taking place in vivo. More recent data show that there are two principally different DNA-histone complexes which can be formed in vitro.

The first type of complexing takes place when individual histones interact with DNA or when all histones are present but the ionic conditions are not suitable for the formation of specific histone complexes. Experiments on this type of histone-DNA interaction have led to the following conclusions:

1.   Histones bind to DNA without respect to DNA base sequences. There is only a slight preference for AT regions of the lysine-rich histones.
2.   Histones protect DNA from thermal denaturation, increasing significantly its melting temperature.
3.   When complexed with DNA, histones strongly inhibit DNA transcription.
4.   These nonspecific artificial histone-DNA complexes behave very differently with respect to nuclease digestion and electron microscopical pictures[157-159] as compared to the native nucleohistone.

The second type of histone-DNA complexes can be formed under special ionic conditions when all four histones H2a, H2b, H3, and H4 are present. They give structures which, in many respects, seem to be identical to native nucleosomes.[157-159] This type of interaction of DNA with preformed histone complexes is also nonspecific with respect to base sequences (see Section VII.E).

VI. POSTTRANSLATIONAL MODIFICATIONS OF HISTONES

A. Phosphorylation

Phosphorylation of histones is catalyzed by specific protein kinases which transfer the γ-phosphate from adenosine triphosphate (ATP) to the seryl and, to a less extent, to the threonyl residues of the protein.[160]

Studies on different cellular systems[161-169] show that the highest level of phosphorylation is observed always in the group of the lysine-rich histones H1 and in H2a, which in all tissues studied is highly phosphorylated at all times of the cell life. Only in trout testis was H2a found to be phosphorylated posttranslationally and then dephosphorylated.[165] H2b, although being a good substrate for phosphorylation in vitro, seems to be very poorly, if at all, phosphorylated in vivo.

The two arginine-rich histones show only a cell-cycle dependent phosphorylation. H3 is transiently phosphorylated in mitosis and is then rapidly dephosphorylated,[167] while H4 is phosphorylated in the cytoplasm immediately after its synthesis and is dephosphorylated in the nucleus.[170]

The most complex pattern of histone phosphorylation is found in the group of the lysine-rich histones.[33,166-169]

H1 is subjected to three types of phosphorylation: (1) after its synthesis when only one serine residue in the C terminal portion of the molecule is modified; (2) during mitosis when four sites are phosphorylated in both halves of the molecule;[167,168] and (3) after hormonal stimulation when only one serine residue in the N terminal fragment is phosphorylated.[171,172] The first two growth-related modifications are cAMP-independent[166,173] while the hormone-related depends on cAMP.[171,172] During erythrocyte maturation, H5 is progressively phosphorylated soon after its synthesis and is then dephosphorylated in the chromatin.[66,174]

No tissue specificity has been found in the phosphorylation pattern of the nucleosomal histones except differences between resting and dividing cells. Similarities were found even between the phosphopeptide bands of H2a and H4 from erythroblasts,[163] regenerating liver,[175] and trout testis.[161]

Only the group of the lysine-rich histones shows some tissue-specificity expressed as preferential phosphorylation of its subfractions.[176-180] This is due, at least in some cases, to a mutation replacing serine by alanine at a major site of hormone-related phosphorylation in the N terminal portion of the molecule.[178] Such a replacement may induce important functional differences between different H1 subfractions.

Several literature data which contradict some of these conclusions may be explained by methodological shortcomings such as nonhistone phosphorus-containing contaminations,[33,170] overlapping of histone fractions due to altered mobility of phosphorylated histones,[175,181] and superimposition of different types of phosphorylation related to different physiological processes.

The most probable functions of phosphorylation seem to be related to three different processes: (1) *correct deposition* of individual histones on the replicating chromatin (phosphorylation of H1 and H5),[66,167] or maybe of the whole histone complex (phosphorylation of H4);[83,170] (2) *condensation and stabilization* of chromatin during mitosis — superphosphorylation of H1[166,168,182-184a] and phosphorylation of H3;[168,184a] during maturation of erythrocytes — dephosphorylation of the highly phosphorylated H5;[66] and during spermatogenesis — dephosphorylation of protamines.[83,185] It was also suggested that the phosphorylation of H2a is involved in the formation of heterochromatin structures.[185a] (3) *transcription* — phosphorylation of Ser-37 of H1 and phosphorylation of H2a (see Section IX.B.1).

B. Acetylation

Acetylation is achieved by specific acetyltransferases, which transfer the acetyl group from acetylcoenzyme A to histone amino acid residues. The incorporated acetyl groups are found as *N*-acetyls and as labile *O*-aceytls,[33,185] but mostly the first type of acetylation was studied.

A specificity of acetyltransferases for different histones and different acetylation sites has been demonstrated.[33,186,187] Multiplicity and organ specificity of these enzymes has also been reported.[188] The presence of enzymes which release the acetyl groups — histone deacetylases — was also shown,[33] and their multiplicity and specificity was demonstrated.[189,190]

Two types of histone *N*-acetylation exist. The first is N terminal and affects the serine residues of histones H1, H2a, and H4. This type of acetylation occurs in the cytoplasm immediately after histone synthesis, very likely on the nascent polypeptide chain.[191] The acetyl groups introduced as a result of this acetylation are metabolically stable.[33,185]

The second type of histone *N*-acetylation affects internal N^6-amino groups of lysine residues, occurs in the nucleus on preexisting histones, and leads to a heterogeneous population of histone molecules differing only in the number of acetylated residues.[33,185] In most studies, the arginine-rich histones H3 and H4 were found to be the major species which were internally acetylated. When protein synthesis was inhibited, only these histones were acetylated.[192,193] Some authors, however, have reported such acetylation in all nucleosomal histones.

The internal *N*-acetylation of the lysine residues is unstable, the acetyl groups showing a turnover rate with different halflife times.

Not all internal lysine residues are acetylated in vivo.[185] In H3, acetylation occurs at lysyl 9, 14, 18, and 23, in H4 at lysyl 5, 8, 12, and 16. One acetylation site (lys-5) was reported for H2a and four for H2b (lysyl 5, 10, 13, and 18). It is seen that acetylation occurs within the highly basic N terminal end of the molecule which is the main region interacting with DNA in chromatin (see Section V.D). For this reason it can be expected that the posttranslational internal acetylation will weaken the ionic interactions between DNA and histones by decreasing the net positive charge of the molecule. In fact, there are some data indicating that acetylation of histones may affect their interaction with DNA.[83,161,194] Thus, although both acetylated and nonacetylated histone H4 bind to DNA, the form monoacetylated at lys-16 was less effective in inducing conformational changes of DNA while the multiacetylated forms caused a different type of circular dichromism (CD) changes.[195]

Acetylation of histones was suggested to play a role in the correct binding of newly synthesized histones to DNA[83,185] and in the process of transcription (see Section IX.B.2).

C. Methylation

This chemical modification affects mainly lysine residues predominantly in arginine-rich histones. In vitro incubation of rat brain and liver nuclei showed methylation of these histones only.[196] It seems that lysyl residues of H1, H2a, and H2b are not accessible to methylases when the histones are organized in the chromatin structure, since the same enzyme which can methylate all isolated histones modifies only the arginine-rich histones when acting on chromatin.[196]

The methylated lysine residues occur as mono-, di-, and trimethylated derivatives,[33] but the highest proportion has been found for dimethyllysine.[197,198]

In contrast to the situation in vivo, rat liver and brain nuclei incubated in vitro contain more monomethyllysine than dimethyllysine and very low content of trimethylated derivatives.[196] This supports the hypothesis that the methyl groups are added sequentially. This is in agreement with data indicating that monomethyllysine in H4 is present as a first modified product after histone synthesis in proliferating cells only.[197] It has also been suggested that protein methylation may be an intermediate step in DNA methylation.[33]

The sites of methylation in calf thymus H4 have been identified as N^6-mono- and dimethyl derivatives of lys-20[199,200] and as N^6-mono-, di-, and trimethyl derivatives of lysyl 9 and 27 in H3.

The enzymes responsible for histone methylation transfer methyl groups from methionine via the intermediate donor S-adenosylmethionine.[33] This modification takes place in the nucleus after DNA synthesis[33] immediately after the arginine-rich histones enter the nucleus.[198] There is some controversy concerning the metabolic stability of the methyl groups of histones. Some data indicated a lack of turnover of these groups, but new results have shown that they turn over independently of the polypeptide backbone.[200a]

Although some differences in the methylation sites have been found between different species, no such tissue differences have been observed. A comparative study of five organs of the rat has shown that the molar content of mono-, di-, and trimethyllysine in H3 and H4 were the same in all tissues studied — cerebrum, cerebellum, kidney, liver, and thymus.[197]

The role of histone methylation is most unclear. It has been supposed to increase the stability of the DNA-histone complex, thus changing the structure of chromatin.[201] No relations between histone methylation and transcription were found, but attempts were made to relate this modification to the structural changes of chromatin during the cell cycle.[201,202] It seems, however, that the higher histone methylation in G2 and mitosis[203] is due to a dimethylation step.[198] The constant molar ratios of different methyl derivatives in histones[197] and their low turnover make less probable the hypothesis that methylation plays a role in mitotic condensation. It seems more probable that the increased methylation of histones during the cell cycles is related to the sequential methylation of newly synthesized histones.

D. Poly-ADP-Ribosylation

When chromatin or isolated nuclei were incubated in vitro with NAD, poly(ADP-ribose) was found associated with histones.[33] Later the existence of this polymer covalently bound to histones in vivo was demonstrated.[204,205]

An enzyme has been found in mammalian cells which can transfer the adenosine diphosphoribose moiety of NAD to chromatin proteins, principally histones.[33,206] Another enzyme — poly(ADP-ribose)-synthetase — was discovered bound to chromatin which catalyzes the elongation of the ADP-ribose polymer chain.[207] The nuclei contain also specific hydrolases which degrade the ADP-ribose polymer.[208]

The lysine-rich histone H1 was found to be a good acceptor of ADP-ribose both in vitro and in vivo.[209] Other histones were also shown to be acceptors in vitro,[210] but there are contradictory results whether this can occur in vivo. In rat liver, poly-ADP-ribosylated H3 was reported,[210] but in trout testis only H1, the trout-specific H6, and protamines were found to be ribosylated.[211] The conclusion was drawn that only proteins which were outside of the nucleosomal particles could be subjected to this chemical modification while the nucleosomal histones were not available for the enzyme. Some data indicated that ADP-ribosylation in histones may occur on serine phosphate.[210]

The polymer chain length of H1 and H6[37,37a] of trout testis was from 3 to 9 monomeric units.[211] In various mammalian cells, the number of such units differ from 15 to 1.5, depending on the level of the enzyme degrading the polymer.[208]

The role of this histone modification is not clear. Ribosylation of histones in vitro did not affect transcription, but it had an inhibitory effect on DNA synthesis.[33] More poly-ADP-ribosylated histones were reported to be present in resting liver than in the S phase of regenerating liver.[204] Thus, it seems possible that this modification may be related to the control of DNA replication. Some data indicate that H1, which is the major acceptor, may form dimers linked by a single chain of poly(ADP-ribose),[208] a process supposed to play a role in chromatin condensation. If serine phosphates are the sites for poly-ADP-ribosylation,[210] histone phosphorylation at specific sites may be an intermediate step in some types of chromatin condensation. The latter may be enzymatically controlled since it has been found that the dimeric form of H1 linked through a poly(ADP-ribose) chain is synthesized when poly(ADP-ribose)-glycohydrolase activity is low, while high activity of this degrading enzyme leads to the formation of modified H1 monomers.[208] The role of this histone modification in chromatin condensation is supported by new data on the stimulatory effect of polyamines and divalent cations on the formation of the H1-poly(ADP-ribose) complex.[208a]

VII. ROLE OF HISTONES IN CHROMATIN STRUCTURE

A. The Concept of Repeating Unit and Nucelosomes

Earlier electron microscopic studies had shown that the chromatin fibers are much thicker (100 to 200 Å) than free DNA.[212] On the basis of X-ray diffraction data, this picture was explained by a supercoiling of DNA induced by interaction between DNA-associated histones.[213] Thus, these earlier data indicated already that histones played an important structural role in the packing of DNA.

A new development started with the discovery that chromatin consisted of repeating units of DNA. Mild digestion of chromatin with nucleases revealed the existence of sites more sensitive to nucleases, leading to the degradation of chromatin DNA into pieces of relatively uniform size of about 200 bp.[214,215] Such a repeating unit was shown to be associated with a fixed number of histones — two each of H2a, H2b, H3, and H4 and one molecule of H1.[155,216-218]

The repeating units appear under the electron microscope as spherical particles about 100 Å in diameter first called ν-bodies[219] and, later, nucleosomes.[157] It is very important that nucleosomes were found in all eukaryotic cells studied — unicellular organisms, plants, and animals.[22,28-32,51,220] They were also present in mitotic[32,221-223] and in polytene chromosomes.[223a]

From the size of the nucleosomes (about 100 Å) and the length of DNA in the repeating unit, it is evident that DNA in this structure should be folded to give a packing ratio of about 1:6. The idea was put forward that DNA in chromatin is on the outside,[224,225] wrapped around a histone core. This model was confirmed by the effect of DNAses and by neutron-scattering studies.[215,226]

It should be pointed out that some misunderstanding may arise by using the terms "repeating unit" and "nucleosome" as synonyms. It should be taken into consideration that the presence of repeating units is detected on the basis of nuclease digestion, and this term should be used without respect to the conformational state of DNA, while nucleosome denotes a special particulate conformation of DNA.

The use of different ionic conditions has shown that the nucleosomes can interact more or less strongly depending on the ionic environment so that they can be tightly packed in thick fibers.[227] This fact tends to reconcile the model of a continuous supercoil of DNA with a discontinuous nucleosomal supercoil.

B. The Core Nucleosome

A more extensive digestion of chromatin with nucleases has revealed that the repeating unit consists of a relatively resistant core containing 140 bp of DNA and a short DNA spacer of about 30 to 70 bp which is easily degraded by the enzyme.[215,228-230] Many data indicate that the core nucleosome contains eight molecules of H2a, H2b, H3, and H4 in equimolar amounts[155,216,217] while the spacer is associated with one molecule of H1.[231,232] In native chromatin, the nucleosomes are closely situated so that no interconnecting spacers are visible under the electron microscope.[226,227] A number of factors such as hydrodynamic and surface forces, stretching, elimination of H1, etc. reveal the spacer and lead to the originally observed "beads-on-a-string" picture, which should be regarded as an artifact of preparation.

Recent studies on nucleosomes of different species have led to a conclusion of fundamental importance. It was found that the size of the core nucleosome (140 bp) did not change in evolution. The lower value for its size reported for the lower eukaryote *D. dictyostelium,*[32d] if not due to core digestion, would indicate that this standard unit may have been different at the early stages of evolution.

In contrast to the core nucleosome, the spacer exhibits large variations in different organisms, in different tissues, and within the same tissue.[28,30,51,230,233-235] Even the three different nuclear types of a ciliate were shown to have spacer regions of different length.[27c] It seems that no correlation exists between the functional activity of the genome and the length of the spacer. During embryonic development, the spacer length of neural chromatin becomes shorter, while that of liver chromatin is enlarged, the size of the core nucleosome remaining unaltered in both cases.[235a] On the other hand, transcribed and nontranscribed regions of chromatin were shown to have the same length of nucleosome-associated DNA.[235b] The variations of the spacer size were correlated with the variable structure of H1 which is associated with the spacer.[30,233] This is, however, contradicted by the fact that chicken erythroid cells which already contain H5 still have a smaller spacer.[236]

All available data indicate that the core nucleosome is a standard eukaryotic structure which has appeared at the epoch of the primitive eukaryotes and has been conserved in evolution. The evolutionary limitation imposed on this structure is an important fact already indicating the functional significance of the core nucleosome.

C. Higher-Order Structures

Electron microscopic studies show that in native chromatin the nucleosomes can be tightly packed to form a second order supercoil with a pitch of about 100 Å and about six nucleosomes per turn.[237,238] This higher-order structure increases further the packing ratio of DNA to about 1:40. Neutron scattering studies have also suggested a coiled-coil model with a major pitch of 500 Å.[239] Other arrangements of nucleosomes were also observed — coiled to give 200-Å fibers[240] or packed in 200-Å large particles containing six to eight nucleosomes.[241-243] It seems probable that different types of coiled or folded arrangements may exist in vivo, all constructed from closely packed particles.

Many data indicate that the mechanism responsible for the formation of such higher-order structures is most probably a process of crosslinking of chromatin fibers by histone H1, but the participation in this process of some nonhistone proteins cannot be excluded. The ion-induced contraction of chromatin gels was shown to depend on the presence of H1,[244] and electron microscopic observations demonstrated that the presence of dense chromatin and particles oganized in globular 200-A structures depended on the presence[245] and on the conditions for cooperative binding of H1.[242] Short-range and long-range chromatin crosslinking by H1 may be achieved due to the possibility of poly-ADP-ribosylation (see Section VI.D). The reversibility of this process may be an important mechanism for the unfolding of these higher-order structures to allow for chromatin replication.

It should be noted, however, that such a structural and functional role may not be related exclusively to H1 since the micronucleus of *Tetrahymena* is able to carry out its chromosome replication and mitotic chromosome condensation in the absence of H1.[27a]

Another mechanism involved in higher-order chromatin organization may be a process of self-assembly of identical nucleosomes into knobs or solenoid structures[246] which are additionally stabilized by H1 crosslinking. The supercoiling of DNA in the nucleosomes may favor especially the binding of H1 which was shown to exhibit a large preference for superhelical DNA.[247] Another possibility for a strong stabilization of nucleosomal supercoils is the binding of some nonhistone proteins as suggested by protein A24 representing a covalently linked complex of a nonhistone protein and H2a.[248] More recent data suggest the interesting possibility that the N-terminal ends of the nucleosomal histones are responsible for the interaction of the spacer DNA with the nucleosomes, thus providing a mechanism for their tight packing.[148b]

The higher-order structures of packed nucleosomes is of utmost importance for the problem of gene control. It raises the question whether such structures can be transcribed and, if not, what is the state of transcribable chromatin. From this point of view, two higher-order arrangements of nucleosomes seem of particular interest — the solenoid structure and the 200-Å large knobs. The first arrangement is interesting because it implies the formation of a strictly ordered structure resembling a microcrystalline state.[246] The mechanisms maintaining such a structure should be of high importance for the blocked state of the chromatin and, therefore, for the determination of a cellular type.

The existence of 200-Å particles representing associations of several nucleosomes is also of interest because it shows a second order of discontinuity in the packing of DNA, the first order being the internucleosomal spacer. These particles seem to indicate that groups of nucleosomes are separated by a much larger spacer which may permit variations in the internucleosomal spacer. Thus, changes in the spacer length may occur with only a short-distance sliding of the nucleosomes which can explain tissue differences in the spacer length. If the spacer size and the sliding of nucleosomes played a role in some control mechanism (see Section X.B), the existence of spare spacers may turn out to be of great importance.

D. The Binary Structure of the Nucleosomes

Evidence that the nucleosome is built of two subunits, or half-nucleosomes, comes from several different methodological approaches. Electron microscopic measurements of the size of *v*-bodies or nucleosomes[157,219,220,249] have resulted in large variations in the estimated size — from 60 to 130 Å — which cannot be explained by the use of different techniques or by shrinkage. On the other hand, it was found that one and the same chromatin can contain two types of particles depending on the ionic conditions and the method of preparation.[227,250]

The conclusion was drawn that each large-size particle consisted of two small particles (subunits), each containing a heterotypic histone tetramer surrounded by a DNA supercoil, and the two supercoils linked by an intranucleosomal spacer.[227] The existence of two half-nucleosomes was strongly supported by experiments with the minichromosome of SV-40. It was shown that this circular structure, which contains about 21 nucleosomes of 110 to 125 Å diameter, can be transformed into a structure with the same contour length but containing 40 to 50 particles of a much smaller diameter of 93 Å.[250]

Results obtained from X-ray, neutron, and laser light scattering and nuclear magneting resonance led to the same binary model of the nucleosome.[251] Evidence for a twofold symmetry of the nucleosome comes also from the finding that under appropriate ionic conditions, DNAse II cuts chromatin DNA in the middle of the 200-bp repeat.[252]

Thus, quite different methodological approaches support a binary structure of the nucleosome characterized by a twofold symmetry. The presence of two interacting histone tetramers with conservative structural parameters determines a standard size of the 140-bp piece of DNA. The existence of an intranucleosomal spacer permits the "opening" of this structure and its transformation into two smaller particles. It is possible that the "closed" state of the nucleosome is maintained by the much stronger interaction between the two arginine-rich pairs belonging to the half-nucleosomes. The basis of this interaction may be a structural complementarity between nucleosomal histones which shows that these proteins are capable of mutual recognition.[148c] The transition between the "closed" and "open" conformational state of the nucleosome may have an important functional role.

E. Formation of the Nucleosomes

It has been shown that nucleosomes with properties identical to the active particles can be reconstituted in vitro from DNA and histones.[57,249,253] Such exeriments have demontrated that in the process of reconstitution, DNA interacts with preformed histone complexes — tetramers or octamers (see Section V.C). Nuclesomes cannot be formed if the assembly of histones into specific protein cores is prevented by high concentrations of urea.[158,254] This shows the leading role of histones in the organizion of DNA into nucleosomes.

This first level of organization proceeds in two steps. The first step involves interactions between histones to form histone cores (see Section V.C), and the second step is an interaction between DNA and histone cores.

It has been show that in the reonstitution process, all four histone species H2a, H2b, H3, and H4 should be present in order to form a nuclosome in vitro. The preformed cores which interact with DNA are most probably tetramers or octamers. More rcent data show that, in vivo, the first histone complex which binds to DNA is a homotypic arginine-rich tetramer followed by the H2a-H2b dimers, while H1 is the last to join chromatin.[254a] In reconstitution experiments in vitro a sequential binding of H3-H4 tetramer and H2a-H2b dimers to DNA was also demonstrated.[254b,c] The particles thus formed in the absence of H1 represent core nucleosomes. This again shows that the lysine-rich histone H1 does not participate in the formation of the core particles.

More recent experiments revealed the central role played by the arginine-rich histone pair H3.H4 in the organization of the core nucleosome. Earlier data had already shown that many physical properties of chromatin, such as melting curves, CD-spectra, and X-ray diffraction pattern, depend mainly on the arginine-rich histones. In reconstitution experiments it was found that particles with properties very similar to the native nuclesomes can be formed in the presence of the H3.H4 pair only.[159,255-257a]

However, these particles differed from the nucleosome — they contained less DNA and one arginine-rich histone tetramer only. The possibility of obtaining these subnucleosmal particles shows the organizing role of the two arginine-rich histones in the format of the nucleosome. This may be correlated with the fact that these histones have also the most conservaive primary structure.

The formation of subnucleosomes containing an arginine-rich histone tetramer is in agreement with the originally proposed model of the nucleosome with a central arginine-rich tetramer and two laterally associated slightly lysine-rich dimers.[217,258] Such a model seems to contradict the binary model discussed above. However, the discrepancy is only apparent. The order of histones in the nucleosome established in recent studies[258a,258b] indicates that upon folding of DNA into two coils around the twoheterotypic tetramers, a homotypic arginine-rich tetramer may remain in the center. Depending on ionic and other factors we can either separate the two heterotypic tetramers and obtain small half-nucleosomes, or eliminate the slightly lysine-rich histone pairs and obtain a subnucleosmal particle containing an arginine-rich tetramer. Thus, the two models reflect different properties of thenucleosome.

The coiling of DNA around the histone core leaves the histones only partly buried in the large groove of DNA as shown by the accessibility of the DNA bases to methylation with dimethylsulfate.[259]

The binding of the histone cores to DNA is also nonspecific with respect to base sequences. Several different tests have shown that the nucleosomes are randomly distributed along DNA,[260,263] although more recent studies show some degree of sequence preference.[263a,b] The absence of sequence-specificity of histone-DNA interactions is an important fact which should be taken into account when discussing the functional role of histones.

F. Heterogeneity of Nucleosomes

In the task of elucidating the functional role of histones it is highly important to discuss the experimental evidence concerning the possible heterogeneity of nucleosomes with respect to their protein complement. It is largely accepted that all nucleosomes are identical. It was recently reported, however, that different nucleosomes are unfolded at different concentrations of urea,[264] an indication that all nucleosomes may not be identical.

The protein moiety of nucleosomes may be heterogeneous with respect to the following characteristics:

1. Histone composition
2. Histone arrangement
3. Histone conformation
4. Chemical modifications of histones
5. Histone variants
6. Presence of nonhistone proteins

Histone composition — Analysis of the histone complement of isolated nucleosomes has shown that all small histone species are present in equimolar amounts.[155,216,217]

Together with the fact that all of these histone species are needed to reconstitute a nucleosome this shows that at least the bulk of these particles contain the same histones. By using antibodies to H2b, it was also found that at least 90% of the nucleosomes contained this histone.[265] Fractionation of such antibody-reacted nucleosomes in a density gradient gave a broad distribution of particles, each fraction of which contained the same histone complement. Thus, it seems reasonable to assume that all nucleosomes are identical with respect to the main histone species.

Histone arrangement — Covalent linking of histones to the 5′ end of DNA[258a,258b,266,267] and crosslinking of histones[268] suggest that the nucleosomes may be also identical with respect to the histone arrangement.

Histone conformation — Evidence for possible differences in the conformation of histones may be deduced from studies on the tryptic digests of nucleosomal histones,[269] on the limit digest with nucleases,[270-272] and on the crosslinking of histones.[273] The data obtained from such studies give indirect evidence that some differences between nucleosomes may exist leading to degradation or crosslinking patterns which are not compatible with identical structures. Other explanations, however, are also possible.

Chemical modifications of histones — It is enough to mention that histone H4 only may give rise to more than 240 different molecules if all possible chemical modifications took place.[56] That such modifications may really cause heterogeneity of nucleosomes in the same tissue is indicated by the finding that not all histone molecules are modified and that transcriptionally active chromatin regions exhibit a higher degree of phosphorylation and acetylation (see Section IX.B).

Histone variants — Although the literature on histone variants (see Section IIIA.2) is very limited and many more studies are needed to reach a final conclusion, the available data clearly show already that nucleosomes must be heterogeneous with respect to the presence of different histone variants. With two variants of H2a and three variants for H3 and for H2b, 144 different nucleosomes can be formed, each containing the same main histones and in the same order. Bearing in mind that the substitutions in different variants affect mainly the evolutionarily most stable hydrophobic regions, the replacement of a variant by another one may strongly influence the histone-histone interactions in the nucleosomal core and, thereby, the ability of the nucleosome to undergo some conformational changes or to interact with other molecules.

Presence of nonhistone proteins — The data on the presence of nonhistone proteins in the nucleosome are still contradictory, but most of the authors have reported their presence.[272,274-276] Both negative and positive results may arise as a result of artifacts due either to dissociation or to association of proteins during digestion of chromatin and isolation of the particles. Immunochemical studies confirm the association of nonhistone proteins with the nucleosomes,[277,278] but it would be difficult to tell whether they are part of the core nucleosome or are associated with the internucleosomal spacer in close contact with the core particle. If the nonhistone proteins were a real component of the nucleosome, the heterogeneity of the latter may be extremely high considering the high number of different nonhistone chromosomal proteins.

An interesting recent discovery was the finding of a new class of nonhistone proteins — the so-called high mobility group (HMG) — associated with nucleosomes and rendering them more sensitive to nucleases,[278a-e] a feature characteristic of the active parts of the genome (see Section VIII.A). It was also found that extraction of these proteins with $0.35 M$ NaCl eliminated the sensitivity of nucleosomes to DNase I, while after their rebinding this sensitivity was restored.[278f] These data indicate that specific binding of nonhistone proteins to nucleosomes may be a mechanism controlling gene activity.

The tentative conclusion from all these data is that the nucleosomes seem to be identical with respect to the four main histone species and their arrangement but must be heterogeneous with respect to their different variants. It may be supposed that the histone variants cause a primary heterogeneity which leads to a secondary one expressed as conformational differences, possibility of chemical modifications and of interaction with nonhistone proteins.

A more direct experimental evidence for heterogeneity of nucleosomes was recently obtained. In addition to the fact that different nucleosomes uncoiled at diffferent urea concentrations,[264] experiments with antibodies against the four individual nucleosomal histones indicated that nucleosomes were heterogeneous with respect to the availability of their histone antigenic determinants.[278g] Our own data show that the nucleosomes differ in their stability toward salt dissociation,[278h] and different types of nucleosomes are separately clustered in chromatin. Nucleosomes containing different variants of H3 as well as different nonhistone proteins were also isolated.[279]

VIII. HISTONES AND DNA REPLICATION

A. Timing of Histone Synthesis

Histone synthesis takes place in the cytoplasm on small polyribosomes[280,281] and is tightly coupled to DNA replication in all eukaryotic cells.[282-283] Some data have suggested that this coupling is realized by the opening of sites for histone mRNA transcription by processes related to DNA replication.[284] All histone species have the same rate of synthesis, some differences reported in the literature being due to contaminations.[285]

It is also well established that once incorporated into chromatin, histones are metabolically stable.[286-288] Only the extranucleosomal H1 has been reported to show a DNA-independent synthesis and continuous replacement in resting cells.[289,290] The other extranucleosomal histone H5 was also shown to be synthesized independently of DNA replication in nondividing avian reticulocytes.[291,292]

The only case of total histone synthesis independent of DNA replication was found during oogenesis.[105,293,294] This synthesis supplies stored histones necessary for the fast chromosomal replication during early development.

An interesting feature of histone synthesis is that they are the only proteins which are coded for by reiterated and clustered genes.[58] It was speculated that reiteration was necessary for the rapid supply of mRNA in rapidly dividing cells, the degree of reiteration in different species showing some correlation between number of gene repeats and amount of histones stored in the egg cytoplasm.[58]

Another important characteristic of histone genes is their specific clustering which seems to have common features in all eukaryotes,[58] with a possible exception in lower eukaryotes where the histone genes of *Stylonychia mytilus* were not located together on the same macromolecular DNA.[27b] It was suggested that the repeat unit of the histone genes may be controlled and transcribed as a single operon in order to ensure histone stoichiometry in chromatin.[58] It was found, however, that the five histone genes in *D. melanogaster*[294a] and in HeLa cells[294b] do not function as a single transcriptional unit.

An important general conclusion can be drawn: under normal conditions, DNA replication requires immediate supply of all histones. A number of mechanisms have evolved to realize this process — clustered and reiterated genes, coupling of their transcription to DNA replication, stored histone mRNA,[295] and stored histones in egg cytoplasm. These facts evidently support the idea that in eukaryotic cells normal DNA replication proceeds simultaneously with, or very closely preceding, the formation of the nucleohistone complex. The rapid assembly of replicating DNA into chromatin subunits was well supported by biochemical[295a] and electron microscopical[295b] data.

B. Distribution of Histones During DNA Replication

The metabolic stability of histones does not show how they behave during replication. However, the constant ratio between the label of histones and of DNA during many cell generations[288] indicates that most probably the histones do not interrupt their close association with DNA during replication. Otherwise, it would be difficult to accept that when old histones are mixed with the pool of newly synthesized molecules, the dilution would be exactly the same as for the semiconservatively replicating DNA.

A more direct indication that histones do not leave DNA during replication was obtained by following the labeled histones after separation of the old from the new DNA strands. Such experiments showed that old histones remained associated with the old DNA strand while newly synthesized histones joined the new strand.[296] This conclusion was contradicted by experiments showing a random distribution of histones in the second generation.[297] More recent experiments, however, gave additional support to a nonrandom distribution of histones during DNA replication.[298,298a]

A nonrandom segregation of old and new histones was found in another type of experiments separating the new from the old histones on the basis of their labeling with heavy isotopes.[299] The results obtained show that the histone unit which is conserved during replication is a histone octamer so that old and new histones do not mix but form new and old octamers. This is in agreement with reconstitution experiments showing that the formation of the nucleosomes requires preformed histone cores.

It would be difficult to describe the exact mechanism of the association of the new histone complexes to the replicating DNA. Some data show that the new histones do not join immediately the newly synthesized DNA, thus indicating some sliding of nucleosomes along DNA towards the replication fork.[300-302]

All these data are not sufficient to draw a final conclusion, but it seems justified to assume that histones do not leave DNA during replication and that old and new histones do not mix.

IX. HISTONES AND TRANSCRIPTION

A. Presence of Histones at the Sites of Transcription

Early hypotheses on the role of histones were based on the assumption that histones should be eliminated in order to make possible the process of transcription. However, many data, both biochemical and electron microscopic, show definitely the presence of histones in transcriptionally active chromatin. More recent methods of separating chromatin into "nonactive" and "active" fractions have shown that such fractions do not differ in their histone content. The decreased amount of H1 in "active" chromatin observed in some experiments was found to be probably due to its proteolytic degradation.[6]

A strong biochemical evidence for the presence of histones in transcriptionally active chromatin was obtained from nuclease digestion studies which have demonstrated that active genes are organized in the same repeating units as genes which are never transcribed in a given tissue.[272,303-308] Since the existence of repeating units of DNA is due to its partial protection by associated histones, these data undoubtedly prove that binding of histones to DNA does not prevent transcription. Direct evidence was also presented recently that in a model system, *Escherichia coli* polymerase was not greatly inhibited in its rate of propagation by the presence of the four histones on the DNA.[308a] Isolated nucleosomes and oligonucleosomes were also shown to be transcribed in vitro by the RNA polymerase.[308b] The same was found also for the nucleosomes of the SV-40 minichromosome.[308c,d] All these data do not show, however, what is the conformation of the repeating unit in transcriptionally active chromatin and cannot be a proof for the existence of nucleosomes in such chromatin, as they were often incorrectly interpreted.

Several studies show that the so-called active chromatin is more easily attacked by nucleases, which indicates that its repeating units have an altered conformation.[6,304,308,309] This is also confirmed by the different physical properties of the nucleoprotein particles isolated from digests of active chromatin.[6]

Electron microscopic studies on the transcription of ribosomal genes have shown that no particles corresponding to nucleosomes could be observed between individual transcripts. The conclusion was drawn that nucleosomes were absent in transcriptionally active sites.[310,311] On the other hand, digestion of ribosomal chromatin with nucleases suggests the presence of repeating units.[306,312] It can be concluded that in the case of ribosomal genes, a completely unfolded conformation of the repeating unit seems to be the reason for the absence of electron microscopically visible particles.

Recent data on the visualization of transcription of nonribosomal genes[313-315] have shown that single or several transcripts at longer distances are observed, in this case indicating a low frequency of initiation of nonribosomal RNA. The 100- to 200-Å large particles between these transcripts have been interpreted as nucleosomes by some authors[313,314] while others did not recognize them as nucleosomes.[315,315a] Our unpublished observations indicate that nucleosomes are present at the sites of nonribosomal transcription but are often easily unfolded completely or into half-nucleosomes under the effect of different concentrations of urea or detergents used to disrupt chromatin.

The positive evidence for the presence of nucleosomes being stronger than the negative one, we can draw the tentative conclusion that not only histones, but also a particulate conformation of the repeating unit, are compatible with transcription. It seems, however, that these particles are more easily unfolded under the effect of different agents, and it may be supposed that they are unfolded also by the RNA polymerase in the natural process of transcription. If the nucleosomes were unfolded during transcription, this may explain why they are not visible under conditions of high frequency of initiation as in the case of rRNA transcription.

It may be that the mechanism which makes some nucleosomes transcribable lies in structural changes of the histone core permitting the separation of the two subunits and their complete unfolding when the RNA polymerase slides along DNA. Thus the capability for conformational changes of the nucleosome from a particulate to a linear state may be the basic requirement for transcription.[315a-315c]

B. Posttranslational Modifications of Histones and Transcription

Some metabolic modifications of histones have been related to the changing protein pattern of the cell. They are often referred to as changes accompanying cell differentiation, but the analysis of the literature data shows that the interrelationship between these two processes is far from being clear.

1. Phosphorylation

A relationship between phosphorylation of histones and activation of genes[33] was supported by experimental evidence showing a correlation between phosphorylation of histone H1 and activation of RNA synthesis after hormonal stimulation. This phosphorylation affects preexisting histones in chromatin, since it is observed in nondividing tissues and proceeds even when protein synthesis is inhibited by cycloheximide.[172] It was shown to be cAMP-dependent and to affect Ser-37.[171,172,316]

Another histone phosphorylated independently of its synthesis is H2a (see Section VI.A), and the continuous turnover of its phosphate groups may also be related to the process of RNA synthesis. This is supported by the finding that dexamethasone which influences transcriptional activity of sensitive cells stimulates phosphorylation of H2a.[316a] In many experiments, however, it is not clear to what extent the histones were contaminated with highly phosphorylated nonhistone proteins which are present in the acid chromatin extracts and interfere even with electrophoretically fractionated histones.[170]

The data on histone phosphorylation are not sufficient to draw a final conclusion, but it may be accepted that activation of genes is probably correlated with an accelerated turnover of phosphate groups in the N terminal region of H1 and possibly also at unidentified sites of H2a. Such a correlation does not prove, however, that histone phosphorylation is a control mechanism in gene activation.

2. Acetylation

The first studies on histone acetylation have already suggested that this chemical modification is necessary to counteract the inhibitory effect of histones on transcription, probably by affecting chromatin compactness.[33,161,170,194] Such a hypothesis is supported by a number of observations showing a correlation between histone acetylation and RNA syntheis as shown by the following typical examples:

1. In thymus lymphocytes, H3 and H4 of the diffuse chromatin which is active in RNA synthesis show a much higher rate of acetylation than the same histones in the dense chromatin.[194]
2. The genetically active maternal chromosomes of the mealybug incorporate seven times more radioactive acetate as compared to the inactive chromatin of the parental heterochromatic chromosomes.[317]
3. *Tetrahymena pyriformis* macronucleus which is active in RNA synthesis contains some acetylated histones, while the histones of the inactive micronucleus are nonacetylated.[24,27a] Similar results were obtained with *Stylonychia mytilus*.[318]
4. The increased RNA synthesis after hormone stimulation in many different target tissues was associated with an increased histone acetylation.[33,319]
5. The histones H3 and H4 of the synthetically active sperm-precursor cells of sea urchin are partially acetylated[170] while in the mature sperm-cells which do not synthesize RNA, these histones are entirely nonacetylated.[110,320]
6. During maturation of erythrocytes, their loss of RNA synthesizing capacity is correlated with a progressive decrease in the proportion of acetylated histones H3 and H4.[319,321]
7. A correlation was found between a pregastrular increase in histone acetylation and gene activation in sea urchin.[322]
8. Inactivation of hepatocyte nuclei by aflatoxin B1 is accompanied by a loss of acetyl groups from acetylated histones H3 and H4 which is followed by a suppresson of RNA synthesis.[323]
9. The transcriptionally active puffs of the polytene chromosomes of *Chironomus tentans* incorporate more acetate than inactive region.[194]
10. Internal acetylation of H4 was found to be minimal in the highly condensed and synthetically inactive mitotic chromatin of prophase and metaphase cells and maximal in interphase chromatin.[324]
11. In isolated and fractionated chromatin, increased acetylation was found in the fraction which was supposed to be transcriptionally more active.[325] This is supported by the finding that the highly acetylated histones were located in the chromatin regions preferentially attacked by DNAse I[325a-e] and DNAse II[325f] as is the case with active genes.[6,304,308,309,325h]

12. Chemical acetylation of calf thymus chromatin was shown to increase its template activity in vitro[326] and to have dramatic effects on some properties of chromatin, making it similar to transcriptionally active chromatin.[327] Similar results were obtained with rat liver chromatin where chemical acetylation led to a two-fold increase in initiation sites.[327a]

In parallel with this positive evidence, data have been obtained which do not show a simple correlation between gene activity and histone acetylation, as for example:

1. There is no quantitative relationship between histone acetylation and gene activity in thymus lymphocytes where half of the H4 molecules are acetylated but only a few percent of the genome is active.[319] The same disproportion was found when acetylation of nuclear and nucleolar histones was compared in normal and regenerating liver and in Novikoff hepatome.[33] More recent data have confirmed the finding that a much larger proportion of the histones is acetylated than would be necessary if this process were involved only in gene activation.[327b]
2. No preferential acetylation of histones was observed in heat-induced puffs of *Drosophila* polytene chromosomes.[328,329]
3. In PHA-stimulated lymphocytes, it was shown that cortisol can uncouple the increase of RNA synthesis from the increased histone acetylation.[330]
4. No correlation was found between histone acetylation and increased RNA-polymerase activity in a system of isolated rat liver nuclei after cortisol stimulation in vitro.[331]
5. Additional acetylation in vitro did not stimulate RNA synthesis in isolated nuclei of calf thymus and chicken embryo.[332]

The controversial literature data led some authors to the conclusion that it cannot be accepted unequivocally that histone acetylation is related to the process of transcription.[33] However, the following two considerations should be taken into account.

The first is that many negative findings can also be explained by methodological defects or inadequate models. For example, the absence of acetylation in polytene puffs[328] was explained by the easier extraction of acetylated histones by the acid fixatives, and the nonpreferential labeling of the same puffs[329] was suggested[317] to be due most likely to the N terminal labeling of newly synthesized histones. In some models — as, for example, the liver, where normally a large number of genes are active — it may be difficult to detect an increased histone acetylation after hormonal treatment. Isolated nuclei or chromatin may also be inadequate models where some normal mechanisms are damaged.

The second consideration is that the relationship between histone acetylation and gene activity may be more complex. It is possible that acetylation itself is not sufficient to induce RNA synthesis, being only one step in a much more complex mechanism.[170,194,330,332] One possibility is that acetylation is only a preparatory step unfolding the tightly packed nucleosomes and thus making them potentially active. This may be achieved by acetylation of N-terminal parts of the nucleosomal histones which interact with the spacer DNA.[148b] On the other hand it seems very probable that acetylation may also have other functions depending on the sites and degree of acetylation.

X. HISTONES AND CONTROL MECHANISMS OF CELL DIFFERENTIATION

The problem of the mechanisms controlling cell differentiation has two aspects — structural and informational. The first aspect concerns the mechanisms leading to the formation of two types of chromatin structures — transcribable (deblocked) and non-transcribable (blocked). The second aspect refers to the mechanisms recognizing the DNA sequences which should be made transcribable in different tissues. The structural aspect raises problems about the role of histones in the formation of blocked and deblocked structures as well as about the mechanisms which permit the transcription of the folded nucleosomal DNA. The informational aspect is more complicated and is related to the possible involvement of histones in mechanisms of gene recognition and transfer of tissue-specific information.

A. Structural Role of Histones and Cell Differentiation

The data on histone-histone and histone-DNA interactions (see Section V.C and D) have shown that histones play a leading role in the folding of DNA and the structural organization of chromatin. It is logical to assume that the function of histones in DNA packing was the first to appear in evolution allowing the condensation of the increasing amount of eukaryotic DNA in a small volume.

The interactions between DNA and histones has resulted in the formation of two main levels of chromatin organization — a first level expressed in the packing of DNA into nucleosomes and a second level realized in the folding of nucleosomal arrays into higher-order structures.

All major histone species are involved in the first level of organization. There is no doubt about the role of the four nucleosomal histones in the formation of the core nucleosome, and it seems very likely that the lysine-rich histones, possibly together with some nonhistone proteins, determine the spacer regions.

The participation of histones in the formation and stabilization of higher-order structures is also very probable. The coiling of the nucleosomes into highly ordered superstructures may be due to specific interactions between the histone cores, while the stabilization of these structures is most probably achieved through the crosslinking ability of H1 (see Section VII.C). However, it is not excluded that both in the formation and in the stabilization of the superstructures some nonhistone proteins take part, too. A long-range crosslinking realized by means of poly-ADP-ribosylation of H1 (see Section VI.D) seems an attractive reversible mechanism for the condensation of large masses of chromatin.

The relationship between various chromatin structures and the transcription of different DNA sequences is a crucial question. From the point of view of transcription, we can distinguish between three types of DNA sequences — sequences which are never transcribed and which represent a substantial portion of the total DNA (tissue nonspecific blocking); sequences which are never transcribed in a given cellular type but can be transcribed in another cellular type (tissue-specific blocking); and sequences which are available for transcription in a given tissue.

It is reasonable to assume that different levels of structural organization of chromatin determine these three different states of DNA. A superstructure of tightly packed nucleosomes may correspond to heterochromatin which is never transcribed; simple solenoids or knobs of several nucleosomes may represent the second structural form which can be regulated for the purpose of cell differentiation, i.e., can be selectively made available for transcription in different tissues by unraveling some of the higher-order arrangements into linear arrays of nucleosomes. The latter may represent the transcribable (deblocked) form of chromatin which is further regulated by another

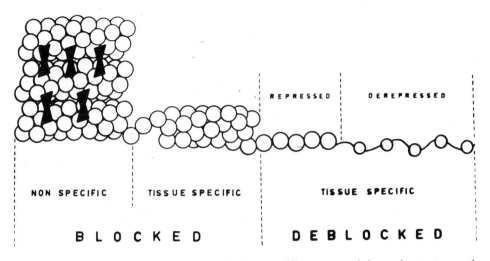

REPRESSED   DEREPRESSED

NON SPECIFIC   TISSUE SPECIFIC   TISSUE SPECIFIC

B L O C K E D   D E B L O C K E D

FIGURE 1.   Tentative scheme of the relationship between different types of chromatin structures and levels of control of cell differentiation.

mechanism into transcribed (derepressed) and nontranscribed (repressed) regions, thus leading to different functional states of the same cellular type (Figure 1).

According to this scheme, the chromatin should represent a highly ordered sequence of these different structural types. It is important that during the cell cycle the information for this structural order is preserved, although the process of DNA replication requires a temporary unfolding of all higher-order structures and during the subsequent mitotic condensation another higher-order structure is formed. It seems that the latter process proceeds in such a way that identically organized structures interact to form different chromosome regions of transcribable and nontranscribable DNA. This is indicated by the finding of a nonrandom and chromosome-specific distribution pattern of nonhistone proteins and newly synthesized RNA along the mitotic chromosomes.[333]

The process of transcription itself should require a complete uncoiling of the nucleosomal DNA in order to permit the sliding of the RNA polymerase along DNA and the separation of the two strands. The presence of nucleosomes at the sites of transcription (see Section IX.A) shows that nucleosomal unfolding must be a reversible process, occurring only at the moment when the enzyme transcribes the nucleosome. This supports the idea that the nucleosomes may be a dynamic structure[306,315b] subjected to reversible conformational changes.[315b,334] Only when the frequency of transcription is very high, as in the case of rRNA transcription, the nucleosomes may remain in a linear conformation, as long as transcription continues.

It would be difficult to speculate on the conformation of the histone core during this process, but it seems necessary to assume that histones should remain temporarily bound to one DNA strand in order to permit the separation of the two strands for the process of transcription. Since this process is asymmetric,[335] it would not be hindered by the histone-asociated antistrand.

In the absence of transcription, the histones cover the large groove of DNA (see Section V.D) and interact most probably with both strands of DNA. However, the interaction between arginine residues and phosphate groups being stronger,[336] histones may be more strongly bound to one of the DNA strands through their arginyl groups, still interacting with the complementary strand through their lysine residues. Such a strand crosslinking will stabilize the double helix and would be a hindrance to strand separation for transcription. An efficient mechanism for counteracting this crosslinking may be acetylation of lysine residues, which, as we have seen (see Section VI.B), affects the main DNA binding sites of histones. This can explain why acetylation is needed as one of the steps leading to transcription. On the other hand, the arginine-dependent asymmetric binding of histones requires a special order in the distribution of arginine and lysine residues along the polypeptide chain. This can explain why, in evolution, lysine and arginine have not been mutually replaced, although both may serve the function of binding histones to DNA.

Thus, all available data show that the structural aspect of cell differentiation — concerning both its stable and labile forms — is closely associated with the histone-dependent structural organization of chromatin permitting a reversible folding of DNA at different levels.

B. Informational Aspect of Cell Differentiation and Histones

The structural mechanisms which underlie cell differentiation do not tell how specific DNA sequences are selected for organization into different chromatin structures. This point is one of the most unclear since the facts which may elucidate it are much less abundant than the hypotheses proposed by different authors. It is widely accepted that the information for the selection of genes to be activated is purely genetic, i.e., entirely based on a simple mechanism of specific recognition of DNA base sequences by chromosomal proteins. However, some considerations show that the transcriptional mechanisms controlling cell differentiation may be more complex.

A first point is that this mechanism operates at two levels — control of the cellular type and control of the functional state — which have almost opposite biological characteristics (see Section II). At the level regulating the functional states, a mechanism relying on protein-DNA recognition seems very probable, both from the point of view of the requirements for the control of single genes and from the point of view of evolution, being the continuation in eukaryotes of a mechanism already existing in prokaryotes.

The situation is different when the regulation of cellular types is concerned. In this case, the control covers large chromatin blocks containing a high number of genes. The regulation actually consists in the organization of all these genes into two different structures — blocked and deblocked — in a tissue-specific manner. The involvement of higher-order structures in this regulation makes more probable that this type of control operates on the basis of protein-protein interactions. Thus, the information for specific recognition in this case may be epigenetic, i.e., expressed as specific protein structures associated with different DNA sequences. This implies that chromosomal proteins and, in particular, histones may not play a structural role only but may also have an important informational function.[5]

Another point is that the process of transcription occurs in the presence of histones, so that all models of regulation based on elimination of histones seem incorrect. It is not excluded that even the mechanism of single-gene control based on protein-DNA recognition may be influenced by the presence of histones. It has been suggested[233] that the initiation sites for transcription can be used only when localized in the spacer region between core nucleosome and will be inefficient when organized in core nucleosomes. A controlled short-distance sliding of core nucleosomes on account of spare spacers may cause a ''dephasing'' of initiation sites, thus operating as a mechanism of transcriptional regulation.[233]

There are also the following facts which suggest that the function of histones may not be structural only:

1. The strictly conserved primary structure of some histones is difficult to explain solely by their role in DNA packing. A comparison of chromatin structures in different cells and species leads to the general conclusion that there is a relationship between the degree of precision in regulating the function of a structure and the degree of evolutionary variability of the histones involved in this structure. Thus, compact chromatin structures such as those in spermatozoa, nucleated erythrocytes, or in micronuclei of ciliates are realized by highly variable basic proteins, most probably derived from histones by gene duplication and mutations (see Section IV.C). In all these cases, the structural function of these basic proteins has not imposed evolutionary restrictions on their primary structure, and at the same time, the "regulation" is restricted to the complete inactivation of DNA functions. The relatively coarse control leading to different cellular types requires a higher precision of regulation, and in this case, the formation of higher-order structures in the chromatin is associated with a limited freedom of mutations as shown by the group of lysine-rich histones. And finally, at the level of linear arrangements of nucleosomes where the most precise controls operate, the primary structure of histones is extremely conservative. Thus, the structural functions of histones are realized by polypeptide chains displaying an order of increasing mutational freedom (nucleosomal histones < extranucleosomal lysine-rich histones < sperm-histones) which is inversely related to the precision of genetic control (single-gene control > control of large portions of the genome > total gene inactivation). This is an evidence, although circumstantial, which indicates that all histones would have exhibited a much higher flexibility in their primary structure if they were to play a structural role only.

2. The existence of nonallelic histone variants (see Section III.A.2) is a strong evidence that nucleosomes are heterogeneous with respect to their histone cores. This heterogeneity, which was also experimentally revealed (see Section VII.F), cannot be explained by structural requirements. The conservation in evolution of these variants, the programmed switch of their synthesis during early embryonic development,[109,113a] and some tissue differences in their content [39] favor the idea that subtle variations in the structure of the histone cores may be an additional information needed for control processes. In this connection it is important to note that the globin genes of H1- and H5-depleted avian red blood cells were nevertheless selectively digested by DNase I, which showed that the enzyme recognized a structural heterogeneity within the core particles rather than higher order structures dependent on lysine-rich histones.[338]

3. The slightly lysine-rich histones H2a and H2b have been allowed to undergo more mutations which occur at their DNA-binding sites while the sites involved in protein-protein interactions are more conservative (see Section V.A). It seems that in the H2a-H2b pair two types of protein binding sites should exist — an inner site for interaction with the H3-H4 tetramer and an external site for interaction with some nonhistone proteins. The latter possibility is indicated by the binding of anti H2b antibodies which shows that part of H2b (peptide 36-50) is at the surface of the nucleosome.[339] The variability of the DNA-binding sites is consistent with the fact that the constraint on DNA for its folding is imposed by the arginine-rich histones H3-H4. The evolutionary conservation of the protein-binding domains in H2a-H2b shows the vital importance for the cell of some specific protein-protein interactions in which the slightly lysine-rich histones are involved. The same holds true for different portions of the molecule of H1 (see Section IV). The existence of several nonallelic histone variants with amino acid substitutions in these conservative sites suggests that the functional significance of the protein-protein interactions in chromatin is not only structural.

4.   The absence of mutations in spite of the reiteration of histone genes (see Section VIII.A) suggests that mutations, even in one single histone gene, must have been lethal because of the parallel synthesis of a false histone species which will form structures providing incorrect information for control processes.

All these considerations support the idea that histones have a double function — structural and informational. We have suggested that the informational role resides in different histone arrangements which mark different chromatin regions.[5] In the light of the present data on the composition of nucleosomes, it may be proposed that the basis of these different histone arrangements are different histone variants.[113a] The two contradictory requirements imposed on nucleosomal histones — to pack DNA in a standard way for structural purposes and to exhibit some variability for the purpose of control — may be one of the reasons for the restricted possibility of variations in the structure of these histone species.

The heterogeneity of the nucleosomal histone complexes may be used in two ways as an additional information for the realization of control mechanisms — in interactions between histones and nonhistone proteins and in histone-histone interactions.

The first type of interactions implies that different nucleosomal structures may be recognized by different nonhistone proteins which in this way can specifically control the functional state of the nucleosomes. Since large portions of the genome may have nucleosomes with identical histone cores, a high number of molecules of a nonhistone protein should be needed for this type of regulation. Such regulatory nonhistone proteins may be operating either to block or to deblock a chromatin region. It is also probable that such specific interactions may be associated with some chemical modifications of the histones necessary for transcription.

The second type are interactions between identical nucleosomes leading to highly ordered structures.[246] The association of lysine-rich histones with these nucleosomal complexes may be also based on specific histone-histone interactions. It is not known how different subspecies of H1 are distributed in the chromatin, but the presence of about five H1 subfractions in the nucleus with only one molecule per nucleosome (see Section VII.A) shows that chromatin should be heterogeneous with respect to different H1 species. A direct evidence was obtained recently that different H1 subfractions were unevenly distributed among the chromatin subunits, one of them, $H1_3$, showing most variations.[339a] It was also found that each H1 subfraction differed from the others in its power to compact DNA.[339b]

An important question is how the information for the distribution of different nucleosomes is transmitted to the daughter cells during the cell cycle. Since histones and histone complexes do not recognize DNA base sequences, the reconstitution of chromatin during replication should also be based on specific interactions between old and newly formed histones. Several data indicate that histones do not leave chromatin during replication (see Section VIII.B) so that they may serve as templates for the reproduction of the same chromatin structure[5] or a different structure during embryonic development when new histone variants are synthesized.[113a] In both cases, the reproduction or the reorganization of the chromatin should be associated with the synthesis of the corresponding nonhistone proteins which specifically interact with the histone complexes. In this connection it is worth mentioning that the $0.35 M$ NaCl extractable nonhistone proteins which were responsible for the DNase I sensitivity of active genes were not found to be tissue specific and probably do not recognize specific DNA sequences.[278f]

Such a control mechanism of cell differentiation, based on information provided by histone-dependent structures, may meet at least two difficulties: the replacement of histones by protamines in spermatozoa and the possibility of chromatin reconstitution in vitro.

The complete replacement of histones by protamines reported in some species (see Section IV.C) means that all information which may be contained in the chromatin structures organized by histones should be lost. In such a case, the restoration of the somatic chromatin structure during embryonic development would be impossible without the use of some information encoded in DNA, i.e., protein-DNA interactions recognizing specific base sequences. However, most of the species preserve at least part of their somatic histones in the male gametes, and in the species where a "complete" replacement is accepted, the experimental evidence does not prove a replacement more than 90%. It is evident that in different species, a variable extent of replacement takes place, and it is possible that in all cases at least some histone complexes are preserved marking different regions of the genome. In the process of chromatin reconstitution during embryonic development, these complexes may serve as initiation centers for a process of self-assembly of nucleosomal structures. Such a mechanism should be regarded as purely hypothetical since no experimental data are available for the mode of reconstruction of somatic chromatin in the embryo. It is also possible that some nonhistone proteins tightly bound to DNA remain in the spermatozoids and provide the necessary information for a faithful reconstitution of the somatic nucleohistone complexes. The existence of such proteins covering 14% of DNA has been demonstrated in herring sperm nuclei[339c] and we have found similar proteins in ram sperm chromatin.[339d]

A second argument against the existence of histone-dependent information may come from experiments on reconstitution of chromatin from DNA, histones, and nonhistone proteins. Several authors have obtained results interpreted as showing a high fidelity of reconstitution with respect to the synthesis of specific mRNAs whose type depended on the nonhistone proteins used.[337,340,341] Many methodological errors may accompany reconstitution experiments, but the most serious objection which was recently raised is the presence of a RNA-dependent RNA polymerase activity of the enzymes used.[342,343] This leads to the synthesis of new RNA complementary to endogeneous mRNA which is always present in chromatin components and serves as a template for the enzyme. These data explain earlier results which have shown failure of functionally correct reconstitution when endogeneous RNA was destroyed[344,345] and have been misinterpreted as indicating the role of chromosomal RNA in the control of transcription. The RNA-directed RNA synthesis greatly complicates the interpretation of results from reconstitution experiments even when mercurated nucleotides are used as precursors.

Thus, the question of whether a functionally faithful reconstitution is possible remains open. If the chromatin structure determined by the chromosomal proteins has an informational significance, functional fidelity of reconstitution would be principally impossible due to the loss of information when proteins are dissociated from DNA.

All these considerations suggest, but do not rigorously prove, the informational role of histone complexes. To elucidate this problem, more experimental evidence is needed on several crucial points in this field — the occurrence and developmental changes of histone variants, the heterogeneity of nucleosomes, the distribution of H1 subspecies in chromatin, the completeness of histone replacement in spermatozoa, the mode of chromatin reconstruction during embryogenesis, the possibility of faithful reconstitution of chromatin in vitro, etc. The results from such experiments may help in the near future to answer more clearly the question what, exactly, histones do in chromatin.

REFERENCES

1. **Stedman, E. and Stedman, E.**, Cell specificity of histones, *Nature (London)*, 166, 780, 1950.
2. **Bullough, W. S.**, Introduction, *The Evolution of Differentiation*, Academic Press, New York, 1967, 3.
3. **Jacob, F. and Monod, J.**, Genetic repression, allosteric inhibition, and cellular differentiation, in *Cytodifferentiation and Macromolecular Synthesis*, Locke, M., Ed., Academic Press, New York, 1963, 30.
4. **Tsanev, R.**, Cell cycle and liver function, in *Results and Problems of Cell Differentiation*, Reinert, J. and Holtzer, H., Eds., Springer-Verlag, Berlin, 1975, 7.
5. **Tsanev, R. and Sendov, Bl.**, Possible molecular mechanism for cell differentiation in multicellular organisms, *J. Theor. Biol.*, 30, 337, 1971.
6. **Gottesfeld, J. M. and Bonner, J.**, Isolation and properties of the expressed portion of the mammalian genome, in *The Molecular Biology of the Mammalian Genetic Apparatus*, Ts'o, P. O. P., Ed., North-Holland, Amsterdam, 1977, 381.
7. **Wallace, R. B., Dube, S. K., and Bonner, J.**, Localization of the globin gene in the template active fraction of chromatin of Friend leukemia cells, *Science*, 198, 1166, 1977.
7a. **Miller, D. M., Turner, P., Nienhuis, A. W., Axelrod, D. E., and Gopalakrishnan, T. V.**, Active conformation of the globin genes in uninduced and induced mouse erythroleukemia cells, *Cell*, 14, 511, 1978.
7b. **Stalder, J., Seebeck, T., and Braun, R.**, Degradation of the ribosomal genes by DNase I in Physarum polycephalum, *Eur. J. Biochem.*, 90, 391, 1978.
7c. **Palmiter, R. D., Mulvihill, E. R., McKnight, G. S., and Senear, A. W.**, Regulation of gene expression in the chick oviduct by steroid hormones, *Cold Spring Harbor Symp. Quant. Biol.*, 42, 639, 1978.
7d. **Wu, C., Wong, Y.- C., and Elgin, S. C. R.**, The chromatin structure of specific genes: II. Description of chromatin structure during gene activity, *Cell*, 16, 807, 1979.
8. **Rizzo, P. J.**, Basic chromosomal proteins in lower eukaryotes: relevance to the evolution and function of histones, *J. Mol. Evol.*, 8, 79, 1976.
8a. **Jardine, N. J. and Leaver, J. L.**, The fractionation of histones isolated from *Euglena gracilis*, *Biochem. J.*, 169, 103, 1978.
9. **Charlesworth, M. C. and Parish, R. W.**, The isolation of nuclei and basic nucleoproteins from the cellular slime mold *Dictyostelium discoideum*, *Eur. J. Biochem.*, 54, 307, 1975.
10. **Leighton, T., Leighton, F., Dill, B., and Stock, J.**, The similarities of ribosomal and basic chromosomal proteins from fungi, *Biochim. Biophys. Acta*, 432, 381, 1976.
11. **Conkel, M. B. and Walker, I. O.**, The basic nuclear proteins of the cellular slime mold *Dictyostelium discoideum*, *Cell Differ.*, 2, 87, 1973.
11a. **Rouvière-Yaniv, J.**, Localization of the HU protein on the *Escherichia coli* nucleoid, *Cold Spring Harbor Symp. Quant. Biol.*, 42, 439, 1978.
11b. **Laine, B., Sautière, P., Biserte, G., Cohen-Solal, M., Gros, F., and Rouvière-Yaniv, J.**, The amino- and carboxy-terminal aminoacid sequences of protein HU from *Escherichia coli*, *FEBS Lett.*, 89, 116, 1978.
11c. **Rouvière-Yaniv, J., Yaniv, M., and Germond, J.- E.**, E. coli DNA binding protein HU forms nucleosomelike structure with circular double-stranded DNA, *Cell*, 17, 265, 1979.
12. **Searcy, D. G.**, Histone-like protein in the prokaryote thermoplasma *Acidophilum*, *Biochim. Biophys. Acta*, 395, 535, 1975.
13. **Gofshtein, L. V., Yurina, N. P., Romashkin, V. J., and Oparin, A. I.**, Comparison of histone-like proteins from blue-green alga with ribosomal basic proteins of alga and wheat germs histones, *Biokhimiya*, 40, 1104, 1975.
13a. **Haselkorn, R. and Rouvière-Yaniv, J.**, Cyanobacterial DNA-binding protein related to *Escherichia coli* HU, *Proc. Natl. Acad. Sci. U.S.A.*, 73, 1917, 1976.
14. **Rizzo, P. J. and Nooden, L. D.**, Partial characterization of dinoflagellate chromosomal proteins, *Biochim. Biophys. Acta*, 349, 415, 1974.
15. **Rizzo, P. J. and Nooden, L. D.**, Chromosomal proteins in the dinoflagellate alga *Gyrodinium cohnii*, *Science*, 176, 796, 1972.
16. **Rizzo, P. J. and Cox, E. R.**, Histone occurrence in chromatin from *Peridinium balticum*, *Nature*, 198, 1258, 1977.
17. **Bradley, D. M., Goldin, H. H., and Claybrook, J. R.**, Histone analysis in *Volvox*, *FEBS Lett.*, 41, 219, 1974.
17a. **Kozlov, A. V., Ivanova, S. B., Lipskaya, A. A., Bers, E. P., and Vodop'yanova, L. G.**, Immunofluorescence study of main chromosomal proteins in some Green algae and Euglena, *Tsitologiya, SSSR*, 21, 459, 1979.

18. **Cohen, R. J. and Stein, G. S.**, Chromosomal proteins of *Phycomyces blakesleeanus*, *Exp. Cell Res.*, 96, 247, 1975.

19. **Goff, C. G.**, Histones of *Neurospora crassa*, *J. Biol. Chem.*, 251, 4131, 1976.

20. **Felden, R. A., Sanders, M. M., and Morris, N. R.**, Presence of histones in *Aspergillus nidulans*, *J. Cell Biol.*, 68, 430, 1976.

21. **Moll, R. and Wintersberger, E.**, Synthesis of yeast histones in the cell cycle, *Proc. Natl. Acad. Sci. U.S.A.*, 73, 1863, 1976.

22. **Nelson, D. A., Beltz, W. R., and Rill, R. L.**, Chromatin subunits from baker's yeast: isolation and partial characterization, *Proc. Natl. Acad. Sci. U.S.A.*, 74, 1343, 1977.

22a. **Suchiliené, S. P., and Gineitis, A. A.**, Histones from *Saccharomyces cerevisiae*, *Exp. Cell Res.*, 114, 454, 1978.

22b. **Sommer, A.**, Yeast chromatin; search for histone H1, *Mol. Gen. Genet.*, 161, 323, 1978.

22c. **Pastink, A., Berkhout, T. A., Mager, W. H., and Planta, R. J.**, Analysis of histones from the yeast *Saccharomyces carlsbergensis*, *Biochem. J.*, 177, 917, 1979.

23. **Osborn, P. J. and Ashworth, J. M.**, Changes in the basic nuclear proteins of the cellular slime mould *Dictyostelium discoideum* during growth and differentiation, *Cell Differ.*, 4, 237, 1975.

23a. **Glover, C. V. C., and Gorovsky, M. A.**, Histone-histone interactions in a lower eukaryote, *Tetrahymena thermophila*, *Biochemistry*, 17, 5705, 1978.

23b. **Jardine, N. J., and Leaver, J. L.**, The isolation of nuclei and histones from *Euglena gracilis*, *Exp. Cell Res.*, 106, 423, 1977.

24. **Gorovsky, M. A., Pleger, G. L., Keevert, J. B., and Johmann, C.**, Studies on histone fraction F2a1 in macro- and micronuclei of *Tetrahymena pyriformis*, *J. Cell Biol.*, 57, 773, 1973.

25. **Johmann, C. A. and Gorovsky, M. A.**, Purification and characterization of the histones associated with the macronucleus of *Tetrahymena*, *Biochemistry*, 15, 1249, 1976.

25a. **Glover, C. V. C. and Gorovsky, M. A.**, Amino-acid sequence of Tetrahymena histone H4 differs from that of higher eukaryotes, *Proc. Natl. Acad. Sci. U.S.A.*, 76, 585, 1979.

26. **Johmann, C. A. and Gorovsky, M. A.**, An electrophoretic comparison of the histones of various strains of *Tetrahymena pyriformis*, *Arch. Biochem. Biophys.*, 175, 694, 1976.

27. **Gorovsky, M. A., Keevert, J. B., and Pleger, G. L.**, Histone F1 of *Tetrahymena* macronuclei. Unique electrophoretic properties and phosphorylation of F1 in an amitotic nucleus, *J. Cell Biol.*, 61, 134, 1974.

27a. **Gorovsky, M. A., Glover, C., Johmann, C. A., Keevert, J. B., Mathis, D. J., and Samuelson, M.**, Histones and chromatin structure in *Tetrahymena* macro- and micronuclei, *Cold Spring Harbor Symp. Quant. Biol.*, 42, 493, 1978.

27b. **Elsevier, S. M., Lipps, H. J., and Steinbrük, G.**, Histone genes in macronuclear DNA of the ciliate *Stylonychia mytilus*, *Chromosoma*, 69, 291, 1978.

27c. **Lipps, H. J. and Morris, N. R.**, Chromatin structure in the nuclei of the ciliate *Stylonychia mytilus*, *Biochem. Biophys. Res. Commun.*, 74, 230, 1977.

28. **Noll, M.**, Differences and similarities in chromatin structure of *Neurospora crassa* and higher eukaryotes, *Cell*, 8, 349, 1976.

29. **Jerzmanowski, A., Staron, K., and Tyniec, B.**, Subunit structure of *Physarum polycephalum* chromatin, *FEBS Lett.*, 62, 251, 1976.

30. **Morris, N. R.**, Nucleosome structure in *Aspergillus nidulans*, *Cell*, 8, 357, 1976.

31. **Lohr, D. and Van Holde, K. E.**, Yeast chromatin subunit structure, *Science*, 188, 165, 1975.

32. **Vogt, V. M. and Braun, R.**, Repeated structure of chromatin in metaphase nuclei of *Physarum*, *FEBS Lett.*, 64, 190, 1976.

32a. **Parish, R. W., Stalder, J., and Schmidlin, S.**, Biochemical evidence for a DNA repeat length in the chromatin of *Dictyostelium discoideum*, *FEBS Lett.*, 84, 63, 1977.

32b. **Prince, D. J., Cummings, D. J., and Seale, R. L.**, Analysis of chromatin repeat units in logarithmically and stationary growing cells of *Paramecium aurelia* and *Tetrahymena pyriformis*, *Biochem. Biophys. Res. Commun.*, 79, 190, 1977.

32c. **Silver, J. C.**, Chromatin organization in the oomycete Achlya ambisexualis, *Biochim. Biophys. Acta*, 561, 261, 1979.

32d. **Widmer, R., Fuhrer, S., and Parish, R. W.**, Biochemical evidence for a distinctive chromatin structure in nucleoli of *Dictyostelium*, *FEBS Lett.*, 106, 363, 1979.

32e. **Lipps, H. J., Nock, A., Riewe, M., and Steinbrük, G.**, Chromatin structure in the macronucleus of the ciliate *Stylonychia mytilus*, *Nucl. Acids Res.*, 5, 4699, 1978.

32f. **Bakke, A. C., Wu, J.- R., and Bonner, J.**, Chromatin structure in the cellular slime mold *Dictyostelium discoideum*, *Proc. Natl. Acad. Sci. U.S.A.*, 75, 705, 1978.

33. **Hnilica, L. S.**, *The Structure and Biological Functions of Histones*, CRC Press, Cleveland, Ohio, 1972.

34. **Elgin, S. C. R. and Weintraub, H.**, Chromosomal proteins and chromatin structure, *Annu. Rev. Biochem.*, 44, 725, 1975.
35. **Johnson, J. D., Douvas, A. S., and Bonner, J.**, Chromosomal proteins, *Int. Rev. Cytol.*, Suppl. 4, 273, 1974.
36. **Bradbury, E. M.**, Foreword: histone nomenclature, in *The Structure and Function of Chromatin*, Ciba Foundation Symposium, 28, Associated Scientific Publishers, Amsterdam, 1975, 1.
37. **Wigle, D. T. and Dixon, G. H.**, A new histone from trout testis, *J. Biol. Chem.*, 246, 5636, 1971.
37a. **Watson, D. C., Wong, N. C. W., and Dixon, G. H.**, The complete amino-acid sequence of a trout-testis non-histone protein, H6, localized in a subset of nucleosomes and its similarity to calf-thymus non-histone proteins HMG-14 and HMG-17, *Eur. J. Biochem.*, 95, 193, 1979.
38. **Franklin, S. G. and Zweidler, A.**, Non-allelic variants of histones 2a, 2b, and 3 in mammals, *Nature (London)*, 266, 273, 1977.
39. **Zweidler, A.**, Complexity and variability of the histone complement, in *Organization and Expression of Chromosomes*, Allfrey, V. G., Bautz, E. K. F., McCarthy, B. J., Schimke, R., and Tissières, A., Eds., Dahlem Konferenzen, Berlin, 1976, 187.
40. **Borun, T. W., Ajiro, K., Zweidler, A., Dolby, T. W., and Stephens, R. E.**, Studies of human histone messenger RNA. II. The resolution of fractions containing individual human histone messenger RNA species, *J. Biol. Chem.*, 252, 173, 1977.
40a. **Van Helden, P., Strickland, W. N., Brandt, W. F., and Von Holt, C.**, Histone H2B variants from the erythrocytes of an amphibian, a reptile and a bird, *Biochim. Biophys. Acta*, 533, 278, 1978.
40b. **Strickland, M., Strickland, W. N., Brandt, W. F., Von Holt, C., Wittmann-Liebold, B., and Lehmann, A.**, The complete amino-acid sequence of histone H2B$_{(3)}$ from sperm of the sea urchin *Parechinus angulosus*, *Eur. J. Biochem.*, 89, 443, 1978.
40c. **Von Holt, C., Strickland, W., Brandt, W. F., and Strickland, M. S.**, More histone structures, *FEBS Lett.*, 100, 201, 1979.
41. **Laine, B., Sautière, P., and Biserte, G.**, Primary structure and microheterogeneities of rat chloroleukemia histone H2a (histone ALK, IIb1 or F2a2), *Biochemistry*, 15, 1640, 1976.
42. **Marzluff, W. F., Jr., Sanders, L. A., Miller, D. M., and McCarthy, K. S.**, Two chemically and metabolically distinct forms of calf thymus histone F3, *J. Biol. Chem.*, 247, 2026, 1972.
43. **Bustin, M., Reeder, R. H., and McKnight, S. L.**, Immunological cross-reaction between calf and *Drosophila* histones, *J. Biol. Chem.*, 252, 3099, 1977.
44. **Alfageme, C. R., Zweidler, A., Mahowald, A., and Cohen, L. H.**, Histones of *Drosophila* embryos. Electrophoretic isolation and structural studies, *J. Biol. Chem.*, 249, 3729, 1974.
45. **Nadeau, P., Pallotta, D., and Lafontaine, J. G.**, Electrophoretic study of plant histones: comparison with vertebrate histones, *Arch. Biochem. Biophys.*, 161, 171, 1974.
46. **Brandt, W. F. and Von Holt, C.**, Isolation and characterization of the histones from cycad pollen, *FEBS Lett.*, 51, 84, 1975.
47. **Spiker, S.**, An evolutionary comparison of plant histones, *Biochim. Biophys. Acta*, 400, 46, 1975.
48. **Spiker, S.**, Expression of parental histone genes in the intergenetic hybrid *Triticale hexaploide*, *Nature (London)*, 259, 418, 1976.
49. **Spiker, S., Key, J. L., and Wakim, B.**, Identification and fractionation of plant histones, *Arch. Biochem. Biophys.*, 176, 510, 1976.
50. **Hayashi, H., Iwai, K., Johnson, J. D., and Bonner, J.**, Pea histones H2a and H2b. Variable and conserved regions in the sequences, *J. Biochem. (Tokyo)*, 82, 503, 1977.
50a. **Rodrigues, J. de A., Brandt, W. F., and Von Holt, C.**, Plant histone 2 from wheat germ, a family of histone H2a variants. Partial amino acid sequences, *Biochim. Biophys. Acta*, 578, 196, 1979.
51. **McGhee, J. D. and Engle, J. O.**, Subunit structure of chromatin is the same in plants and animals, *Nature (London)*, 254, 449, 1975.
52. **Philipps, G. and Gigot, C.**, DNA associated with nucleosomes in plants, *Nucleic Acids Res.*, 4, 3617, 1977.
53. **DeLange, R. J., Fambrough, D. M., Smith, E. L., and Bonner, J.**, Calf and pea histone IV. III. Complete amino acid sequence of pea seedling histone IV; comparison with the homologous calf thymus histone, *J. Biol. Chem.*, 244, 5669, 1969.
54. **Pathy, L., Smith, E. L., and Johnson, J.**, Histone III. V. The amino acid sequence of pea embryo histone III, *J. Biol. Chem.*, 248, 6834, 1973.
55. **Brandt, W. F., Strickland, W. N., Morgan, M., and Von Holt, C.**, Comparison of N-terminal amino acid sequences of histone F3 from a mammal, a bird, a shark, an echinoderm, a mollusc and a plant, *FEBS Lett.*, 40, 167, 1974.
56. **DeLange, R. J. and Smith, E. L.**, Histone function and evolution as viewed by sequence studies, in *The Structure and Function of Chromatin*, Ciba Foundation Symposium, 28, Associated Scientific Publishers, Amsterdam, 1975, 59.
56a. **Roland, B., and Pallota, D.**, An immunological comparison of rye and calf histones, *Can. J. Biochem.*, 56, 1021, 1978.

57. **Wuilmar, C. and Wyns, L.,** An evolutionary scheme for the histones as derived from a study of internal repetitions and homologies among the different classes, *J. Theor. Biol.,* 65, 231, 1977.

57a. **Reek, G. R., Swanson, E., and Teller, D. D.,** The evolution of histones, *J. Mol. Evol.,* 10, 309, 1978.

58. **Kedes, L. H.,** Histone messengers and histone genes, *Cell,* 8, 321, 1976.

59. **Blankstein, L. A. and Levy, S. B.,** Changes in histone F2a2 associated with proliferation of Friend leukaemic cells, *Nature (London),* 260, 638, 1976.

59a. **Hohmann, Ph.,** The H1 class of histone and diversity in chromosomal structure, *Sub Cell. Biochem.,* 5, 87, 1978.

60. **Kinkade, J. M., Jr.,** Quantitative species differences and quantitative tissue differences in the distribution of lysine-rich histones, *J. Biol. Chem.,* 244, 3375, 1969.

61. **Hohmann, P., Cole, R. D., and Bern, H. A.,** Comparison of lysine-rich histones in various normal and neoplastic mouse tissues, *J. Natl. Cancer Inst.,* 47, 337, 1971.

62. **Panyim, S. and Chalkley, R.,** A new histone found only in mammalian tissues with little cell division, *Biochem. Biophys. Res. Commun.,* 37, 1042, 1969.

63. **Sherod, D., Panyim, S., Balhorn, R., and Chalkley, R.,** A comparison of histones from tumor cells and normal somatic tissue, *Fed. Proc.,* 29, 730, 1970.

63a. **Bustin, M. and Stollar, B. D.,** Immunological relatedness of thymus and liver F1 histone subfractions, *J. Biol. Chem.,* 248, 3506, 1973.

64. **Stellwagen, R. H., Reid, B. R., and Cole, R. D.,** Degradation of histones during the manipulation of isolated nuclei and deoxyribonucleoprotein, *Biochim. Biophys. Acta,* 155, 581, 1968.

65. **Destrée, O. H. J., D'Adelhart-Toorop, H. A., and Charles, R.,** Analysis of histones from different tissues and embryos of *Xenopus laevis* (Daudin). I. Technical problems in the purification of undegraded native total histone preparation, *Acta Morphol. Neerl. Scand.,* 10, 233, 1972.

66. **Sung, M. T.,** Phosphorylation and dephosphorylation of histone V (H5): controlled condensation of avian erythrocyte chromatin, *Biochemistry,* 16, 286, 1977.

67. **Adams, G. H. M. and Neelin, J. M.,** The absence of cell-specific histone in erythroid cells from rabbit marrow, *Can. J. Biochem.,* 54, 571, 1976.

68. **Sheridan, W. F. and Stern, H.,** Histones of meiosis, *Exp. Cell Res.,* 45, 323, 1967.

69. **Subirana, J. A., Cozcolluela, C., Palau, J., and Unzeta, M.,** Protamines and other basic proteins from spermatozoa of molluscs, *Biochim. Biophys. Acta,* 317, 364, 1973.

70. **Palau, J., Ruiz-Carrillo, A., and Subirana, J. A.,** Histones from sperm of the sea urchin *Arbacia lixula, Eur. J. Biochem.,* 7, 209, 1969.

71. **Thaler, M. M., Cox, M. C. L., and Villee, C. A.,** Histones in early embryogenesis. Developmental aspects of composition and synthesis, *J. Biol. Chem.,* 245, 1479, 1970.

72. **Easton, D. and Chalkley, R.,** High resolution electrophoretic analysis of the histones from embryos and sperm of *Arbacia punctulata, Exp. Cell Res.,* 72, 502, 1972.

73. **Spadafora, C., Noviello, L., and Geraci, G.,** Chromatin organization in nuclei of sea urchin embryos. Comparison with the chromatin organization of the sperm, *Cell Differ.,* 5, 225, 1976.

74. **Strickland, W. N., Strickland, M., Brandt, W. F., Morgan, M., and Von Holt, C.,** Partial amino acid sequence of two new arginine-serine rich histones from male gonads of the sea urchin, *FEBS Lett.,* 40, 161, 1974.

75. **Strickland, M., Strickland, W. N., Brandt, W. F., and Von Holt, C.,** The complete amino-acid sequence of histone H2b$_{(1)}$ from sperm of the sea urchin *Parechinus angulosus, Eur. J. Biochem.,* 77, 263, 1977.

76. **Strickland, W. N., Strickland, M., Brandt, W. F., and Von Holt, C.,** The complete amino-acid sequence of histone H2b($_2$) from sperm of the sea urchin *Parechinus angulosus, Eur. J. Biochem.,* 77, 277, 1977.

77. **Black, J. A. and Dixon, G. H.,** Evolution of protamine: a further example of partial gene duplication, *Nature (London),* 216, 152, 1967.

78. **Tessier, A. and Pallotta, D.,** Analysis on basic proteins during spermatogenesis in the cricket, *Acheta domestica, Exp. Cell Res.,* 82, 103, 1973.

79. **Pallotta, D. and Tessier, A.,** Amino acid composition of sperm histones in the house cricket *Acheta domestica, Can. J. Biochem.,* 54, 56, 1976.

80. **Kaye, J. S. and McMaster-Kaye, R.,** Histones of spermatogenous cells in the house cricket, *Chromosoma,* 46, 397, 1974.

81. **McMaster-Kaye, R. and Kaye, J. S.,** Basic protein changes during the final stages of sperm maturation in the house cricket, *Exp. Cell Res.,* 97, 378, 1976.

82. **Ando, T., Yamasaki, M., and Suzuki, K.,** Protamines. Isolation, characterization, structure and function, in *Molecular Biology, Biochemistry and Biophysics,* Kleinzeller, A., Springer, G. F., and Wittmann, H. G., Eds., Springer-Verlag, Berlin, 1973, 12.

82a. **Sakai, M., Fujii-Kuriyama, Y., and Muramatsu, M.,** Number and frequency of protamine genes in rainbow trout testis, *Biochemistry,* 17, 5510, 1978.

83. **Louie, A. J., Candido, E. P. M., and Dixon, G. H.**, Enzymatic modifications and their possible roles in regulating the binding of basic proteins to DNA and in controlling chromosomal structure, *Cold Spring Harbor Symp. Quant. Biol.*, 38, 803, 1973.

83a. **Iatrou, K. and Dixon, G. H.**, Protamine messenger RNA: its life history during spermatogenesis in rainbow trout, *Fed. Proc.*, 37, 2526, 1978.

84. **Subirana, J. A., Puigjaner, L. C., Roca, J., Llopis, R., and Suau, P.**, X-ray diffraction of nucleo-histones from spermatozoa, in *The Structure and Function of Chromatin,* Ciba Foundation Symposium, 28, Associated Scientific Publishers, Amsterdam, 1975, 157.

85. **Honda, B. M., Baillie, D. L., and Candido, E. P. M.**, The subunit structure of chromatin: characteristics of nucleohistone and nucleoprotamine from developing trout testis, *FEBS Lett.*, 48, 156, 1974.

86. **Adler, D. and Gorovsky, M. A.**, Electrophoretic analysis of liver and testis histones of the frog *Rana pipiens, J. Cell Biol.*, 64, 389, 1975.

86a. **Kasinsky, H. E., Huang, S. Y., Kwauk, S., Mann, M., Sweeney, M. A. J., and Yee, B.**, On the diversity of sperm histones in the vertebrates. III. Electrophoretic variability of testis-specific histone patterns in Anura contrasts with relative constancy in Squamata, *J. Exp. Zool.*, 203, 109, 1978.

87. **Bols, N. C., Byrd, E. W., Jr., and Kasinsky, H. E.**, On the diversity of sperm histones in the vertebrates. I. Changes in basic proteins during spermiogenesis in the newt *Notophthalamus viridescens, Differentiation*, 7, 31, 1976.

88. **Nakano, M., Tobita, T., and Ando, T.**, Fractionation of galline, a protamine from fowl sperm, and some characterization of the components, *Biochim. Biophys. Acta*, 207, 553, 1970.

89. **Mezquita, C. and Teng, C. S.**, Studies on sex-organ development. Changes in nuclear and chromatin composition and genomic activity during spermatogenesis in the maturing rooster testis, *Biochem. J.*, 164, 99, 1977.

90. **Coelingh, J. P., Rozijn, T. H., and Monfoort, C. H.**, Isolation and partial characterization of a basic protein from bovine sperm heads, *Biochim. Biophys. Acta*, 188, 353, 1969.

91. **Monfoort, C. H., Schiphof, R., Rozijn, T. H., and Steyn-Parve, E. P.**, Amino acid composition and carboxyl-terminal structure of some basic chromosomal proteins of mammalian spermatozoa, *Biochim. Biophys. Acta*, 322, 173, 1973.

92. **Kistler, W. S., Geroch, M. E., and Williams-Ashman, H. G.**, Specific basic proteins from mammalian testes. Isolation and properties of small basic proteins from rat testes and epididymal spermatozoa, *J. Biol. Chem.*, 248, 4532, 1973.

92a. **Grimes, S. R., Jr., Meistrick, M. L., Platz, R. D., and Hnilica, L. S.**, Nuclear protein transions in rat testis spermatids, *Exp. Cell Res.*, 110, 31, 1977.

93. **Marushige, Y. and Marushige, K.**, Properties of chromatin isolated from bull spermatozoa, *Biochim. Biophys. Acta*, 340, 498, 1974.

94. **Puwaravutipanich, T. and Panyim, S.**, The nuclear basic proteins of human testes and ejaculated spermatozoa, *Exp. Cell Res.*, 90, 153, 1975.

95. **Kumaroo, K. K., Jahnke, G., and Irvin, J. L.**, Changes in basic chromosomal proteins during spermatogenesis in the mature rat, *Arch. Biochem. Biophys.*, 168, 413, 1975.

96. **Kolk, A. H. J. and Samuel, T.**, Isolation, chemical and immunological characterization of two strongly basic nuclear proteins from human spermatozoa, *Biochim. Biophys. Acta*, 393, 307, 1975.

96a. **Svasti, J. and Talupphet, N.**, Improvement in the resolution of human sperm protamines by use of iodoacetamide as alkylating agent, *Biochim. Biophys. Acta*, 577, 221, 1979.

97. **Platz, R. D., Grimes, S. R., Meistrich, M. L., and Hnilica, L. S.**, Changes in nuclear proteins of rat testis cells separated by velocity sedimentation, *J. Biol. Chem.*, 250, 5791, 1975.

98. **Calvin, H. J.**, Comparative analysis of the nuclear basic proteins in rat, human, guinea pig, mouse and rabbit, *Biochim. Biophys. Acta*, 434, 377, 1976.

98a. **Grimes, S. R., Jr., Meistrich, M. L., Platz, R. D., and Hnilica, L. S.**, Nuclear protein transitions in rat testis spermatids, *Exp. Cell Res.*, 110, 31, 1977.

99. **Lam, D. M. K. and Bruce, W. R.**, The biosynthesis of protamine during spermatogenesis of the mouse: extraction, partial characterization, and site of synthesis, *J. Cell. Physiol.*, 78, 13, 1971.

100. **Grimes, S. R., Jr., Platz, R. D., Meistrich, M. L., and Hnilica, L. S.**, Partial characterization of a new basic nuclear protein from rat testis elongated spermatids, *Biochem. Biophys. Res. Commun.*, 67, 182, 1975.

100a. **Loir, M. and Lanneau, M.**, Partial characterization of ram spermatidal nuclear proteins, *Biochem. Biophys. Res. Commun.*, 80, 975, 1978.

100b. **Loir, M. and Lanneau, M.**, Transformation of ram spermatid chromatin, *Exp. Cell Res.*, 115, 231, 1978.

101. **Grimes, S. R., Jr., Meistrich, M. L., Platz, R. D., and Hnilica, L. S.**, Nuclear protein transitions in rat testis spermatids, *Exp. Cell Res.*, 110, 31, 1977.

102. **Goldberg, R. B., Geremia, R., and Bruce, W. R.**, Histone synthesis and replacement during spermatogenesis in the mouse, *Differentiation*, 7, 167, 1977.

102a. **Samuel, T.**, Differentiation between antibodies to protamines and somatic nuclear antigens by means of a comparative fluorescence study on swollen nuclei of spermatozoa and somatic cells, *Clin. Exp. Immunol.*, 32, 290, 1978.

102b. **Samuel, T., Kolk, A. H. J., and Rümke, P.**, Studies on the immunogenicity of protamines in humans and experimental animals by means of a micro-complement fixation test, *Clin. Exp. Immunol.*, 33, 252, 1978.

103. **Marushige, Y. and Marushige, K.**, Enzymatic unpacking of bull sperm chromatin, *Biochim. Biophys. Acta*, 403, 180, 1975.

104. **Hnilica, L. S., McClure, M. E., and Spelsberg, T. C.**, Histone biosynthesis and the cell cycle, in *Histones and Nucleohistones*, Phillips, D. M. P., Ed., Plenum Press, New York, 1971, 187.

105. **Cognetti, G., Platz, R. D., Meistrich, M. L., and DiLiegro, J.**, Studies on protein synthesis during sea urchin oogenesis. I. Synthesis of histone F2b, *Cell Differ.*, 5, 283, 1977.

105a. **Woodland, H. R.**, The modification of stored histones H3 and H4 during the oogenesis and early development of Xenopus laevis, *Develop. Biol.*, 68, 360, 1979.

106. **Shutt, R. H. and Kedes, L. H.**, Synthesis of histone mRNA sequences in isolated nuclei of cleavage stage sea urchin embryos, *Cell*, 3, 283, 1974.

107. **Kano, K. and Mano, Y.**, Synthesis of the acid-soluble proteins in early cleaving embryos of the sea urchin. Cyclic synthesis of histones, *J. Biochem.*, 80, 625, 1976.

108. **Seale, R. L. and Aronson, A. I.**, Chromatin-associated proteins of the developing sea urchin embryo. II. Acid-soluble proteins, *J. Mol. Biol.*, 75, 647, 1973.

109. **Cohen, L. H., Newrock, K. M., and Zweidler, A.**, Stage-specific switches in histone synthesis during embryogenesis of the sea urchin, *Science*, 190, 994, 1975.

109a. **Ord, M. G. and Stocken, L. A.**, Histones in the first cleavage cycle of fertilized sea urchin eggs, *Cell Differ.*, 7, 271, 1978.

110. **Ruiz-Carrillo, A. and Palau, J.**, Histones from embryos of the sea urchin *Arbacia lixula*, *Dev. Biol.*, 35, 115, 1973.

111. **Gineitis, A. A., Stankevicute, Y. V., and Vorob'ev, V. J.**, Chromatin proteins from normal, vegetalized and animalized sea urchin embryos, *Dev. Biol.*, 52, 181, 1976.

112. **Byrd, W. E., Jr. and Kasinsky, H. E.**, Nuclear accumulation of newly synthesized histones in early Xenopus development, *Biochim. Biophys. Acta*, 331, 430, 1973.

113. **Holmgreen, P., Rasmuson, B., Johanson, T., and Sundquist, G.**, Histone content in relation to amount of heterochromatin, and developmental stage in three species of *Drosophila*, *Chromosoma*, 54, 99, 1976.

113a. **Newrock, K. M., Alfageme, C. R., Nardi, R. V., and Cohen, L. H.**, Histone changes during chromatin remodeling in embryogenesis, *Cold Spring Harbor Symp. Quant. Biol.*, 42, 421, 1978.

113b. **Newrock, K. M., Cohen, L. H., Hendricks, M. B., Donelly, R. J., and Weinberg, E. S.**, Stage-specific mRNAs coding for subtypes of H2A and H2B histones in the sea urchin embryo, *Cell*, 14, 327, 1978.

113c. **Carroll, A. G. and Ozaki, H.**, Changes in the histones of the sea urchin Strongylocentrotus purpuratus at fertilization, *Exp. Cell Res.*, 119, 307, 1979.

113d. **Brandt, W. F., Strickland, W. N., Strickland, M., Carlisle, L., Woods, D., and Von Holt, C.**, A histone programme during the life cycle of the sea urchin, *Eur. J. Biochem.*, 94, 1, 1979.

113e. **Spinelli, G., Gianuzza, F., Casano, C., Acierno, P., and Burckhardt, J.**, Evidences of two different sets of histone genes active during embryogenesis of the sea urchin Paracentrotus lividus, *Nucl. Acids Res.*, 6, 545, 1979.

114. **Yoshida, K. and Sasaki, K.**, Changes of template activity and proteins of chromatin during wheat germination, *Plant Physiol.*, 59, 497, 1977.

115. **Ruderman, J. V., Baglioni, C., and Gross, P.**, Histone mRNA and histone synthesis during embryogenesis, *Nature (London)*, 247, 36, 1974.

116. **Ruderman, J. V. and Gross, P. R.**, Histones and histone synthesis in sea urchin development, *Dev. Biol.*, 36, 286, 1976.

117. **Trevithick, J. B.**, Patterns of incorporation of (^{32}P) orthophosphate and (^{3}H) acetate into histones of rainbow trout during early development, *Can. J. Biochem.*, 52, 399, 1974.

117a. **Senger, D. R., Arceci, R. J., and Gross, P. R.**, Histones of sea urchin embryos, *Dev. Biol.*, 65, 416, 1978.

117b. **Koster, J. G., Kasinsky, H. E., and Destreé, O. H. J.**, Newly synthesized histones in chromatin of early embryos of Xenopus laevis, *Cell Diff.*, 8, 93, 1979.

118. **Arceci, R. J., Senger, D. R., and Gross, P. R.**, The programmed switch in lysine-rich histone synthesis at gastrulation, *Cell*, 9, 171, 1976.

119. **Adamson, E. D. and Woodland, H. R.**, Changes in the rate of histone synthesis during oocyte maturation and very early development of *Xenopus laevis*, *Dev. Biol.*, 57, 136, 1977.

120. **Hnilica, L. S., Taylor, C. W., and Busch, H.,** Analysis of peptides of the moderately lysine-rich histone fraction, F2b, of the Walker tumor and other tissues, *Exp. Cell Res.,* Suppl. 9, 367, 1963.

121. **Desai, L., Ogawa, Y., Mauritzen, C. M., Taylor, C. W., and Starbuck, W. C.,** Carboxyl-terminal sequence of the glycine-arginine-rich histone from bovine lymphosarcoma, Novikoff hepatoma and fetal calf thymus, *Biochim. Biophys. Acta,* 181, 146, 1969.

122. **Sluyser, M. and Hermes, Y.,** A rat-specific lysine-rich histone, *Biochim. Biophys. Acta,* 295, 605, 1973.

123. **Sluyser, M.,** High multiplicity of H1 histones from mouse mammary tumors, *Cancer Lett.,* 2, 147, 1977.

123a. **Balhorn, R., Balhorn, M., Morris, H. P., and Chalkley, R.,** Comparative high-resolution electrophoresis of tumor histones; variation in phosphorylation as a function of cell replication rate, *Cancer Res.,* 32, 1775, 1972.

124. **Sluyser, M. and Bustin, M.,** Immunological specificity of lysine-rich histones from tumors, *J. Biol. Chem.,* 249, 2507, 1974.

125. **Lea, M. A., Koch, M. R., and Morris, H. P.,** Nuclear protein changes in rat hepatomas correlating with growth rate, *Cancer Res.,* 35, 1693, 1975.

126. **Balhorn, R., Chalkley, R., and Granner, D.,** Lysine-rich histone phosphorylation. A positive correlation with cell replication, *Biochemistry,* 11, 1094, 1972.

127. **Marsh, W. H. and Fitzgerald, P. J.,** Pancreas acinar cell regeneration. XIII. Histone synthesis and modification, *Fed. Proc.,* 32, 2119, 1973.

128. **Marks, D. B., Kanefsky, T., Keller, B. J., and Marks, A. D.,** The presence of histone H1⁰ in human tissues, *Cancer Res.,* 35, 886, 1975.

129. **Varicchio, F.,** Postnatal increase in histone H1a in the rat pancreas, *Arch. Biochem. Biophys.,* 179, 715, 1977.

130. **Tsanev, R. and Hadjiolov, D.,** Chromosomal proteins in hepatocarcinogenesis, *Z. Krebsforsch.,* 91, 237, 1978.

131. **Bradbury, E. M. and Crane-Robinson, C.,** Physical and conformational studies of histones and nucleohistones, in *Histones and Nucleohistones,* Phillips, D. M. P., Ed., Plenum Press, New York, 1971, 85.

132. **Bradbury, E. M., Hjelm, R. P., Carpenter, B. G., Baldwin, J. P., Kneale, G. G., and Hancock, R.,** Histones and chromatin structure, in *The Molecular Biology of the Mammalian Genetic Apparatus,* Ts'o, P. O. P., Ed., North-Holland, Amsterdam, 1977, 53.

133. **Kornberg, R. D.,** Structure of chromatin, *Annu. Rev. Biochem.,* 46, 931, 1977.

133a. **McLaughlin, P. J. and Dayhoff, M. O.,** Evolution of species and proteins: a time scale, in *Atlas of Protein Sequence and Structure,* Vol. 4, Dayhoff, M. O., Ed., National Biomedical Research Foundation, Silver Spring, Maryland, 1969, 39.

133b. **King, J. L. and Jukes, T. H.,** Non-Darwinian evolution. Most evolutionary changes in proteins may be due to neutral and genetic drift, *Science,* 164, 788, 1969.

133c. **Kimura, M. and Ohta, T.,** On the rate of molecular evolution, *J. Mol. Evol.,* 1, 1, 1971.

134. **Subirana, J. A.,** Specific aggregation products of histone fractions. (Presence of cysteine in F2a1 from echinoderms), *FEBS Lett.,* 16, 133, 1971.

135. **DeLange, R. J., Hooper, J. A., and Smith, E. L.,** Histone III. III. Sequence studies on the cyanogen bromide peptides; complete amino acid sequence of calf thymus histone III, *J. Biol. Chem.,* 248, 3261, 1973.

136. **Hooper, J. A., Smith, E. L., Sommer, K. R., and Chalkley, R.,** Histone III. IV. Amino acid sequence of histone III of the testes of the carp, *Letiolus bubalus, J. Biol. Chem.,* 248, 3275, 1973.

137. **Brandt, W. F. and Von Holt, C.,** The determination of the primary structure of histone F3 from chicken erythrocytes by automatic Edman degradation. II. Sequence analysis of histone F3, *Eur. J. Biochem.,* 46, 419, 1974.

138. **Koostra, A. and Bailey, G. S.,** The primary structure of histone H2b from brown trout (*Salmo trutta*) testes, *FEBS Lett.,* 68, 76, 1976.

138a. **Van Helden, P. D., Strickland, W. N., Brandt, W. F., and Von Holt, C.,** The complete amino-acid sequence of histone H2b from the mollusc Patella granatina, *Eur. J. Biochem.,* 93, 71, 1979.

138b. **Ohe, Y., Hayashi, H., and Iwai, K.,** Human spleen histone H2b, *J. Biochem.,* 85, 615, 1979.

139. **Sautière, P., Wouters-Tyrou, D., Laine, B., and Biserte, G.,** Structure of histone H2a (histone ALK, IIb1 or F2a2), in *The Structure and Function of Chromatin,* Ciba Foundation Symposium 28, Associated Scientific Publishers, Amsterdam, 1975, 77.

140. **Bailey, G. S. and Dixon, G. H.,** Histone IIb1 from rainbow trout. Comparison in amino acid sequence with calf thymus IIb1, *J. Biol. Chem.,* 248, 5463, 1973.

140a. **Laine, B., Kmiecik, D., Sautière, P., and Biserte, G.,** Primary structure of chicken erythrocyte histone H2A, *Biochimie,* 60, 147, 1978.

140b. **Wouters, D., Sautière, P., and Biserte, G.,** Primary structure of histone H2A from gonad of the sea urchin *Psammechinus miliaris, Eur. J. Biochem.,* 90, 231, 1978.

140c. **Spiker, S. and Isenberg, I.,** Evolutionary conservation of histone-histone binding sites: Evidence from interkingdom complex formation, *Cold Spring Harbor Symp. Quant. Biol.,* 42, 157, 1978.

140d. **Wilhelm, M. L., Langenbuch, J., Wilhelm, F. X., and Gigot, C.,** Nucleosome core particles can be reconstituted using mixtures of histones from two eukaryotic kingdoms, *FEBS Lett.,* 103, 126, 1979.

141. **Rall, S. C. and Cole, R. D.,** Amino acid sequence and sequence variability of the amino-terminal regions of lysine-rich histones, *J. Biol. Chem.,* 246, 7175, 1971.

142. **Arutyunyan, A. A., Shlyapnikov, S. V., and Severin, E. S.,** Investigation of the variability of amino acid residues in subfractions of calf thymus histone F1, *Bioorg. Chem.,* 1, 1188, 1975.

143. **Smith, E. L.,** Discussion, in *The Structure and Function of Chromatin,* Ciba Foundation Symposium 28, Associated Scientific Publishers, Amsterdam, 1975.

144. **Moss, T., Cary, P. D., Abercombie, B. D., Crane-Robinson, C., and Bradbury, E. M.,** A pH-dependent interaction between histones H2a and H2b involving secondary and tertiary folding, *Eur. J. Biochem.,* 71, 337, 1976.

145. **Crane-Robinson, C., Hayashi, H., Cary, P. D., Briand, G., Sautière, P., Krieger, D., Vidali, G., Lewis, P. N., and Tom-Kun, J.,** The location of secondary structure of histone H4, *Eur. J. Biochem.,* 79, 535, 1977.

146. **Hartman, P. G., Chapman, G. E., Moss, T., and Bradbury, E. M.,** Studies on the role and mode of operation of the very-lysine rich histone H1 in eukaryote chromatin, *Eur. J. Biochem.,* 77, 45, 1977.

147. **Pardon, J. F., Worcester, D. L., Woooley, J. C., Cotter, R. I., Lilley, D. M. J., and Richards, B. M.,** The structure of the chromatin core particle in solution, *Nucleic Acids Res.,* 4, 3199, 1977.

148. **Lilley, D. M. J., Pardon, J. F., and Richards, B. M.,** Structural investigation of chromatin core protein by nuclear magnetic resonance, *Biochemistry,* 16, 2853, 1977.

148a. **Whitlock, J. P., Jr. and Stein, A.,** Folding of DNA by histones which lack their NH_2-terminal regions, *J. Biol. Chem.,* 253, 3857, 1978.

148b. **Pospelov, V. A., Svetlikova, S. B. and Vorob'ev, V. I.,** Nucleosome interaction in chromatin, *FEBS Lett.,* 99, 123, 1979.

148c. **Ohlenbusch, H. H.,** Structural complementarity in chromatin subunits, *Naturwissenschaften,* 66, 206, 1979.

149. **Sperling, R. and Bustin, M.,** Histone dimers: fundamental unit in histone assembly, *Nucleic Acids Res.,* 3, 1263, 1976.

150. **Kelley, R. I.,** Isolation of a histone IIb1-IIb2 complex, *Biochem. Biophys. Res. Commun.,* 54, 1588, 1973.

151. **Hyde, J. E. and Walker, I. O.,** Covalent cross-linking of histones in chromatin, *FEBS Lett.,* 50, 150, 1975.

152. **Lewis, P. N.,** Histone-histone interactions. I. An electrophoretic study, *Can. J. Biochem.,* 54, 641, 1976.

153. **Weintraub, H., Palter, K., and Van Lente, F.,** Histones H2a, H2b, H3 and H4 form a tetrameric complex in solutions of high salt, *Cell,* 6, 85, 1975.

154. **Roark, D. E., Geoghegan, T. E., and Keller, G. H.,** A two-subunit histone complex from calf thymus, *Biochem. Biophys. Res. Commun.,* 59, 542, 1974.

155. **Thomas, J. O. and Kornberg, R. D.,** An octamer of histones in chromatin and free in solution, *Proc. Natl. Acad. Sci. U.S.A.,* 72, 2626, 1975.

155a. **Ruiz-Carrillo, A. and Jorcano, J. L.,** An octamer of core histones in solution: central role of the H3.H4 tetramer in the self-assembly, *Biochemistry,* 18, 760, 1979.

156. **Kato, Y. and Iwai, K.,** DNA-binding segments of four histone sequences identified in trypsin-treated H1-depleted chromatin, *J. Biochem.,* 81, 621, 1977.

157. **Oudet, P., Gross-Bellard, M., and Chambon, P.,** Electron microscopic and biochemical evidence that chromatin structure is a repeating unit, *Cell,* 4, 281, 1975.

158. **Woodcock, C. L. F.,** Reconstitution of chromatin subunits, *Science,* 195, 1350, 1977.

159. **Camerini-Otero, R. D. and Felsenfeld, G.,** Supercoiling energy and nucleosome formation: the role of the arginine-rich histone kernel, *Nucleic Acids Res.,* 4, 1159, 1977.

160. **Rubin, C. S. and Rosen, O. M.,** Protein phosphorylation, *Annu. Rev. Biochem.,* 44, 831, 1975.

161. **Sung, M. T. and Dixon, G. H.,** Modification of histones during spermiogenesis in trout: a molecular mechanism for altering histone binding to DNA, *Proc. Natl. Acad. Sci. U.S.A.,* 67, 1616, 1970.

162. **Rickwood, D., Riches, P. G., and MacGillivray, A. J.,** Studies of the in vitro phosphorylation of chromatin non-histone proteins in isolated nuclei, *Biochim. Biophys. Acta,* 299, 162, 1973.

163. **Seligy, V. L. and Neelin, J. M.,** Phosphorylation of histones in avian erythroblasts, *Can. J. Biochem.,* 51, 1316, 1973.

164. **Louie, A. J. and Dixon, G. H.,** Kinetics of phosphorylation and dephosphorylation of testis histones and their possible role in determining chromosomal structure, *Nature (London) New Biol.,* 243, 164, 1973.

165. **Louie, A. J., Sung, M. T., and Dixon, G. H.,** Modification of histones during spermatogenesis in trout. III. Levels of phosphohistone species and kinetics of phosphorylation of histone IIb1, *J. Biol. Chem.,* 248, 3335, 1973.

166. **Lake, R. S.,** Further characterization of the F1 histone phosphokinase of metaphase arrested animal cells, *J. Cell Biol.,* 58, 317, 1973.

167. **Gurley, L. R., Walters, R. A., and Tobey, R. A.,** Sequential phosphorylation of histone subfractions in Chinese hamster cell cycle, *J. Biol. Chem.,* 250, 3936, 1975.

168. **Hohmann, P., Tobey, R. A., and Gurley, L. R.,** Phosphorylation of distinct regions of F1 histone. Relationship to the cell cycle, *J. Biol. Chem.,* 251, 3685, 1976.

169. **Garrard, W. T., Kidd, G. H., and Bonner, J.,** Histone phosphorylation during regeneration, *Biochem. Biophys. Res. Commun.,* 70, 1219, 1976.

170. **Ruiz-Carrillo, A., Wangh, L. J., and Allfrey, V. G.,** Processing of newly synthesized histone molecules. Nascent histone H4 chains are reversibly phosphorylated and acetylated, *Science,* 190, 117, 1975.

171. **Langan, T. A.,** Cyclic AMP and histone phosphorylation, *Ann. N.Y. Acad. Sci.,* 185, 166, 1971.

172. **Lamy, F., Lecocq, R., and Dumont, J. E.,** Thyrotropin stimulation of the phosphorylation of serine in the N-terminal region of thyroid H1 histones, *Eur. J. Biochem.,* 73, 529, 1977.

173. **Sherod, D., Johnson, G., Balhorn, R., Jackson, V., Chalkley, R., and Granner, D.,** The phosphorylation region of lysine-rich histone in dividing cells, *Biochim. Biophys. Acta,* 381, 337, 1975.

174. **Tobin, R. S. and Seligy, V. L.,** Characterization of chromatin-bound erythrocyte histone V (F2c). Synthesis, acetylation and phosphorylation, *J. Biol. Chem.,* 250, 358, 1975.

175. **Sung, M. T., Dixon, G. H., and Smithies, O.,** Phosphorylation and synthesis of histones in regenerating rat liver, *J. Biol. Chem.,* 246, 1358, 1971.

176. **Panyim, S., Bilek, D., and Chalkley, R.,** An electrophoretic comparison of vertebrate histones, *J. Biol. Chem.,* 246, 4206, 1971.

177. **Buckingham, R. H. and Stocken, L. A.,** Histone F1. Purification and phosphorus content, *Biochem. J.,* 117, 157, 1970.

178. **Langan, T. A., Rall, S. C., and Cole, R. D.,** Variation on primary structure of a phosphorylation site in lysine-rich histones, *J. Biol. Chem.,* 246, 1942, 1971.

179. **Jergil, B., Sung, M., and Dixon, G. H.,** Species- and tissue-specific patterns of phosphorylation of very lysine-rich histones, *J. Biol. Chem.,* 245, 5867, 1970.

180. **Sherod, D., Johnson, G., and Chalkley, R.,** Phosphorylation of mouse ascites tumor cells lysine-rich histone, *Biochemistry,* 9, 4611, 1970.

181. **Gurley, L. R. and Walters, R. A.,** Evidence from triton X-100 polyacrylamide gel electrophoresis that histone F2a2, not F2b, is phosphorylated in Chinese hamster cells, *Biochem. Biophys. Res. Commun.,* 55, 697, 1973.

182. **Marks, D. B., Paik, W. K., Borun, T. W.,** The relationship of histone phosphorylation to deoxyribonucleic acid replication and mitosis during the HeLa S-3 cell cycle, *J. Biol. Chem.,* 248, 5660, 1973.

183. **Bradbury, E. M., Inglis, R. J., and Matthews, H. R.,** Molecular basis of control of mitotic cell division in eukaryotes, *Nature (London),* 249, 553, 1974.

184. **Bradbury, E. M.,** Histones in chromosomal structure and control of cell division, in *The Structure and Function of Chromatin,* Ciba Foundation Symposium, 28, Associated Scientific Publishers, Amsterdam, 1975, 131.

184a. **Gurley, L., D'Anna, J. A., Barham, S. S., Deaven, L. L., and Tobey, R. A.,** Histone phosphorylation and chromatin structure during mitosis in Chinese hamster cells, *Eur. J. Biochem.,* 84, 1, 1978.

185. **Dixon, G. H., Candido, E. P. M., Honda, B. M., Louie, A. J., Macleod, A. R., and Sung, M. T.,** The biological roles of postsynthetic modifications of basic nuclear proteins, in *The Structure and Function of Chromatin,* Ciba Foundation Symposium, 28, Associated Publishers, Amsterdam, 1975, 229.

185a. **Gurley, L. R., Walters, R. A., Barham, S. S., and Deaven, L. L.,** Heterochromatin and histone phosphorylation, *Exp. Cell Res.,* 111, 373, 1978.

186. **Lue, P. F., Gornall, A. G., and Liew, C. C.,** Two forms of histone-acetyltransferase in high salt extracts of rat liver nuclei, *Can. J. Biochem.,* 51, 1177, 1973.

187. **Candido, E. P. M.,** Partial characterization of a histone acetyltransferase from trout testis, *Can. J. Biochem.,* 53, 796, 1975.

188. **Gallwitz, D.,** Organ specificity of histone acetyltransferase, *FEBS Lett.,* 13, 306, 1971.

189. **Vidali, G., Boffa, L. C., and Allfrey, V. G.,** Properties of an acidic histone-binding protein fraction from cell nuclei, *J. Biol. Chem.,* 247, 7365, 1972.

190. **Kikuchi, H. and Fujimoto, D.,** Multiplicity of histone deacetylase from calf thymus, *FEBS Lett.,* 29, 280, 1973.

191. **Pestana, A. and Pitot, H. C.,** N-terminal acetylation of histone-like nascent peptides on rat liver polyribosomes in vitro, *Nature (London),* 247, 200, 1974.

192. **Grimes, S. R., Jr., Chae, C. B., and Irvin, J. L.**, Acetylation of histones of rat testes, *Arch. Biochem. Biophys.*, 168, 425, 1975.

193. **Krause, M. O. and Stein, G. S.**, Arginine-rich histone synthesis and acetylation in WI38-cells stimulated to proliferate, *Exp. Cell Res.*, 100, 63, 1976.

194. **Allfrey, V. G.**, Functional and metabolic aspects of DNA-associated proteins, in *Histones and Nucleohistones*, Phillips, D. M. P., Ed., Plenum Press, New York, 1971, 241.

195. **Adler, A. J. and Fasman, G. D.**, Altered conformational effects of naturally acetylated histone F2a1 (IV) in F2a1-deoxyribonucleic acid complexes, *J. Biol. Chem.*, 249, 2911, 1974.

196. **Lee, C. T. and Duerre, J. A.**, Changes in histone methylase activity of rat brain and liver with ageing, *Nature (London)*, 251, 240, 1974.

197. **Duerre, J. A. and Chakrabarty, S.**, Methylated basic amino acid composition of histones from the various organs from the rat, *J. Biol. Chem.*, 250, 8457, 1975.

198. **Thomas, G., Lange, H. W., and Hempel, K.**, Kinetics of histone methylation in vivo and its relation to the cell cycle in Ehrlich ascites tumor cells, *Eur. J. Biochem.*, 51, 609, 1975.

199. **DeLange, R. J., Fambrough, D. M., Smith, E. L., and Bonner, J.**, Calf and pea histone IV. II. The complete amino acid sequence of calf thymus histone IV, presence of ε-N-acetyllysine, *J. Biol. Chem.*, 244, 319, 1969.

200. **Ogawa, Y., Quagliarotti, G., Jordan, J., Taylor, C. W., Starbuck, W. C., and Busch, H.**, Structural analysis of the glycine-rich, arginine-rich histone. III. Sequence of the amino-terminal half of the molecule containing the modified lysine residues and the total sequence, *J. Biol. Chem.*, 244, 4387, 1969.

200a. **Hempel, K., Thomas, G., Roos, G., Stocker, W., and Lange, H.- W.**, Nᶜ-methyl groups on the lysine residues in histones turn over independently of the polypeptide backbone, *Hoppe-Seyler's Z. Physiol. Chem.*, 360, 869, 1979.

201. **Paik, W. K. and Kim, S.**, Enzymatic methylation of proteins after translation may take part in control of biological activities of proteins, *Science*, 174, 114, 1971.

202. **Tidwell, T., Allfrey, V. G., and Mirsky, A. E.**, The methylation of histones during regeneration of the liver, *J. Biol. Chem.*, 243, 707, 1968.

203. **Borun, T. W., Pearson, D., and Paik, W. K.**, Studies on histone methylation during the HeLa S-3 cell cycle, *J. Biol. Chem.*, 247, 4288, 1972.

204. **Smith, J. A. and Stocken, L. A.**, Identification of poly (ADP-ribose) covalently bound to histone F1 in vivo, *Biochem. Biophys. Res. Commun.*, 54, 297, 1973.

205. **Ueda, K., Omachi, A., Kawaichi, M., and Hayashi, O.**, Natural occurrence of poly (ADP-ribosyl) histones in rat liver, *Proc. Natl. Acad. Sci. U.S.A.*, 72, 205, 1975.

206. **Sigimura, T.**, Poly (adenosine diphosphate ribose), *Prog. Nucleic Acid Res. Mol. Biol.*, 13, 127, 1973.

207. **Ueda, K., Okayama, H., Fukushima, M., and Hayashi, O.**, Seminar on poly (ADP-ribose) and ADP-ribosylation of protein, *J. Biochem.*, 77, 1p, 1975.

208. **Lorimer, W. S., III, Stone, P. R., and Kidwell, W. R.**, Control of histone H1 dimer-poly (ADP-ribose) complex formation by poly (ADP-ribose) glycohydrolase, *Exp. Cell Res.*, 106, 261, 1977.

208a. **Byrne, R. H., Stone, P. R., and Kidwell, W. R.**, Effect of polyamines and divalent cations on histone H1-poly(adenosine diphosphate ribose) complex formation, *Exp. Cell Res.*, 115, 277, 1978.

209. **Roberts, J. H., Stark, P., Giri, C. P., and Smulson, M.**, Cytoplasmic poly (ADP-ribose) polymerase during the HeLa cell cycle, *Arch. Biochem. Biophys.*, 171, 305, 1975.

210. **Ord, M. G. and Stocken, L. A.**, Adenosine diphosphate ribosylated histones, *Biochem. J.*, 161, 583, 1977.

211. **Wong, N. C. W., Poirier, G. G., and Dixon, G. H.**, Adenosine diphosphorybosylation of certain basic chromosomal proteins in isolated trout testis nuclei, *Eur. J. Biochem.*, 77, 11, 1977.

212. **Ris, H.**, Chromosomal structure as seen by electron microscopy, in *The Structure and Function of Chromatin*, Ciba Foundation Symposium, 28, Associated Scientific Publishers, Amsterdam, 1975, 7.

213. **Pardon, J. F., Wilkins, M. H. F., and Richards, B. M.**, Molecular structure. Super-helical model for nucleohistone, *Nature (London)*, 215, 508, 1967.

214. **Hewish, D. R. and Burgoyne, L. A.**, Chromatin substructure. The digestion of chromatin DNA at regularly spaced sites by a nuclear deoxyribonuclease, *Biochem. Biophys. Res. Commun.*, 52, 504, 1973.

215. **Noll, M.**, Differences and similarities in chromatin structure of *Neurospora crassa* and higher eukaryotes, *Cell*, 8, 349, 1976.

216. **Joffe, J., Keene, M., and Weintraub, H.**, Histones H2a, H2b, H3 and H4 are present in equimolar amounts in chick erythroblasts, *Biochemistry*, 16, 1236, 1977.

217. **Kornberg, R. D.**, Chromatin structure: a repeating unit of histones and DNA, *Science*, 184, 868, 1974.

218. **Goodwin, G. H., Nicolas, R. H., and Johns, E. W.,** A quantitative analysis of histone H1 in rabbit thymus nuclei, *Biochem. J.,* 167, 485, 1977.
219. **Olins, A. L. and Olins, D. E.,** Spheroid chromatin units (ν-bodies), *Science,* 183, 330, 1974.
220. **Woodcock, C. L. F., Safer, J. P., and Stanchfield, J. E.,** Structural repeating units in chromatin, *Exp. Cell Res.,* 97, 101, 1976.
221. **Rattner, J. B., Branch, A., and Hamkalo, B. A.,** Electron microscopy of whole mount metaphase chromosomes, *Chromosoma,* 52, 329, 1975.
222. **Compton, J. L., Hancock, R., Oudet, P., and Chambon, P.,** Biochemical and electron-microscopic evidence that the subunit structure of Chinese-hamster-ovary interphase chromatin is conserved in mitotic chromosomes, *Eur. J. Biochem.,* 70, 555, 1976.
223. **Howze, G. B., Hsie, A. W., and Olins, A. L.,** ν-bodies in mitotic chromatin, *Exp. Cell Res.,* 100, 424, 1976.
223a. **Sorsa, V.,** Beaded organization of chromatin in the salivary gland chromosome bands of *Drosophila melanogaster, Hereditas,* 84, 213, 1976.
224. **Noll, M.,** Internal structure of the chromatin subunit, *Nucleic Acids Res.,* 1, 1573, 1974.
225. **Van Holde, K. E., Sahsrabuddhe, C. G., and Shaw, B. R.,** A model for particulate structure of chromatin, *Nucleic Acids Res.,* 1, 1579, 1974.
226. **Richards, B., Cotter, R., Lilley, D., Pardon, J., Wooley, J., and Worcester, D.,** The molecular structure of chromosomes, in *Current Chromosomal Research,* Jones, K. and Brandham, P. E., Eds., Elsevier, North-Holland, Amsterdam, 1976, 7.
227. **Tsanev, R. and Petrov, P.,** The substructure of chromatin and its variations as revealed by electron microscopy, *J. Microsc. Biol. Cell.,* 27, 11, 1976.
228. **Sollner-Webb, B. and Felsenfeld, G.,** A comparison of the digestion of nuclei and chromatin by staphylococcal nuclease, *Biochemistry,* 14, 2915, 1975.
229. **Shaw, B. R., Herman, T. M., Kovacic, R. T., Beaudreau, G. S., and Van Holde, K. E.,** Analysis of subunit organization in chicken erythrocyte chromatin, *Proc. Natl. Acad. Sci. U.S.A.,* 73, 505, 1976.
230. **Compton, J. L., Bellard, M., and Chambon, P.,** Biochemical evidence of variability in the DNA repeat length in the chromatin of higher eukaryotes, *Proc. Natl. Acad. Sci. U.S.A.,* 73, 4382, 1976.
231. **Varshavsky, A. J., Bakayev, V. V., and Georgiev, G. P.,** Heterogeneity of chromatin subunits in vitro and location of histone H1, *Nucleic Acids Res.,* 3, 477, 1976.
232. **Noll, M. and Kornberg, R. D.,** Action of micrococcal nuclease on chromatin and the location of histone H1, *J. Mol. Biol.,* 109, 393, 1977.
233. **Morris, N. R.,** A comparison of the structure of chicken erythrocyte and chicken liver chromatin, *Cell,* 9, 627, 1976.
234. **Lohr, D., Cordene, J., Tatchell, K., Kovacic, R. T., and Van Holde, K. E.,** Comparative subunit structure of HeLa, yeast and chicken erythrocyte chromatin, *Proc. Natl. Acad. Sci. U.S.A.,* 74, 79, 1977.
235. **Rill, R. L., Nelson, D. A., Oosterhof, D. K., and Hozier, J. C.,** Structural repeat units of Chinese hamster ovary chromatin. Evidence for variations in repeat unit DNA size in higher eukaryotes, *Nucleic Acids Res.,* 4, 771, 1977.
235a. **Ermini, M. and Kuenzle, C. C.,** The chromatin repeat length of cortical neurons shortens during early postnatal development, *FEBS Lett.,* 90, 167, 1978.
235b. **Gottesfeld, J. M. and Melton, D. A.,** The length of nucleosome-associated DNA is the same in both transcribed and nontranscribed regions of chromatin, *Nature (London),* 273, 317, 1978.
236. **Wilhelm, M. L., Mazen, A., and Wilhelm, F. X.,** Comparison of the repeat length in H1- and H5-containing chromatin, *FEBS Lett.,* 79, 404, 1977.
237. **Carpenter, B. G., Baldwin, J. P., Bradbury, E. M., and Ibel, K.,** Organization of subunits in chromatin, *Nucleic Acids Res.,* 3, 1739, 1976.
238. **Finch, J. T. and Klug, A.,** Solenoidal model for superstructure in chromatin, *Proc. Natl. Acad. Sci. U.S.A.,* 73, 1897, 1976.
239. **Bram, S., Butler-Browne, G., Baudy, P., and Ibel, K.,** Quaternary structure of chromatin, *Proc. Natl. Acad. Sci. U.S.A.,* 72, 1043, 1975.
240. **Brasch, K.,** Studies on the role of histones H1 (F1) and H5 (F2c) in chromatin structure, *Exp. Cell Res.,* 101, 396, 1976.
241. **Kiryanov, G. I., Manamshjan, T. A., Polyakov, V. Yu., Fais, D., and Chentsov, Yu. S.,** Levels of granular organization of chromatin fibres, *FEBS Lett.,* 67, 323, 1976.
242. **Renz, M., Nehls, P., and Hozier, J.,** Involvement of histone H1 in the organization of the chromosome fiber, *Proc. Natl. Acad. Sci. U.S.A.,* 74, 1879, 1977.
243. **Hozier, J., Renz, M., and Nehls, P.,** The chromosome fiber: evidence for an ordered superstructure of nucleosomes, *Chromosoma,* 62, 301, 1977.
244. **Bradbury, E. M., Carpenter, B. G., and Rattle, H. W. E.,** Magnetic resonance studies of deoxyribonucleoprotein, *Nature (London),* 241, 123, 1973.

245. Tanaka, T. and Oda, T., Configurational changes in rat liver nuclear chromatin and nucleoli caused by dissociation and reassociation of F1 histone, *Exp. Cell Res.*, 103, 143, 1976.

246. Alberts, B., Worcel, A., and Weintraub, H., On the biological implications of chromatin structure, in *The Organization and Expression of the Eukaryotic Genome*, Bradbury, E. M. and Javaherian, K., Eds., Academic Press, New York, 1977.

247. Vogel, T. and Singer, M. F., Interaction of F1 histone with superhelical DNA, *Proc. Natl. Acad. Sci. U.S.A.*, 72, 2597, 1975.

248. Olson, M. O. J., Goldknopf, I. L., Guetzow, K. A., James, G. T., Hawkins, T. C., Mays-Rotberg, C. J., and Busch, H., The NH_2-and COOH-terminal amino acid sequence of nuclear protein A24, *J. Biol. Chem.*, 251, 5901, 1976.

249. Olins, A. L., Senior, M. B., and Olins, D. E., Ultrastructural features of chromatin *v*-bodies, *J. Cell Biol.*, 68, 787, 1976.

250. Oudet, P., Spadafora, C., and Chambon, P., Nucleosome structure. II. Strucure of SV40 minichromosome and electron microscopic evidence for reversible transition of the nucleosome structure, *Cold Spring Harbor Symp. Quant. Biol.*, 42, 301, 1978.

251. Richards, B., Pardon, J., Lilley, D., Cotter, R., Wooley, J., and Worcester, D., The sub-structure of nucleosomes, *Cell Biol. Int. Rep.*, 1, 107, 1977.

252. Altenburger, W., Hörz, W., and Zachau, H. G., Nuclease cleavage of chromatin at 100-nucleotide pair intervals, *Nature (London)*, 264, 517, 1976.

253. Axel, R., Melhior, W., Jr., Sollner-Webb, B., and Felsenfeld, G., Specific sites of interaction between histone and DNA in chromatin, *Proc. Natl. Acad. Sci. U.S.A.*, 71, 4101, 1974.

254. Yaneva, M., Tasheva, B., and Dessev, G., Nuclease digestion of reconstituted chromatin, *FEBS Lett.*, 70, 67, 1976.

254a. Worcel, A., Han, S., and Wong, M. L., Assembly of newly replicated chromatin, *Cell*, 15, 969, 1978.

254b. Ruiz-Carrillo, A. and Jorcano, J. L., Nucleohistone assembly: sequential binding of histone H3-H4 tetramer and histone H2a-H2b dimer to DNA, *Cold Spring Harbor Symp. Quant. Biol.*, 42, 165, 1978.

254c. Wilhelm, F. X., Wilhelm, M. L., Erard, M., and Daune, M. P., Reconstitution of chromatin: Assembly of the nucleosome, *Nucl. Acids Res.*, 5, 505, 1978.

255. Sollner-Webb, B., Camerini-Otero, R. D., and Felsenfeld, G., Chromatin structure as probed by nucleases and proteases: evidence for central role of histones H3 and H4, *Cell*, 9, 179, 1976.

256. Oudet, P., Germond, J. E., Sures, M., Gallwitz, D., Bellard, M., and Chambon, P., Nucleosome structure. I. All four histones H2a, H2b, H3 and H4 are required to form a nucleosome, but H3-H4 nucleosomal particle is formed with H3-H4 alone, *Cold Spring Harbor Symp. Quant. Biol.*, 42, 287, 1978.

257. Moss, T., Stephens, R. M., Crane-Robinson, C., and Bradbury, E. M., A nucleosome-like structure containing DNA and the arginine-rich histones H3 and H4, *Nucleic Acids Res.*, 4, 2477, 1977.

257a. Bina-Stein, M., Folding of 140-base pair length DNA by a core of arginine-rich histones, *J. Biol. Chem.*, 253, 5213, 1978.

258. Kornberg, R. D. and Thomas, J. O., Chromatin structure: oligomers of the histones, *Science*, 184, 865, 1974.

258a. Mirzabekov, A. D., Shick, V. V., Belyavsky, A. V., and Bavykin, S. G., Primary organization of nucleosome core particle of chromatin: sequence of histone arrangement along DNA, *Proc. Natl. Acad. Sci. U.S.A.*, 75, 4184, 1978.

258b. Mirzabekov, A. D., Shick, V. V., Belyavsky, A. V., Karpov, V. L., and Bavykin, S. G., The structure of nucleosomes: the arrangement of histones in the DNA grooves and along the DNA chain, *Cold Spring Harbor Symp. Quant. Biol.*, 42, 149, 1978.

259. Mirzabekov, A. D., San'ko, D. F., Kolchinsky, A. M., and Melnikova, A. F., Protein arrangement in the DNA grooves in chromatin and nucleoprotamine in vitro and in vivo revealed by methylation, *Eur. J. Biochem.*, 75, 379, 1977.

260. Zimmerman, S. B. and Levin, C. J., Do histones bind to a specific group of DNA sequences in chromatin? A test based on DNA ligase action on reconstituted chromatin, *Biochem. Biophys. Res. Commun.*, 62, 357, 1975.

261. Steinmetz, M., Streeck, R. E., and Zachau, H. G., Nucleosome formation abolishes base-specific binding of histones, *Nature (London)*, 258, 447, 1975.

262. Polisky, B. and McCarthy, B. J., Location of histones on simian virus 40 DNA, *Proc. Natl. Acad. Sci. U.S.A.*, 72, 2895, 1975.

263. Cremisi, C., Pignatti, P. F., and Yaniv, M., Random location and absence of movement of the nucleosomes on SV40 nucleoprotein complex isolated from infected cells, *Biochem. Biophys. Res. Commun.*, 73, 548, 1976.

263a. Chao, M. V., Gralla, J., and Martinson, H. G., DNA sequence directs placement of histone cores on restriction fragments during nucleosome formation, *Biochemistry*, 18, 1068, 1979.

263b. **Wasylyk, B., Oudet, P., and Chambon, P.,** Preferential in vitro assembly of nucleosome cores on some AT-rich regions of SV40 DNA, *Nucl. Acids Res.,* 7, 705, 1979.

264. **Woodcock, C. L. F. and Frado, L-L. Y.,** Ultrastructure of chromatin subunits during unfolding, histone depletion and reconstitution, *Cold Spring Harbor Symp. Quant. Biol.,* 42, 43, 1978.

265. **Simpson, R. T. and Bustin, M.,** Histone composition of chromatin subunits studied by immunosedimentation, *Biochemistry,* 15, 4305, 1976.

266. **Simpson, R. T.,** Histones H3 and H4 interact with ends of nucleosome DNA, *Proc. Natl. Acad. Sci. U.S.A.,* 73, 4400, 1976.

267. **Mirzabekov, A. D., Shik, V. V., Belyavsky, A. V.,** Preliminary sequence of histone arrangement on DNA in nucleosome. A new method of protein molecule localization on DNA, *Dokl. Akad. Nauk SSSR,* 235, 710, 1977.

268. **Martinson, H. G. and McCarthy, B. J.,** Histone-histone interactions within chromatin. Preliminary characterization on presumptive H2b-H2a and H2b-H4 binding sites, *Biochemistry,* 15, 4126, 1976.

269. **Weintraub, H.,** Release of discrete subunits after nuclease and trypsin digestion of chromatin, *Proc. Natl. Acad. Sci. U.S.A.,* 72, 1212, 1975.

270. **Camerini-Otero, R. D., Sollner-Webb, B., and Felsenfeld, G.,** The organization of histones and DNA in chromatin: evidence for an arginine-rich histone kernel, *Cell,* 8, 333, 1976.

271. **Axel, R.,** Cleavage of DNA in nuclei and chromatin with staphylococcal nuclease, *Biochemistry,* 14, 2921, 1975.

272. **Lacy, E. and Axel, R.,** Analysis of DNA of isolated chromatin subunits, *Proc. Natl. Acad. Sci. U.S.A.,* 72, 3978, 1975.

273. **Hardison, R. C., Eichner, M. E., and Chalkley, R.,** An approach to histone nearest neighbours in extended chromatin, *Nucleic Acids Res.,* 2, 1751, 1975.

274. **Lieu, C. C. and Chan, P. K.,** Identification of nonhistone chromosomal proteins in chromatin subunits, *Proc. Natl. Acad. Sci. U.S.A.,* 73, 3458, 1976.

275. **Paul, J. and Malcolm, S.,** A class of chromatin particles associated with nonhistone proteins, *Biochemistry,* 15, 3510, 1976.

276. **Goodwin, G. H., Woodhead, L., and Johns, E. W.,** The presence of high mobility group nonhistone chromatin proteins in isolated nucleosomes, *FEBS Lett.,* 73, 85, 1977.

277. **Bustin, M.,** Chromatin structure and specificity revealed by immunological techniques, *FEBS Lett.,* 70, 1, 1976.

278. **Bustin, M., Goldblatt, D., and Sperling, R.,** Chromatin structure visualization by immuno-electron microscopy, *Cell,* 7, 297, 1976.

278a. **Levy-Wilson, B. and Dixon, G. H.,** Limited action of micrococcal nuclease on trout testis nuclei generates two mononucleosome subset enriched in transcribed DNA sequences, *Proc. Natl. Acad. Sci. U.S.A.,* 76, 1682, 1979.

278b. **Levy-Wilson, B., Connor, W., and Dixon, G. H.,** A subset of trout testis nucleosomes enriched in transcribed DNA sequences contains high mobility group proteins as major structural components, *J. Biol. Chem.,* 254, 609, 1979.

278c. **Mathew, C. G. P., Goodwin, G. H., and Johns, E. W.,** Studies on the association of the high mobility group non-histone chromatin proteins with isolated nucleosomes, *Nucl. Acids Res.,* 6, 167, 1979.

278d. **Defer, N., Crepin, M., Terrioux, C., Kruh, J., and Gros, F.,** Comparison of non histone proteins selectively associated with nucleosomes with proteins released during limited DNase digestions, *Nucl. Acids Res.,* 6, 953, 1979.

278e. **Walker, J. M., Goodwin, G. H., and Johns, E. W.,** The primary structure of the nucleosome-associated chromosmal protein HMG 14, *FEBS Lett.,* 100, 394, 1979.

278f. **Weisbrod, S., and Weintraub, H.,** Isolation of a subclass of nuclear proteins responsible for conferring a DNase I-sensitive structure on globin chromatin, *Proc. Natl. Acad. Sci. U.S.A.,* 76, 630, 1979.

278g. **Goldblatt, D., Bustin, M., and Sperling, R.,** Heterogeneity in the interaction of chromatin subunits with anti-histone sera visualized by immuno-electron microscopy, *Exp. Cell Res.,* 112, 1, 1978.

278h. **Russev, G., Vassilev, L., and Tsanev, R.,** Salt-induced structural changes in nucleosomes, *Molec. Biol. Rep.,* 6, 45, 1980.

279. **Sanders, M. M. and Hsu, J. T.,** Fractional of purified nucleosomes on the basis of aggregation properties, *Biochemistry,* 16, 1690, 1977.

280. **Gallwitz, D. and Mueller, G. C.,** Histone synthesis in vitro on HeLa cell microsomes, *J. Biol. Chem.,* 244, 5947, 1969.

281. **Moav, B. and Nemer, M.,** Histone synthesis. Assignment to a special class of polyribosomes in sea urchin embryos, *Biochemistry,* 10, 881, 1971.

282. **Robbins, E. and Borun, T. W.,** The cytoplasmic synthesis of histones inHeLa cells and its temporal relationship to DNA replication, *Proc. Natl. Acad. Sci. U.S.A.,* 57, 409, 1967.

283. **Stein, G. S., Park, W. D., Thrall, C. L., Mans, R. J., and Stein, J. L.,** Cell cycle stage-specific transcription of histone genes, *Biochem. Biophys. Res. Commun.,* 63, 945, 1975.

284. **Butler, W. B. and Mueller, G. C.,** Control of histone synthesis in HeLa cells, *Biochim. Biophys. Acta,* 294, 481, 1973.

285. **Dick, C. and Johns, E. W.,** The biosynthesis of the five main histone fractions of rat thymus, *Biochim. Biophys. Acta,* 174, 380, 1969.

286. **Byvoet, P.,** Metabolic integrity of deoxyribonucleohistones, *J. Mol. Biol.,* 17, 311, 1966.

287. **Piha, R. S., Cuénod, M., and Waelsch, H.,** Metabolism of histones of brain and liver, *J. Biol. Chem.,* 241, 2397, 1966.

288. **Hancock, R.,** Conservation of histones in chromatin during growth and mitosis in vitro, *J. Mol. Biol.,* 40, 457, 1969.

289. **Appels, R. and Ringertz, N. R.,** Metabolism of F1 histone in G_1 and G_0 cells, *Cell Differ.,* 3, 1, 1974.

290. **Ohba, Y., Hayashi, K., Nakagawa, Y., and Yamaguchi, Z.,** Metabolic activities of histones in rat liver and spleen, *Eur. J. Biochem.,* 56, 343, 1975.

291. **Appels, R. and Wells, J. R. E.,** Synthesis and turnover of DNA-bound histone during maturation of avian red blood cells, *J. Mol. Biol.,* 70, 425, 1972.

292. **Sung, M. T., Harford, J., Bundman, M., and Vidalakas, G.,** Metabolism of histones in avian erythroid cells, *Biochemistry,* 16, 279, 1977.

293. **Woodland, H. R. and Adamson, E. D.,** The synthesis and storage of histones during the oogenesis of *Xenopus laevis, Dev. Biol.,* 57, 118, 1977.

294. **Adamson, E. D. and Woodland, H. R.,** Changes in the rate of histone synthesis during oocyte maturation and very early development of *Xenopus laevis, Dev. Biol.,* 57, 136, 1977.

294a. **Lifton, R. P., Goldberg, M. L., Karp, R. W., and Hogness, D. S.,** The organization of the histone genes in Drosophila melanogaster: functional and evolutionary implications, *Cold Spring Harbor Symp. Quant. Biol.,* 42, 1047, 1978.

294b. **Hackett, P. B., Traub, P., and Gallwitz, D.,** The histone genes in HeLa cells are on individual transcriptional units, *J. Mol. Biol.,* 126, 619, 1978.

295. **Ruderman, J. V. and Gross, P. R.,** Histones and histone synthesis in sea urchin development, *Dev. Biol.,* 36, 286, 1974.

295a. **Hildebrand, C. E. and Walters, R. A.,** Rapid assembly of newly synthesized DNA into chromatin subunits prior to joining of small DNA replication intermediates, *Biochem. Biophys. Res. Commun.,* 73, 157, 1976.

295b. **McKnight, S. and Miller, O. L.,** Electron microscopic analysis of chromatin replication in the cellular blastoderm *Drosophila melanogaster* embryo, *Cell,* 12, 795, 1977.

296. **Tsanev, R. and Russev, G.,** Distribution of newly synthesized histones during DNA replication, *Eur. J. Biochem.,* 43, 257, 1974.

297. **Jackson, V., Granner, D. K., and Chalkley, R.,** Deposition of histones onto replicating chromosomes, *Proc. Natl. Acad. Sci. U.S.A.,* 72, 4440, 1975.

298. **Freedlender, E., Taichman, L., and Smithies, O.,** Nonrandom distribution of chromosomal proteins during cell replication, *Biochemistry,* 16, 1802, 1977.

298a. **Russev, G. and Tsanev, R.,** Nonrandom segregation of histones during chromatin replication, *Eur. J. Biochem.,* 93, 123, 1979.

299. **Leffak, I. M., Grainer, R., and Weintraub, H.,** Conservative assembly and segregation of nucleosomal histones, *Cell,* 12, 837, 1977.

300. **Jackson, V., Granner, D., and Chalkley, R.,** Deposition of histone onto replication chromosomes: newly synthesized histone is not found near replicating fork, *Proc. Natl. Acad. Sci. U.S.A.,* 73, 2266, 1976.

301. **Seale, R. L.,** Temporal relationship of chromatin protein synthesis, DNA synthesis, and assembly of deoxyribonucleoprotein, *Proc. Natl. Acad. Sci. U.S.A.,* 73, 2270, 1976.

302. **Hancock, R.,** Assembly of new nucleosomal histones and new DNA into chromatin, *Proc. Natl. Acad. Sci. U.S.A.,* 75, 2130, 1978.

303. **Kuo, M. T., Sahasrabuddhe, C. G., and Saunders, G. F.,** Presence of messenger specifying sequences in DNA of chromatin subunits, *Proc. Natl. Acad. Sci. U.S.A.,* 73, 1572, 1976.

304. **Axel, R. and Garel, A.,** Structure of the ovalbumin gene in chromatin, *Ann. N.Y. Acad. Sci.,* 286, 135, 1977.

305. **Mathis, D. J. and Gorovsky, M. A.,** Subunit structure of rDNA-containing chromatin, *Biochemistry,* 15, 750, 1976.

306. **Reeves, R.,** Ribosomal genes of *Xenopus laevis:* evidence of nucleosomes in transcriptionally active chromatin, *Science,* 194, 529, 1976.

307. **Reeves, R. and Jones, A.,** Genomic transcriptional activity and the structure of chromatin, *Nature (London),* 260, 495, 1976.

308. **Bellard, M., Gannon, F., and Chambon, P.,** Nucleosome structure. III. The structure and transcriptional activity of the chromatin containing the ovalbumin and globin genes in chick oviduct nuclei, *Cold Spring Harbor Symp. Quant. Biol.,* 42, 779, 1978.

308a. **Camerini-Otero, R. D., Sollner-Webb, B., Simon, R. H., Williamson, P., Zasloff, M., and Felsenfeld, G.,** Nucleosome structure, DNA folding and gene activity, *Cold Spring Harbor Symp. Quant. Biol.,* 42, 57, 1978.

308b. **Shaw, Ph. A., Sahasrabuddhe, Ch. G., Hodo, H. G., III, and Saunders, G. F.,** Transcription of nucleosomes from human chromatin, *Nucleic Acids Res.,* 5, 2999, 1978.

308c. **Meneguzzi, G., Chenciner, N., and Milanesi, G.,** Transcription of nucleosomal DNA in SV40 minichromosomes by eukaryotic and prokaryotic RNA polymerases, *Nucleic Acids Res.,* 6, 2947, 1979.

308d. **Gariglio, P., Llopis, R., Oudet, P., and Chambon, P.,** The template of the isolated native simian virus 40 transcriptional complexes is a minichromosome, *J. Mol. Biol.,* 131, 75, 1979.

309. **Weintraub, H. and Groudine, M.,** Chromosomal subunits in active genes have an altered conformation. Globin genes are digested by deoxyribonuclease I in red blood cell nuclei but not in fibroblast nuclei, *Science,* 193, 848, 1976.

310. **Woodcock, C. L. F., Frado, L.- L. Y., Hatch, C. L., and Ricciardiello, L.,** Fine structure of active ribosomal genes, *Chromosoma,* 58, 33, 1976.

311. **Franke, W. W., Sheer, W., Frendelenburg, M. F., Spring, H., and Zentgraf, H.,** Absence of nucleosomes in transcriptionally active chromatin, *Cytobiology,* 13, 401, 1976.

312. **Reeves, R.,** Analysis and reconstitution of *Xenopus* ribosomal chromatin nucleosomes, *Eur. J. Biochem.,* 75, 545, 1977.

313. **Laird, C. D., Wilkinson, L. E., Foe, V. E., and Chooi, W. Y.,** Analysis of chromatin-associated fiber arrays, *Chromosoma,* 58, 169, 1976.

314. **McKnight, S. L., Bustin, M., and Miller, O. L., Jr.,** Electron microscopic analysis of chromosome metabolism in the *Drosophila melanogaster* embryo, *Cold Spring Harbor Symp. Quant. Biol.,* 42, 741, 1978.

315. **Puvion-Dutilleul, F., Bernadac, A., Puvion, E., and Bernhard, W.,** Visualization of two different types of nuclear transcriptional complexes in rat liver cells, *J. Ultrastruct. Res.,* 58, 108, 1977.

315a. **Franke, W. W. and Scheer, U.,** Morphology of transcriptional units at different states of activity, *Philos. Trans. R. Soc. London Ser. B,* 283, 333, 1978.

315b. **Tsanev R.,** The substructure of nucleosomes, in *The Cell Nucleus,* Vol. 4, Busch, H., Ed., Academic Press, New York, 1978, 107.

315c. **Oudet, P., Germond, J. E., Bellard, M., Spadafora, C., and Chambon, P.,** Nucleosome structure, *Philos. Trans. R. Soc. London Ser. B,* 283, 241, 1978.

316. **Langan, T. A.,** Histone phosphorylation: stimulation by adenosine 3′,5′-monophosphate, *Science,* 162, 579, 1968.

316a. **Prentice, D. A., Taylor, S. E., Newmark, M. Z., and Kitos, P. A.,** The effect of dexamethasone on histone phosphorylation in L cells, *Biochem. Biophys. Res. Commun.,* 85, 541, 1978.

317. **Berlowitz, L. and Pallotta, D.,** Acetylation of nuclear protein in the heterochromatin and euchromatin of mealy bugs, *Exp. Cell Res.,* 71, 45, 1972.

318. **Lipps, H. J.,** Histone acetylation in the nuclei of the hypotrichous ciliate *Stylonychia mytilus, Cell Differ.,* 4, 123, 1975.

319. **Ruiz-Carrillo, A., Wangh, L. J., and Allfrey, V. G.,** Selective synthesis and modification of nuclear proteins during maturation of avian erythroid cells, *Arch. Biochem. Biophys.,* 174, 273, 1976.

320. **Wangh, L., Ruiz-Carrillo, A., and Allfrey, V. G.,** Separation and analysis of histone subfractions differing in their degree of acetylation: some correlation with genetic activity in development, *Arch. Biochem. Biophys.,* 150, 44, 1972.

321. **Sanders, L. A., Schechter, N. M., and McCarty, K. S.,** A comparative study of histone acetylation, histone deacetylation, and ribonucleic acid synthesis in avian reticulocytes and erythrocytes, *Biochemistry,* 12, 783, 1973.

322. **Burdick, C. J. and Taylor, B. A.,** Histone acetylation during early stages of sea urchin (*Arbacia punctulate*) development, *Exp. Cell Res.,* 100, 428, 1976.

323. **Edwards, G. S. and Allfrey, V. G.,** Aflatoxin B1 and actinomycin D effects on histone acetylation and deacetylation in the liver, *Biochim. Biophys. Acta,* 299, 354, 1973.

324. **D'Anna, J. A., Tobey, R. A., Barham, S. S., and Gurley, L. R.,** A reduction in the degree of H4 acetylation during mitosis in Chinese hamster cells, *Biochem. Biophys. Res. Commun.,* 77, 187, 1977.

325. **Lewy-Wilson, B., Gjerset, R. A., and McCarthy, B. J.,** Acetylation and phosphorylation of *Drosophila* histones. Distribution of acetate and phosphate groups in fractionated chromatin, *Biochim. Biophys. Acta,* 475, 168, 1977.

325a. **Nelson, D. A., Perry, W. M., and Chalkley, R.,** Sensitivity of regions of chromatin containing hyperacetylated histones to DNAse I, *Biochem. Biophys. Res. Commun.,* 82, 356, 1978.

325b. **Vidali, G., Boffa, L. C., Bradbury, E. M., and Allfrey, V. G.,** Butyrate suppression of histone deacetylation leads to accumulation of multiacetylated forms of H3 and H4 and increased DNAse I sensitivity of the associated DNA sequences, *Proc. Natl. Acad. Sci. U.S.A.,* 75, 2239, 1978.

325c. **Simpson, R. T.,** Structure of chromatin containing extensively acetylated H3 and H4, *Cell,* 13, 691, 1978.

325d. **Davie, J. R. and Candido, E. P. M.,** Acetylated histone H4 is preferentially associated with template-active chromatin, *Proc. Natl. Acad. Sci. U.S.A.,* 75, 3574, 1978.

325e. **Shewmaker, C. K., Cohen, B. N., and Wagner, T. E.,** Chemically induced gene activation: Selective increase in DNase I susceptibility in chromatin acetylated with acetyl adenylate, *Biochem. Biophys. Res. Commun.,* 84, 342, 1978.

325f. **Davie, J. R. and Candido, E. P. M.,** Acetylated histone H4 is preferentially associated with template-active chromatin, *Proc. Natl. Acad. Sci. U.S.A.,* 75, 3574, 1978.

325g. **Levy-Wilson, B., Watson, D. C., and Dixon, G. H.,** Multiacetylated forms of H4 are found in a putative transcriptionally component chromatin fraction from trout testis, *Nucl. Acids Res.,* 6, 259, 1979.

325h. **Tata, J. R. and Baker, B.,** Enzymatic fractionation of nuclei: Polynucleosomes and RNA polymerase II as endogenous transcriptional complexes, *J. Mol. Biol.,* 118, 249, 1978.

326. **Marushige, K.,** Activation of chromatin by acetylation of histone side chains, *Proc. Natl. Acad. Sci. U.S.A.,* 73, 3937, 1976.

327. **Wallace, R. B., Sargent, T. D., Murphy, R. F., and Bonner, J.,** Physical properties of chemically acetylated rat liver chromatin, *Proc. Natl. Acad. Sci. U.S.A.,* 74, 3244, 1977.

327a. **Oberhauser, H., Csordas, A., Puschendorf, B., and Grunicke, H.,** Increase in initiation sites for chromatin = directed RNA synthesis by acetylation of chromosomal proteins, *Biochem. Biophys. Res. Commun.,* 84, 110, 1978.

327b. **Moore, M., Jackson, V., Sealy, L., and Chalkley, R.,** Comparative studies on highly metabolically active histone acetylation, *Biochim. Biophys. Acta,* 561, 248, 1979.

328. **Ellgaard, E. G.,** Gene activation without histone acetylation in *Drosophila melanogaster, Science,* 157, 1070, 1967.

329. **Clever, U. and Ellgaard, E. G.,** Puffing and histone acetylation in polytene chromosomes, *Science,* 169, 373, 1970.

330. **Ono, T., Terayama, H., Takaku, F., and Nakao, K.,** Hydrocortisone effect upon the phytohemagglutinin-stimulated acetylation of histones in human lymphocytes, *Biochim. Biophys. Acta,* 179, 214, 1969.

331. **Gallwitz, D. and Sekeris, C. E.,** Stimulation of RNA polymerase activity of rat liver nuclei by cortisol in vitro independent of effects on the acetylation and methylation of histones, *FEBS Lett.,* 3, 99, 1969.

332. **Tischenko, L. I., Mülberg, A. A., and Ashmarin,ome I. P.,** Investigation of interrelations between histone acetylation and RNA synthesis in isolated nuclei, *Biokhimiya,* 36, 595, 1971.

333. **Djondjurov, L., Markov, G., and Tsanev, R.,** Distribution of tryptophan-containing proteins and of newly synthesized RNA in metaphase chromosomes, *Exp. Cell Res.,* 75, 442, 1972.

334. **Weintraub, H., Worcel, A., and Alberts, B.,** A model for chromatin based upon two symmetrically paired half-nucleosomes, *Cell,* 9, 409, 1976.

335. **Wilson, G. N., Steggles, A. W., and Nienhuis, A. W.,** Strand-selective transcription of globin genes in rabbit erythroid cells and chromatin, *Proc. Natl. Acad. Sci. U.S.A.,* 72, 4835, 1975.

336. **Lewin, S.,** Ionic linkages in protein interactions, *J. Theor. Biol.,* 23, 279, 1969.

337. **Gilmour, R. S., Windass, J. D., Affara, N., and Paul, J.,** Control of transcription of the globin gene, *J. Cell. Physiol.,* 85, 449, 1975.

338. **Villeponteaux, B., Lasky, L., and Harary, I.,** Lysine-rich histones and the selective digestion of the globin gene in avian red blood cells, *Biochemistry,* 17, 5532, 1978.

339. **Absolom, D. and Van Regelmortel, M. H. V.,** Nucleosome structure studied with purified antibodies of histones H2b, H3 and H4, *FEBS Lett.,* 85, 61, 1978.

339a. **Gorka, C. and Lawrence, J. J.,** The distribution of histone H1 subfractions in chromatin subunits, *Nucl. Acids Res.,* 7, 347, 1979.

339b. **Welch, S. L. and Cole, R. D.,** Differences between subfractions of H1 histone in their interactions, *J. Biol. Chem.,* 254, 662, 1979.

339c. **Kawashima, S. and Ando, T.,** Deoxyribonucleoproteins of herring sperm nuclei, *J. Biochem.,* 83, 1117, 1978.

339d. **Avramova, Z., Dessev, G., and Tsanev, R.,** Chromosomal proteins of mature ram spermatozoids (to be published).

340. **Chiu, J.-F., Tsai, Y.-H., Sakuma, K., and Hnilica, L. S.,** Regulation of in vitro mRNA transcription by a fraction of chromosomal proteins, *J. Biol. Chem.,* 250, 9431, 1975.

341. **Stein, G. S., Mans, R. J., Gabbay, E. J., Stein, J. L., Davis, J., and Adawadkar, P.D.,** Evidence for fidelity of chromatin reconstitution, *Biochemistry*, 14, 1859, 1975.

342. **Zasloff, M. and Felsenfeld, G.,** Use of mercury-substituted ribonucleoside triphosphates can lead to artefacts in the analysis of in vitro chromatin transcripts, *Biochem. Biophys. Res. Commun.*, 75, 598, 1977.

343. **Giesecke, K., Sippel, A. E., Nguyen-Huu, M. C., Groner, B., Hynes, N. E., Wurtz, T., and Schütz, G.,** A RNA-dependent RNA polymerase activity: implications for chromatin transcription experiments, *Nucleic Acids Res.*, 4, 3943, 1977.

344. **Bekhor, I., Kung, G. M., and Bonner, J.,** Sequence-specific interaction of DNA and chromosomal proteins, *J. Mol. Biol.*, 39, 351, 1969.

345. **Huang, R. C. C. and Huang, P. C.,** Effect of protein-bound RNA associated with chick embryo chromatin on template specificity of the chromatin, *J. Mol. Biol.*, 39, 365, 1969.

Chapter 3

ROLE OF NONHISTONE CHROMOSOMAL PROTEINS IN SELECTIVE GENE EXPRESSION

I. R. Phillips, E. A. Shephard, J. L. Stein, and G. S. Stein

TABLE OF CONTENTS

I. INTRODUCTION

It is becoming increasingly apparent that chromosomal proteins — histones and nonhistone chromosomal proteins — play an important role in dictating structural and functional properties of the eukaryotic genome. The histones, or basic chromosomal proteins, have been shown to function as repressors of DNA-dependent RNA synthesis as well as to be involved in packaging of the genome. Components of the nonhistone chromosomal proteins may also be involved in the maintenance of genome structure, but additionally several lines of evidence suggest that amongst this complex and heterogeneous class of chromosomal proteins are macromolecules which are responsible for rendering defined genetic sequences transcribable.

In this chapter we will attempt to characterize the nonhistone chromosomal proteins, particularly with respect to their structural and functional properties. Understanding the manner in which these proteins interact with the information encoded in the nucleotide sequences of the DNA double helix and with other genome-associated macromolecules undoubtedly will enhance our comprehension of a broad spectrum of normal biological processes, such as growth, development, differentiation, and maintenance of cellular phenotype. Furthermore, it is reasonable to anticipate that elucidation of the mechanisms by which gene readout is controlled will facilitate deciphering the basis for the aberrations in gene expression which accompny disease processes such as neoplasia.

There are several levels at which gene expression in eukaryotic cells may be controlled. Within the nucleus, regulation may reside at the level of the genome. Such transcriptional control may involve the interactions of chromosomal proteins with DNA sequences and/or the specificity of RNA polymerases which are responsible for the transcription of genetic information. Processing of RNA transcripts also occurs within the nucleus and is a potential level of regulation. Within the cytoplasm, regulation of gene expression may involve further processing of RNA transcripts or any of the complex steps required for protein synthesis. Additionally, posttranslational modifications of proteins, either in the nucleus or in the cytoplasm, may influence gene expression. In any specific biological situation, control of gene expression may reside at any one level or at several levels. Furthermore, the level of control of a given genetic sequence may vary depending upon the biological circumstances. In the present article we will focus attention on transcriptional control and on genome-associated macromolecules potentially involved with control of gene readout, since it appears that regulation of gene expression, at least in part, resides at this level.

A viable model for transcriptional control of gene expression in eukaryotic cells must effectively deal with three fundamental phenomena. First is the quantitative as well as qualitative similarity of DNA in all diploid nuclei of an organism. Thus, every somatic cell presumably possesses a complete and identical set of genetic information. Second is the restricted availability of genetic information for transcription. In differentiated eukaryotic cells, only 2 to 20% of the genome is transcribable at any time, and the specific genetic sequences expressed are different in each cell type, reflecting the metabolic requirements of the cell. That is not to say that all cells express a totally distinct set of genes unexpressed in other cell types. Rather, in addition to expression of genes which are shared in common by many cells, e.g., genes which code for "general housekeeping enzymes", restricted expression of certain genes which often define unique cellular phenotype occurs on a cell- or tissue-specific basis. For example, globin genes are expressed only in erythroid cells, and the expression of ovalbumin genes is observed only in the oviduct. Third is the ability of cells to modulate gene expression in response to specific demands. Such modifications in gene readout occur during development and differentiation, during the cell cycle, in response to hormones, and in general provide a cell with the flexibility required to deal with changes in the intracellular and extracellular environment.

The question which, therefore, arises is how specific regions of the genome are rendered transcribable — or how genes are "turned on" and "turned off". In microbial systems, significant inroads have been made toward understanding the mechanism by which genes are regulated. Specific repressor proteins have been isolated which interact with defined genetic sequences and render genes nontranscribable.[1,2] Specific activators have been shown to modify the interactions of these repressors with DNA and, hence, permit transcription.[3,4] The two prokaryotic systems which have been most extensively characterized are the lac operon[5] and the bacteriophage lambda.[6] While our understanding of prokaryotic gene regulation has progressed to a sophisticated level, caution must be exercised in assuming that analogous mechanisms are operative in eukaryotic cells.

In eukaryotic cells, the problem of gene regulation has been considerably more difficult to approach for several reasons. (1) In comparison with the prokaryotic genome, the eukaryotic genome is considerably more complex. A human cell contains 10^3 times the amount of DNA present in the bacterium *Escherichia coli*. However, it is not clear if all the DNA sequences in eukaryotic cells function as genetic information. In addition to the vast increase in the amount of DNA present in eukaryotic cells, genetic sequences are represented as single copies or, in certain cases, as repeated sequences. Single-copy DNA sequences make up the majority of the genome, and most proteins are coded for by these unique sequences. A small percentage of the DNA of most eukaryotic cells consists of highly repeated sequences which are not transcribed. The function of these highly reiterated sequences is, at present, undetermined. The eukaryotic genome also contains moderately reiterated sequences which include those that code for ribosomal and transfer RNA and for the histones. It has been observed that other short, moderately reiterated sequences are interspersed with unique sequences, and these short, moderately reiterated sequences have been proposed to function as regulatory elements. (2) Availability of large numbers of mutants has facilitated implementation of genetic approaches for studying the regulation of gene expression in prokaryotic cells. However, mutants of eukaryotic cells are difficult to isolate and characterize because of the diploid nature of the genome. Progress has recently been made in genetic analysis of eukaryotic cells by use of the technique of somatic cell hybridization, and this approach offers considerable promise. (3) In contrast to the direct transcription of functional mRNAs in prokaryotes, it has recently been observed that the protein coding regions of at least two eukaryotic genes, those coding for globin and ovalbumin, contain interspersed sequences which are not represented in the functional mRNA molecules.[7,8] Unlike the prokaryotic genome which consists primarily of DNA, the eukaryotic genome is associated with large quantities of heterogeneous proteins. Although specific regulatory proteins in eukaryotic cells have to date not been identified, evidence is rapidly accumulating which suggests that chromosomal proteins play a key role in dictating the structural properties of the genome and in determining the availability of genetic sequences for transcription.

II. HISTONES: THEIR ROLE IN GENOME STRUCTURE AND FUNCTION

Five defined chromosomal proteins have historically been designated as histones. The histones are metabolically stable, positively charged chromosomal proteins enriched in arginine and lysine residues and completely lacking the amino acid tryptophan. These proteins undergo posttranslational acetylation, phosphorylation, and methylation — acetylation and phosphorylation being reversible reactions. Histones as a total class are associated with DNA in a 1:1 (w/w) ratio and are intimately involved in structural and functional properties of the genome. With respect to the involvement of histones in gene regulation, a considerable body of evidence suggests that histones restrict the capacity of the genome of differentiated cells to serve as a template for RNA synthesis. While it is evident that histones are structural as well as regulatory macromolecules, their limited heterogeneity and lack of specificity suggest that histones do not by themselves possess the ability to recognize defined gene loci.

III. GENERAL PROPERTIES OF THE NONHISTONE CHROMOSOMAL PROTEINS

A. Amino Acid Composition

As a class, the nonhistone chromosomal proteins are enriched in acidic amino acid residues. The ratio of acidic to basic amino acids in nonhistone proteins from various sources varies from 1.2 to 1.9,[11-14] and these proteins contain high levels of aspartic and glutamic acid, and sometimes of serine and glycine.[11,15-19] They also possess some sulfur-containing amino acids and, in contrast to histones, they contain tryptophan.[20] Considerable variation in amino acid composition has been found between isolated nonhistone chromosomal proteins from the same tissue.[14] Amino acid sequencing data from nonhistone chromosomal proteins demonstrate that the few proteins so far sequenced have irregular charge distribution[21-23] including long series of acidic amino acid residues,[21,23] some of which are 20 or 30 residues in length.[24] Such clusterings of acidic amino acid residues raises intriguing possibilities with regard to interactions of these proteins with DNA and/or other chromosomal proteins.

B. Synthesis and Turnover

Nonhistone chromosomal proteins are synthesized in the cytoplasm.[25] Unlike the histones, whose synthesis is tightly coupled with DNA replication, various classes of nonhistone chromosomal proteins are synthesized throughout the cell cycle, both in continuously dividing cells [26-30] and in quiescent cells stimulated to proliferate,[16,31-34] and their synthesis is generally unaffected by inhibition of DNA replication.[28,34] The rate of synthesis, however, has been reported to increase in the G1 (prereplicative) phase in mammalian tissue culture cells,[28,35] and, in HeLa cells, specific nonhistone chromosomal proteins are synthesized during different phases of the cell cycle.[28,29,36,37] However, this was not found to be the case in slime mold[38] or hamster fibroblasts.[39]

Early experiments showed that the rate of turnover of nonhistone chromosomal proteins as a total class was far greater than that of histones.[40-44] and that they have a spectrum of stabilities with halflives ranging from a few minutes to several cell generations.[29,45-47] In the cell cycle, the highest rate of turnover of most molecular weight classes of the nonhistone chromosomal proteins occurs during mitosis, and the lowest during S phase.[29] However, this situation is quite complex, with the relatively high molecular weight proteins turning over more rapidly than the lower molecular weight species in G2 phase, and more slowly in G1 phase.[29] Although the messenger RNAs for specific nonhistones have not been identified or isolated, metabolism studies indicate that the stabilities of these mRNAs also cover a broad range.[30] The use of selective inhibitors of protein synthesis has provided evidence for the coordinate synthesis of some nonhistones.[48]

C. Postsynthetic Modifications
1. Acetylation, Methylation, and Glycosylation

Nonhistone chromosomal proteins can undergo several types of postsynthetic modification. Radioactive labeling and composition analysis experiments have shown that they can be acetylated[49-51] and methylated.[52-54] Acetyl CoA serves as the prinicipal acetate donor and S-adenosyl methionine as the primary source of methyl groups. There is also evidence that the thiol groups of nonhistone proteins can undergo rearrangements.[55-57] These proteins can also undergo amino-terminal arginylation by arginyl-tRNA.[58]

Glycoproteins have been found in the nonhistone chromosomal proteins of sea urchin.[59] The polysaccharide moiety was hyaluronic acid and was associated with very low molecular weight proteins. However, it is not certain whether these glycoproteins are of chromatin or membrane origin as fucose labeling experiments have shown that only 0.5% of the total cell glycoprotein is in the chromatin pellet after sedimentation through two sucrose barriers.[37] Stein et al.[60] examined the problem of membrane contamination by adding labeled plasma membranes to unlabeled HeLa cells before isolating chromatin from nuclei which had been washed with nonionic detergent Triton® X-100; the nonhistone chromosomal proteins had no incorporated label. Using these isolation techniques, these workers found that HeLa nonhistone chromosomal proteins contained glycoproteins and glycosaminoglycans. However, Jackson[61] found that even after detergent treatment of erythrocyte nuclei, the nonhistone chromosomal protein fraction was still contaminated with membrane proteins. Recently, three major nonhistone chromosomal proteins have been identified as glycoproteins by virtue of their ability to bind the lectin concanavalin A.[62]

Uncertainty also surrounds the question of the presence of lipoproteins in chromatin. Phospholipids have been found to be attached to nonhistone chromosomal proteins from brain[63] and lymphocytes.[64] When brain chromatin was isolated by a salt dissociation method which excluded membrane material,[63] it was found to contain far more phospholipid than chromatin isolated from detergent-treated liver nuclei;[65] this either could be due to contamination by extrachromosomal phospholipid resulting from the high phospholipid content of brain or may genuinely reflect a higher phospholipid content in brain chromatin.[66,67] Several groups have found RNA to be loosely associated with nonhistone chromosomal protein fractions. In contrast, Huang and Huang[68] reported the existence of a species of RNA (chromosomal RNA) which is covalently bound to chromatin proteins. Similarly, Bhorjee and Pederson[69] have reported that nonhistone chromosomal proteins contain tenaciously associated nucleic acid, DNA, and RNA; the nature of the association and the biological significance of these complexes are to date unresolved. A discussion of chromosomal protein-associated nucleic acid is contained in a review article by MacGillivray and Rickwood.[70]

2. Poly ADP Ribosylation

In nuclei, the ADP-ribose moiety of nicotinamide adenine dinucleotide is polymerized into a homopolymer composed of repeating ADP-ribose units linked by ribose $(1';\rightarrow2')$ bonds.[71-73] The chain length ranges from 1 to 50 units. It has been shown that poly(ADP-ribose) is linked to chromosomal proteins;[74,75] however, it is not yet clear whether most, if not all, of the poly(ADP-ribose) is attached covalently to acceptor molecules[76,77] or if a large proportion exists in a free form.[78] Histones H1, H2A, H2B, H3, and H4 have all been reported to be ADP-ribosylated.[74,75,78-80] Several nonhistone chromosomal proteins also serve as acceptors for ADP-ribose units,[78,81-83] and one of these proteins has been identified as a Ca^{2+}, Mg^{2+}-dependent endonuclease.[82] The modification can take the form of mono-, oligo-, and poly-ADP-ribosylation, and one nonhistone protein species seems to exist in several forms with different numbers of ADP-ribose residues.[78] Poly ADP-ribosylated nonhistone proteins have recently been isolated by covalent chromatography on a dihydroxyboryl polacrylamide bead column, but the amino acid residues which are modified are not well established.[83]

The synthesis of acceptor-bound poly(ADP-ribose) is catalyzed from the ADP-ribosyl moiety of nicotinamide adenine dinucleotide (NAD) by poly(ADP-ribose) synthetase (or polymerase) which is tightly associated with chromatin. Some workers have found that the enzyme is preferentially associated with euchromatin,[84] but others have not found this to be the case.[85] The polymerization reaction exhibits an absolute requirement for DNA, and the presence of histones increases the average chain length but has no effect on chain number.[86] The polymer is degraded by the chromatin-associated enzyme poly(ADP-ribose) glycohydrolase which cleaves the $1'\rightarrow2'$-glycosidic bond between adjacent riboses to yield ADP-ribose.[87]

The functions of poly ADP-ribosylation of nuclear proteins are not clear, but there are indications that it may be involved in DNA replication and alterations of chromatin structure. In isolated nuclei, poly(ADP-ribose) formation is associated with a decrease in DNA synthesis. This effect has been found in nuclei from rat liver,[88,89] *Physarum polycephalum*,[90] regenerating rat liver,[91] Ehrlich carcinoma and HeLa cells[89] and may be mediated by the ADP-ribosylation of a Ca^{2+}, Mg^{2+}-dependent endonuclease that is inhibited upon modification.[82] This inhibition may result in a reduction of the primer sites available to DNA polymerases. However, another group of workers has found that poly ADP-ribosylation leads to an increase in the number of DNA polymerase primer sites.[92,93] Poly(ADP-ribose) synthetase activities, as well as concentrations of poly(ADP-ribose) and poly ADP-ribosylated proteins, have been shown to be higher in the nuclei of dividing cells compared with those of resting cells,[94-97] and the synthetase activity varies during the cell cycle in a way that suggests that this enzyme may be involved in the regulation of DNA replication.[98,99] In addition to a postulated role in DNA replication, poly(ADP-ribose) has been suggested to be involved in changes in chromatin struture; for example, as a bridge between two histone H1 molecules it may be involved in chromatin condensation.[100]

The α-polypeptides of *Escherichia coli* RNA polymerases are modified by an enzyme from T4 bacteriophage.[101,102] A mono-ADP-ribose unit is linked to a specific arginine residue, and this may alter the specificity of the enzyme. Although this phenomenon has not yet been found in eukaryotes, it suggests the possibility that ADP-ribosylation is involved in the control of RNA synthesis.

Even though the functions of ADP-ribosylation are not clear, it is evident that this form of modification can result in a large number of negatively charged groups being placed on a single amino acid residue, and this would presumably have far-reaching effects on chromatin structure and function.

3. Phosphorylation of Nonhistone Chromosomal Proteins

The most widespread and best studied postsynthetic modification of nonhistone chromosomal proteins is their phosphorylation. Early studies showed that nuclear proteins rapidly incorporated radioactive phosphate in vivo.[103,104] A phosphoprotein fraction was isolated from nonhistone chromosomal proteins and was found to contain about 1.0 to 1.3% phosphorus by weight,[105-107] which is sufficient to phosphorylate 4 to 5% of the amino acid residues.

a. Phosphorylation and Dephosphorylation Reactions

The major site of alkali-labile phosphorylation is the hydroxyl group of serine residues, which accounts for about 90% of the phosphorylation, and the remaining 10% of the phosphate is attached to threonine.[106] Phosphate is linked to both these amino acids through a phosphoester bond.[106] In addition to these phosphorylation sites, small amounts of phosphoarginine, phospholysine, and phosphohistidine have also been detected;[108,109] however, the phosphate group is attached to these amino acid residues via a P-N bond, and the acid-labile nature of this linkage[109] may have led to the removal of the phosphates during many studies of nonhistone chromosomal protein phosphorylation. Consequently, current knowledge of the importance of this type of nonhistone chromosomal protein phosphorylation is limited. The phosphorylation reaction is energy-dependent but independent of protein synthesis.[106] Pulse-chase experiments show that 70 to 80% of the incorporated phosphate is lost from the proteins during a 2-hr chase while essentially no breakdown of protein occurs.[106] These findings indicate that nonhistone chromosomal proteins are continually being phosphorylated and dephosphorylated at high rates within the nucleus, and they have been confirmed by several groups using in vitro systems involving nuclei, chromosomes, or chromatin.[108,110-115]

The phosphate groups of nonhistone proteins are derived from the terminal phosphate of various nucleoside and deoxynucleoside triphosphates, with the most efficient sources being ATP and dATP.[107] Phosphate is released from the phosphoproteins as inorganic phosphate,[116] suggesting that the enzyme(s) responsible for the dephosphorylation reaction is a phosphatase (not a phosphorylase) and that the phosphoproteins are not involved merely as intermediates in the metabolic transfer of phosphate groups from one molecule to another.

b. Protein Kinases

The kinase activity responsible for phosphorylating the nonhistone chromosomal proteins is located in the chromatin.[105,106,116] Using a variety of techniques — such as chromatography on phosphocellulose, DEAE-cellulose, or DEAE-Sephadex®, gel filtration, sucrose gradient centrifugation, and DNA affinity chromatography — nuclear protein kinases have been separated into from 2 to 12 fractions in rat liver,[117-127] beef liver,[128] human lymphocytes,[129] calf thymus,[130,131] chick oviduct,[132] pig ovary,[133] rat mammary gland,[120] hepatoma,[126] and HeLa cells.[134] The 12 protein kinase fractions recovered by Kish and Kleinsmith[128] were further resolved, by polyacrylamide gel electrophoresis, into multiple components, thus demonstrating a remarkable degree of enzyme heterogeneity. However, the multiplicity of nuclear protein kinases may be due, in part, to the dissociation, aggregation, or degradation of kinases during isolation or electrophoresis. The fractionation pattern of nuclear protein kinases exhibited some tissue specificity,[128] and each fraction phosphorylated a different complement of nonhistone chromosomal proteins.[126,128,134] These protein kinases have also been shown to differ in activity and substrate specificity between normal and neoplastic tissues[126] and between different stages of the cell cycle.[135]

Kish and Kleinsmith[128] found that five of the beef liver nuclear protein kinases were stimulated by cAMP; however, most workers did not find any cAMP stimulation of the kinases, and some of those who did, found that the nuclear cAMP-dependent kinases were similar to those found in the cytoplasm. This suggested the possibility that the nuclear cAMP-dependent kinases were merely a result of cytoplasmic contamination.[136] However, when nuclei were isolated in nonaqueous media, which precluded the exchange of water-soluble molecules between the cytoplasm and nucleus, two nuclear cAMP-dependent protein kinases were isolated.[133] These kinases were chemically, physically, and antigenically identical to cytoplasmic enzymes. It thus seems that cAMP-dependent protein kinases do occur in nuclei and are very similar, if not identical, to cytoplasmic enzymes. Several groups have found evidence for the hormone or cAMP-mediated dissociation of cytoplasmic cAMP-dependent protein kinase into its catalytic and regulatory subunits and the subsequent translocation of the catalytic subunit into the nucleus. The chromatin acceptor site is a nonhistone protein(s) and the translocation is followed by a selective phosphorylation of nonhistone (not histone) protein.[137,138] This translocation may explain the discrepancy between the cAMP-stimulated phosphorylation of specific nuclear proteins in vivo and the cAMP insensitivity of the nuclear kinases in isolated nuclei.[138]

c. Phosphatases

The phosphatase(s) responsible for dephosphorylating the nonhistone chromosomal proteins is located in the nucleoplasm and not in the chromatin,[139] and this activity has been separated into multiple fractions by DEAE-Sephadex® column chromatography.[139,140]

IV. ISOLATION AND FRACTIONATION OF NONHISTONE CHROMOSOMAL PROTEINS

A. Preparation of Chromatin

Chromatin should be viewed as being operationally defined. Hence, the proteins found associated with the isolated genome reflect the methods used to prepare the chromatin. It is necessary to consider both the loss of genome-associated proteins and the adherence of cytoplasmic, membrane, and nucleoplasmic components during chromatin preparation. Chromatin extracted from purified nuclei[141] contains less cytoplasmic contaminants than chromatin isolated directly from whole tissue.[142] Cytoplasmic and membrane contamination of chromatin can be reduced by washing nuclei in solutions containing nonionic detergents such as Triton® X-100 or by centrifuging the chromatin through heavy sucrose. When chromatin was prepared by these techniques, in the presence of radioactively labeled cytoplasmic extracts, less than 5% of HeLa cell chromatin proteins were due to cytoplasmic contaminants.[36,47] The use of cytoplasmic ''marker enzymes'' revealed less than 10% cytoplasmic contamination of chromatin.[143] When considering this problem, it should be remembered that proteins can migrate in vivo from the cytoplasm to the chromatin, e.g., chromosomal proteins are synthesized in the cytoplasm and are then transported into the nucleus,[25] and hormonal stimulation[144] or cell fusion[145] causes the migration of some cytoplasmic proteins into the nucleus. During the isolation of nuclei in aqueous media proteins can be lost from, or absorbed into, the nucleus. This problem can be overcome by isolating nuclei in nonaqueous media.[146] The presence of proteins common to both nucleoplasm and chromatin fractions need not necessarily be interpreted as an artifact of preparation. Rather, this similarity may reflect a nucleoplasmic pool of macromolecules which exists in a dynamic equilibrium with the chromatin.[147] This movement of molecules between cytoplasm, nucleoplasm, and chromatin most likely has some functional importance.

B. Isolation of Nonhistone Chromosomal Proteins

Some nonhistone chromosomal proteins are difficult to isolate because of their tight binding to DNA and their tendency to aggregate with each other and with histones. A variety of isolation methods has been used in an attempt to overcome this problem, but none has met all the ideal requirements: a total yield; recovery of all the protein species; complete separation of the nonhistone proteins from nucleic acid and histones; avoidance of harsh denaturing conditions which may alter the structural and functional properties of the proteins; widespread applicability and the possibility of further fractionation of the proteins.

Methods for the isolation of nonhistone proteins fall into three general categories: (1) those involving selective extraction of histones followed by dissociation and separation of nonhistones from nucleic acids; (2) those involving the dissociation of macromolecules from total chromatin and their subsequent fractionation; and (3) selective extraction of nonhistone chromosomal proteins directly from chromatin.

1. Isolation of Nonhistone Chromosomal Proteins from Dehistonized Chromatin

Histones are first extracted from the chromatin, usually with dilute HCl or H_2SO_4; then the nonhistone chromosomal proteins are separated from the nucleic acid by various techniques. In early experiments in which the objectives were merely to determine the quantity, chemical composition, or isotope content of the nonhistones, nucleic acids were hydrolyzed with 5% trichloroacetic acid or 0.5 N $HClO_4$ at 90°C and the nonhistones solubilized in strong alkali.[148-151] This method completely denatures the proteins and makes them unsuitable for further investigation. To enable the nonhistones to be analyzed by techniques such as gel electrophoresis, less drastic methods of extraction were developed (Table 1). It should be noted that ''dehistonization'' of chromatin by dilute mineral acid extraction may alter the nonhistone proteins, such that their extractibility and biological properties may be irreversibly modified. Therefore, there is considerable advantage to dehistonization by milder conditions such as urea-NaCl at pH 6.0.[152]

Table 1
EXTRACTION OF NONHISTONE CHROMOSOMAL PROTEINS FROM DEHISTONIZED CHROMATIN

Solubilization of dehistonized chromatin	Removal of nucleic acid	Comments	Ref.
4 M CsCl (pH 11.6)	Equilibrium density gradient centrifugation	40% yield	11
4 M CsCl (pH 14.0)	Equilibrium density gradient centrifugation	Increased yield	153
0.1 to 1% SDS	DNA pelleted by ultracentrifugation	90 to 95% yields; all the major nonhistone chromosomal proteins were recovered; detergent causes denaturation and is difficult to remove	12 154
1% SDS, 8 M urea (pH 11.5), 5 mM 2-mercaptoethanol			155
Histones (together with 15% of the nonhistones) removed with 2 M NaCl, 5 M urea (pH .6); nonhistones extracted from residue by increasing pH to 8.5			152
	DNase I treatment	Yield 95%; nonhistone chromosomal proteins were then precipitated in 0.4 M HC10$_4$ and dissolved in SDS	156
		Dissolved precipitate in 10 M urea, 0.9 M acetic acid, 1% 2-mercaptoethanol	157
0.1 M Tris-HCl (pH 8.4), 0.01 M EDTA, 0.14 M 2-mercaptoethanol	Nonhistone chromosomal proteins partitioned into phenol	Some of residual protein solubilized by reextracting with phenol at pH 9.5; nonhistone chromosomal proteins reconstituted into aqueous media by dialyses	158—161
	Nonhistone chromosomal proteins partitioned into phenol	Phenol-soluble proteins precipitated and then dissolved in 3% SDS, 1% 2-mercaptoethanol	19, 162, 163
	Nonhistone chromosomal proteins partitioned into phenol	Phenol extracts dialyzed directly against electrophoresis sample buffer; residual protein extracted with 5% SDS, 0.14 M 2-mercaptoethanol at 100°C.	14, 164
	Phenol saturated with 0.1 M H$_2$SO$_4$		165

2. Isolation of Nonhistone Chromosomal Proteins from Whole Chromatin

In procedures of this type, the chromatin is dissociated and solubilized; then the DNA and histones are separated from the nonhistone proteins (Table 2).

Methods that involve the coextraction of histones and nonhistone chromosomal proteins result in a reduced yield of nonhistone proteins because (1) before the histones

Table 2
ISOLATION OF NONHISTONE CHROMOSOMAL PROTEINS FROM WHOLE CHROMATIN

Dissociation of chromatin	Removal of DNA	Removal of histones	Comments	Ref.
1 to 3 M NaCl	Reduced salt concentration to 0.14 M		Leaves majority of nonhistone chromosomal proteins in solution	166, 167
	Bio-gel® A-50m	Urea/polyacrylamide gels (pH 2.7) cation exchange resins	Recovery 30 to 60%	15
				17, 168
Guanidine hydrocloride	Gel filtration with Sepharose® 4B	Adsorption to CM-Sephadex®	Yield 60 to 70%	18
	Bio-gel® A-5m	Adsorption to CM-Sephadex®	Yield 60 to 70%; disadvantage: gel filtration methods result in cross-contamination of DNA and protein and dilution of protein	169
Guanidine-HCl	Ultracentrifugation	Ion-exchange chromatography		170
Guanidine-HCl + urea	Ultracentrifugation	Ion-exchange chromatography	90% yield	170, 172
	Pelleted by ultracentrifugation		Introduction of urea into the salt solution enabled chromatin to be dissociated without extensive shearing; >90% recovery	15, 173
		Ion-exchange chromatography		
	Pelleted by ultracentrifugation	Nonhistone chromosomal proteins adsorbed to anion exchange resins		174, 175 176, 177
	Precipitation with LaCl₃ (0.0135 M)	Ion-exchange chromatography		178
	Column chromatography on hydroxylapatite using a phosphate buffer gradient		60 to 70% recovery	13, 179
	Column chromatography on hydroxylapatite using a guanidine hydrochloride gradient		Almost 100% recovery	180
1% SDS	Ultracentrifugation	Ion-exchange chromatography	Difficult to remove histone from SDS solutions	181
25% formic acid, 0.2 M NaCl, 8 M urea	Ultracentrifugation	Ion-exchange chromatography		182

can be removed by ion-exchange chromatography, the salt concentration of the sample must be reduced to less than 0.5 M (usually by dialysis) which results in considerable losses of the nonhistone chromosomal proteins due to precipitation,[170,172] and (2) about 10% of the nonhistone proteins cochromatograph with the histones.[170,172,176]

3. Selective Extraction Procedures

The methods discussed in this section have been used to selectively extract fractions of the nonhistone chromosomal proteins. Gronow and co-workers extracted 70% of the total nuclear proteins with 8 M urea, 50 mM phosphate buffer (pH 7.6),[56,183,184] and other groups have used this technique for selectively extracting a fraction of nonhistone proteins from chromatin.[185] A group of nonhistone chromosomal proteins enriched in phosphoproteins was extracted by Langan[105] using a method similar to that of Wang.[167] Modifications to this method were introduced by Gershey and Kleinsmith[186] and Kleinsmith and Allfrey.[107] Histones were removed using BioRex® 70, and phosphoproteins were adsorbed to calcium phosphate gel. This phosphoprotein-enriched fraction comprised <30% of the total nonhistone chromosomal proteins, and because of the low solubility of these proteins in dilute buffer, they were usually solubilized in sodium dodecyl sulfate (SDS) solutions.[187,188]

Treatment of chromatin with 0.35 M NaCl was first introduced as a method of removing contaminating cytoplasmic proteins from chromatin.[142] Later, it became evident that the proteins extracted by this procedure were of chromosomal origin, and several groups have since used this method to isolate a group of relatively loosely bound nonhistone chromosomal proteins[189-194] which may be important in the maintenance of both chromatin structure and gene expression. The salt/urea extraction method has been adapted to extract several different fractions of nonhistone chromosomal proteins by the sequential treatment of chromatin with a series of 5 M urea solutions, containing progressively more NaCl.[195] Nonhistone chromosomal proteins have also been selectively extracted from chromatin by the use of alkaline reagents.[196,197] The proteins extracted were significantly different from those which remained bound to the chromatin, and their rate of metabolism was higher.

C. Fractionation of Nonhistone Chromosomal Proteins

Due to the complex and heterogeneous nature of the nonhistone chromosomal proteins, fractionation is a prerequisite for examination of the chemical, metabolic, and biological properties of the individual proteins. This group of proteins has proved to be difficult to fractionate, partly because the hydrophobic nature of many of these macromolecules results in their low solubility in the low ionic strength buffers commonly used for protein fractionation.

1. Anaytical Fractonation

Analytical techniques are used for identification, quantitation, and studies on the metabolic properties of the nonhistone chromosomal proteins. These methods usually accommodate only small amounts of protein and result in the irreversible denaturation of most of the proteins, thus precluding the study of their biological functions. The most important technique is that of polyacrylamide gel electrophoresis.

a. Electrophoretic Analysis of Nonhistone Chromosomal Proteins

Initial attempts at separating nonhistone chromosomal proteins by electrophoresis in starch[166,167,198,199] or agarose-polyacrylamide gels[200] were not very successful and resulted in a large proportion of the sample precipitating at the origin and considerable streaking in the gels. The solubility and resolution of the proteins was increased by the use of polyacrylamide gels at alkaline pH[201] or by introducing urea into the gel.[11,15,18,182] However, due to aggregation, large amounts of protein did not enter these gels. Electrophoresis in the presence of SDS prevents protein aggregation and results in much better resolution. The first method used was that of Shapiro et al.[202] (See, for example Elgin and Bonner[154] and Teng et al.[161]) MacGillivray et al.[179] introduced urea into an SDS-containing system. These systems resolved up to 30 peptides ranging in molecular weight from 5,000 to 200,000 daltons, and the introduction of the discontinuous SDS-containing system of Laemmli[203] improved resolution still further[164,204,205] with up to 50 bands being visible on gels.

b. Isoelectric Focusing in Polyacrylamide Gels

Nonhistone chromosomal proteins have also been separated according to their isoelectric points. They focus over a wide range of pH from 3 to 10[170,182,184,206,207] but tend to predominate between pH 5 and 7.[182] Thus, several of these proteins are, in fact, basic; therefore, the use of the term "acidic nuclear fractions" to describe the nonhistone chromosomal proteins can be misleading. An example of such a basic nonhistone chromosomal protein is the BA protein reported by Busch's laboratory.[208]

c. Two-Dimensional Gel Electrophoresis

The introduction of two-dimensional electrophoretic systems greatly increased the resolution of nonhistone proteins. Busch's group have used a system involving electrophoresis at an acid pH in polyacrylamide gels containing urea, followed by a second electrophoretic separation in SDS-polyacrylamide slab gels.[157,209] The potential resolving power of this electrophoretic procedure is limited because proteins are separated in both dimensions largely according to molecular weight differences and, hence, are displayed in a relatively restricted area running diagonally across the slab gel. Yet, this fractionation procedure has permitted isolation of specific nucleolar nonhistone chromosomal proteins which have subsequently been characterized.

By combining the isoelectric focusing system of Gronow and Griffiths[184] with SDS-polyacrylamide slab-gel electrophoresis, Barrett and Gould[210] and MacGillivray and Rickwood[211] have been able to distribute the proteins more evenly over the second dimension slab gel. In the second dimension, Barrett and Gould[210] and Tsitilou and Mathias[207] used the SDS-electrophoresis system of Shapiro et al.,[202] whereas MacGillivray and Rickwood[211] used the discontinuous SDS-electrophoretic system of Laemmli.[203] These techniques have resolved over 50 polypeptide species and have the advantage of separating proteins according to two different criteria (namely, isoelectric point and molecular weight). Peterson and McConkey[212,213] have used the high-resolution two-dimensional electrophoretic system of O'Farrell[214] to resolve nonhistone proteins into several hundred distinct species. In this system, the isoelectric focusing gel contains a nonionic detergent, and proteins can be loaded in low concentrations of SDS, thus improving their solubility

One of the most important consequences of the use of gel electrophoretic systems with ever more powerful resolving abilities has been the realization of the extremely heterogeneous nature of the nonhistone chromosomal proteins. The first attempts to analyze these proteins revealed only about a half dozen or so species, whereas the most recent attempts have demonstrated that this group of proteins contains at least several hundred components.

2. Preparative Methods

For assessment of structural and biological properties of nonhistone chromosomal proteins, in most situations, large amounts of proteins are required, necessitating fractionation by preparative procedures.

a. Gel Filtration

Fractionation of nonhistone chromsomal proteins by gel filtration techniques is particularly affected by the low solubility of these proteins. Nevertheless, some degree of fractionation has been obtained on columns of Sepharose®,[18] Sephadex®,[174,182,215,216] and agarose[15] and polyacrylamide[174] Bio-Gels®.

b. Ion-Exchange Chromatography

Work on the fractionation of nonhistones using DEAE-cellulose was performed by Wang and co-workers.[198,199,217] However, in mild conditions, these proteins tend to form insoluble aggregates, and Levy et al.[171] and Chaudhuri[176] fractionated them on DEAE-cellulose in the presence of 3 to 5 M urea. Using a linear NaCl gradient, Levy et al.[171] found two major peaks of proteins from rabbit chromatin, and with a more complex gradient, these were separated into several distinct peaks.

Several workers[175,176,211,218-220] have used QAE-Sephadex® with a NaCl gradient to fractionate nonhistones in the presence of 5 M urea. Up to 70% of the protein was recovered from the column, but Augenlicht and Baserga[172] obtained 85 to 90% recovery when they used a final elution step involving 4 M guanidine hydrochloride, 6 M urea; and Rickwood and MacGillivray[180] obtained almost complete recovery by using guanidine hydrochloride, instead of NaCl, as the gradient. Elgin and Bonner[182] recovered four fractions of nonhistones using the cation exchanger SE-Sephadex® C-25 at acid pH. CM-Sephadex® has also been used to fractionate the nonhistone chromosomal proteins.[18,221]

The main disadvantage of fractionating nonhistones by ion-exchange chromatography is the low yields obtained. However, as already mentioned, these can be improved by using a guanidine hydrochloride gradient.

c. Affinity Techniques

The ability of some nonhistone chromosomal proteins to bind to DNA has been exploited as a method of fractionating these proteins. Teng et al.[161] extracted nonhistone proteins in high-salt solutions and allowed them to bind to DNA during gradient dialysis to reduce the salt concentration to 0.01 M. One of the problems associated with this procedure is that low-salt concentrations cause some of the proteins to aggregate and precipitate. Some workers have overcome this dilemma by performing the binding reaction in the presence of 5 M urea.[222] The DNA-protein complexes were recovered by sucrose density-gradient centrifugation.[160,161,223] DNA-binding proteins have also been isolated by affinity chromatography on DNA bound to cellulose,[168,224,225] agarose-polyacrylamide,[226] or agarose.[227] However, in the low-salt concentrations used in these experiments, many proteins bind to DNA in a nonspecific manner. This can be avoided either by carrying out the binding reaction in higher salt concentrations, such as 0.2 to 0.25 M,[228] or by prerunning the proteins through a column of heterologous DNA.[168,225] Allfrey and co-workers[229-231] bound single- or double-stranded DNA of different $C_o t$ values to various types of Sephadex® and Sepharose® columns. Nonhistones were adsorbed to the DNA in low-salt concentrations, and a series of different DNA-binding protein fractions was eluted with an increasing step-wise salt gradient. Another method which has been used to isolate DNA-nonhistone complexes is nitrocellulose filtration.[208,232,233]

The hydrophobic nature of several of the nonhistone chromosomal proteins has been utilized as a means of fractionation. A complex group of proteins was separated from the remaining proteins by affinity chromatography, in the presence of high-salt concentrations, to daunomycin-CH-Sepharose® 4B.[234] Another method of fractionating a specific group of nonhistones is by affinity chromatography to other chromosomal proteins, especially histones.[235] Similarly to DNA-affinity chromatography, this method has the advantage of separating the nonhistones on a possible functional basis.

d. Purification of Individual Nonhistone Chromosomal Proteins

Many of the nonhistone chromosomal proteins have enzymic activities, and consequently, their purification can be monitored by assaying for the particular enzyme of interest. Many enzymes, such as the DNA and RNA polymerases, have been purified from chromatin. However, many of the nonhistone chromosomal proteins have structural and regulatory functions which are, as yet, unknown, and there are no simple assays by which their purification can be monitored. An attempt at partial purification of a gene regulatory protein has been undertaken by Stein's group.[215] These workers have suggested that the S phase nonhistone chromosomal proteins of HeLa S₃ cells contain a species which activates histone gene transcription in vitro. The protein(s) responsible for this activation was purified several hundredfold by standard fractionation techniques, and the ability of the species to activate histone gene transcription was used to monitor its purification. Busch's group has used two-dimensional gel electrophoresis to monitor the purification of several nonhistone chromosomal proteins.[236] Assuming that some of the molecules which regulate the expression of a particular gene will be able to bind specifically to a sequence of DNA associated with that gene, it should be possible to further purify these proteins by affinity chromatography using recombinant DNA molecules containing specific sequences. This method should enable specific regulatory proteins to be isolated from a heterogeneous mixture in one step and would circumvent the need to monitor purification by assaying a biological function.

V. FUNCTIONAL ROLES OF NONHISTONE CHROMOSOMAL PROTEINS

Approximately half of the total chromosomal proteins are nonhistones, and current levels of resolution have shown that this group of proteins contains several hundred different species. Such a large, heterogeneous group of proteins might be expected to be involved in many of the metabolic and regulatory functions of the nucleus, and extensive research has shown that this group of proteins contains species which function as enzymatic, structural, or regulatory molecules.

A. Enzymes

Several nuclear enzymes are nonhistone chromosomal proteins (Table 3). These include enzymes involved in DNA replication, repair, and unwinding; RNA synthesis and processing; modification of nucleic acids; postsynthetic modification of proteins by the addition or removal of acetate, methyl, phosphate, and ADP-ribose groups; and processing and degradation of chromosomal proteins.

B. Nonhistone Chromosomal Proteins and the Structure of Chromatin

The repeat structure of chromatin and the structure of nucleosome core particles involved in this have been extensively reviewed by others.[9,10] Almost all the results obtained so far have pertained to the arrangement of DNA and histones, and consequently, little is known about the possible contributions of the nonhistone chromosomal protens to chromatin structure. As these proteins are present in chromatin in similar quantities to histone, models of chromatin structure must eventually take them into account.

The contractile proteins actin, myosin, and tropomyosin have been identified in the chromatin of the lower eukaryotes *Physarum polycephalum*[278,279] and *Dictyostelium discoideum*[280,281] and also in mammalian cells such as HeLa,[279] rat liver,[282] and mouse embryo fibroblasts.[283] However, there is currently a controversy about the possibility

Table 3
ENZYME COMPONENTS OF THE NONHISTONE CHROMOSOMAL PROTEINS

Nucleic acids as substrates	Function	Ref.
DNA polymerases	Polymerization of deoxyribonucleotides into DNA	237—241
RNA polymerases	Polymerization of ribonucleotides into RNA	242—248
Nucleases	Processing or degradation of DNA and/or RNA	249—251
Nucleotide ligase	Joining DNA segments during DNA replication and repair	252
Nucleotide exotransferases		
DNA	Addition of nucleotides to the ends of nucleic acids	253—255
RNA (poly[A] polymerase)		
DNA methylase	Methylation of DNA	256
DNA-untwisting, unwinding, or relaxing enzymes (helix-destabilizing proteins)	Unwind DNA double helix and stabilize the resulting single-stranded DNA	257—263
Chromosomal proteins as substrates		
Proteases	Processing or degradation of proteins	264—267
Acetylases	Acetylation of proteins	268—271
Deacetylases	Removal of acetate groups from proteins	272, 273
Kinases	Phosphorylation of proteins	
Histone		109, 274
Nonhistone		124, 126, 128
Histone methylases	Methylation of histones	275, 276
Poly(ADP-ribose) synthetase	Addition of ADP-ribose moieties to chromosomal proteins	84—86, 277
Poly(ADP-ribose) glycohydrolase	Removal of ADP-ribose moieties from chromosomal proteins	87

that the nuclear actin may be due to cytoplasmic contamination during nuclear preparation[194] or to the random distribution of actin within the cell.[284] If these contractile proteins are true components of chromatin, they may well have a role in chromatin condensation. Other possible roles for these proteins are the transport of RNA from the nucleus to the cytoplasm or, through the ability of actin to specifically bind and inactivate DNase I,[285] the long-term preservation of the genome in cysts or spores.

Adolph and co-workers have investigated the possible role of nonhistone proteins in chromosome structure by dissecting the structural contributions of histones and nonhistone proteins.[286] By competition with dextran sulfate and heparin, all the histones and many nonhistone proteins were gently removed from HeLa metaphase chromosomes. The histone-depleted chromosomes had a DNA to protein ratio of 6:1. The protein component consisted of 6 major and 25 minor nonhistone proteins which were all resistant to removal by 2 M NaCl and 0.2 N H$_2$SO$_4$.[286] Electron microscopic analysis of these histone-depleted chromosomes showed that they retained the characteristic shape of metaphase chromosomes and consisted of a central structure or "scaffold" surrounded by loops of DNA which were attached to adjacent points on the scaffold.[287] When DNA was removed from chromosomes by micrococcal nuclease prior to histone depletion, the nonhistone protein scaffold could still be isolated. It retained the general shape and size of intact chromosomes.[288] This result rules out the possibility that the scaffold structure is an artifactual product caused by the rearrangement or trapping of nonhistone proteins during the removal of histones. These experiments demonstrate that by providing a scaffold to which loops of DNA are attached, the nonhistone proteins play an important role in defining the basic shape of chromosomes. It has been proposed that the long DNA loops are condensed by histones into shorter, possibly twisted loops which are arranged around the scaffold.[289] Similar scaffold structures have also been isolated from histone-depleted chicken erythroid interphase chromosomes.[286]

Although it seems likely that nonhistone proteins play a role in the general organization of chromosome shape (discussed above), it is not yet known whether any of these proteins are involved in the many levels of DNA folding which exist in chromosomes. For example, are nonhistones involved in the folding of DNA around nucleosomes, either through direct interaction with the core particles themselves or through association with the spacer regions of DNA between the nucleosome cores? Most studies on nucleosomes have concentrated on the histones, and, in fact, one study found that there were no nonhistone proteins associated with the nucleosome.[290] However, several groups have since presented evidence indicating that nonhistones may indeed be associated with nucleosomes.[291-295] Goodwin et al.[293] have found four of the high-mobility group (HMG) nonhistone proteins associated with isolated nucleosomes. However, the HMG proteins were bound to only a proportion of the nucleosomes, and, whereas two of these proteins are bound to the core particle itself, the other two seem to be associated with DNA in the internucleosomal spacer region.[23] Another HMG protein (HMG-T) has also been found to be localized in the spacer region.[296] One of the functions of these internucleosomal HMG proteins may be to interact with histone H1[297] which is also localized in the spacer region. The protein designated A24 by Busch's group has been reported to be composed of histone 2A joined by an isopeptide linkage to the protein ubiquitin.[298,299] A24 has recently been shown, along with another protein, Bu, to be contained in nucleosome monomers.[295] Because these proteins are present in smaller amounts than the histones, they may be associated with a subset of the nucleosomes. This corresponds to the findings of several other groups[292-294] suggesting that various nonhistone proteins are associated with only some nucleosomes. For example, when chromatin was digested exhaustively with staphylococcal nuclease, two populations of nucleosomal particles with different densities were observed;[292,300,512] the dense particle may represent a subclass of nucleosomes, and nonhistone proteins were found to be preferentially associated with it.[292] Nonhistone proteins associated with nucleosomes may be involved in the general folding of DNA chains and/or in the control of selective gene expression.

The technique of immunofluorescence[301-304] should help to elucidate the distribution of specific nonhistone proteins within chromatin.

C. Nonhistone Chromosomal Proteins in Ribonucleoprotein Particles

During transcription, several nonhistone proteins are deposited on nascent nonribosomal RNA[305,306] forming a repeating subunit structure of 200- to 300-Å (30- to 55-S) spherical particles connected by RNA strands.[307-310] Depending on the method of extraction, varying amounts of these particles are sometimes extracted along with nonhistone chromosomal proteins.[37] Although the proteins contained in these particles may be involved in the packaging, processing, and transport of the RNA, they will not be discussed in this review, as they have been described in some detail in several recent papers.[311-315]

VI. CORRELATIVE EVIDENCE FOR NONHISTONE CHROMOSOMAL PROTEINS AS REGULATORY MOLECULES

There are several general requirements that a group of molecules would be expected to meet if they were involved in selective gene expression, viz., to have considerable heterogeneity, to exhibit some tissue and species specificity, to vary in their distribution between transcriptionally active and inactive chromatin, to be able to interact with specific DNA sequences and certain hormone-receptor complexes, and to undergo quantitative and qualitative changes at time of alteration of gene expression. The evidence discussed in this section indicates that the nonhistone chromosomal proteins meet many of these requirements and, as such, provide correlative evidence for the involvement of nonhistone chromosomal proteins in the control of gene readout.

A. Heterogeneity of Nonhistone Chromosomal Proteins

With present levels of resolution attainable on two-dimensional gels, the nonhistone proteins in chromatin have been shown to contain several hundred distinct species.[115,212] At this level of resolution, their complexity rivals that of cytoplasmic proteins[212] and contrasts markedly with the general lack of heterogeneity of the histones. When analyzed by ion-exchange chromatography and isoelectric focusing, one of the HMG proteins appears to have a form of microheterogeneity similar to that found in histone H1.[316]

B. Tissue and Species Specificity

Histones display little tissue specificity.[317] In contrast, several groups have analyzed nonhistone proteins by one-dimensional electrophoresis and found tissue-specific differences.[13,15,18,19,56,154,161,175,179,200,318-323] Interpretations of these findings are complicated by the different extraction methods used by the various groups. For example, methods which extract only a fraction of the total nonhistone chromatin proteins tend to give considerable qualitative differences between tissues,[161,318,320] whereas methods which extract a more representative fraction of the proteins show far less tissue specificity.[154,205] The conclusion that nonhistone proteins have only limited tissue specificity was supported by the finding that most of the major proteins were present in most tissues examined.[204,324]

Tissue specificity has also been demonstrated by immunological techniques involving, in particular, DNA-protein complexes of low molecular weight proteins with a high affinity for DNA.[152,226,325-330] This argues against the possibility that differential extractibility is the main reason for the observed tissue-specific differences in the electrophoretic patterns of the proteins.

Wu et al.[331] compared liver and kidney nonhistone proteins from such diverse species as rat, cat, cow, chicken, turtle, and frog and found that the protein pattern had changed a great deal during evolution. Nevertheless, each tissue contained a tissue-specific subset of proteins that appeared to have been conserved.

The introduction of two-dimensional electrophoretic techniques for the separation of nonhistone proteins resulted in better resolution than was possible using one-dimensional electrophoresis, and initial results obtained using these techniques did not change the general concept of the limited tissue and species specificity of these proteins.[157,207,210,211] However, with the introduction of the high-resolution two-dimensional electrophoretic system of O'Farrell[214] (discussed previously), it was found that as many as half the nonhistone chromosomal proteins of Friend and HeLa cells differed.[213] This degree of divergence was less than that observed for the cytoplasmic proteins (three fourths of which differed) indicating that, as suggested by the early studies, many of the nonhistone chromosomal proteins may be under relatively strict evolutionary conservation. The tissue- and/or species-specific chromosomal proteins presumably include those involved in the control of cell-type-specific gene expression, whereas the remainder of the proteins may be conserved because they have to interact with DNA or other molecules in general processes, such as the maintenance of chromosomal structure, DNA replication, or transcription, that are common to both cell types. One group of nonhistone proteins that has little or no tissue or species specificity is the HMG proteins,[23] and these proteins have been shown to bind DNA.[221,332,333] Other workers have also presented evidence of the evolutionary conservation of a group of DNA-binding nonhistone proteins.[334]

A disadvantage of comparing nonhistone chromosomal protein patterns derived from whole tissues is that tissues usually consist of several different cell types, and consequently different chromatins, which complicates results concerning the tissue specificity of nonhistone proteins. Fujitani and Holoubek[335] went some way toward overcoming this problem by comparing nonhistone proteins from the different anatomical regions of brain. However, the anatomical regions still contained various nuclear types. Another approach to this problem has been to compare nonhistone chromosomal proteins extracted from fractions enriched in a particular nuclear type, for example, neuronal and glial nuclei,[336-338] and more recently these proteins have been extracted from three to five types of brain nuclei prepared by isopycnic zonal centrifugation.[115,207] Although these nuclear types were not pure, this approach, which reveals cell-specific variations in nonhistone chromosomal proteins, goes a considerable way toward overcoming the problem of cross-contamination of nuclear types.

C. Quantitative Differences in Nonhistone Chromosomal Proteins of Various Tissues

Although histones are present in chromatin from most tissues at about a 1:1 ratio to DNA, the proportion of nonhistone proteins in chromatin from different tissues varies considerably. This was first noted by Mirsky and Ris.[339] Although many tissues have a nonhistone protein to DNA ratio of about 1 or slightly less,[154,340] the ratio can be as low as 0.13 in sea urchin sperm[341] or as high as 9.1 in slime mold,[342] and the amount of nonhistone proteins in chromatin has been correlated with the RNA synthetic activity of that chromatin.[149,335,343] The nonhistone protein content of chromatin has been found to change with the biological state of a tissue; for example, the levels declined (along with DNA template activity) during the maturation of sperm,[344] increased during sea urchin embryo development,[18,345] and paralleled chromatin template activity during the estrogen-induced differentiation of chick oviduct.[165]

D. Differences in Nonhistone Chromosomal Proteins of Active and Inactive Chromatin

Quantitative variations in the nonhistone chromosomal protein content of active and inactive tissues suggest that chromatin template activity is influenced by the nonhistone chromosomal proteins, and this hypothesis is supported by the finding that when chromatin was fractionated, by several different methods, into eu- and heterochromatin, the nonhistone to DNA ratio was greater in the euchromatin fraction.[148,150,346-352] Electrophoretic analysis demonstrated that there were qualitative and quantitative differences between the nonhistone proteins from the different chromatin fractions, with each fraction possessing unique species.[351,353-358] These differences have been confirmed by immunological techniques.[359] Certain specific nonhistone proteins with defined enzyme activities, such as nuclear protein kinase[360] and poly(ADP-ribose) synthetase,[84] have been found to be preferentially localized in the active fraction of chromatin. The euchromatin fractions were transcriptively active and more diffuse in structure, whereas the heterochromatin fractions were inactive and condensed. These results indicate that some nonhistone proteins may be involved in transcriptional activity and/or maintenance of a diffuse chromatin structure, whereas others may be involved in the inhibition of transcriptional activity or in the condensation of chromatin structure. However, the legitimacy of these chromatin fractions is controversial, and although there is evidence that genes that are in a transcriptionally "active" configuration are associated with the active fraction of chromatin,[349,361,362] other workers found that this was not the case.[363]

E. Changes in Nonhistone Chromosomal Proteins Associated with Modifications in Gene Activation

A regulatory role for components of the nonhistone chromosomal proteins is suggested by changes in these macromolecules associated with modifications of gene expression in a number of biological situations. For example, such changes in nonhistone proteins have been observed following the stimulation of resting cells to proliferate; during differentiation and development; after hormone and drug stimulation; during the transformation of cells; and with aging.

1. Changes in Nonhistone Chromosomal Proteins Associated with Cell Proliferation

When nondividing cells are stimulated to proliferate, an increase in nonhistone chromosomal protein synthesis has been observed in many different systems: salivary glands stimulated by isoproterenol[16]; WI-38 human fibroblasts stimulated by changing the growth medium;[31,32,364] lymphocytes stimulated by phytohemagglutinin,[33] concanavalin A,[365,366] leucoagglutinin,[367] or anti-immunoglobulin[366]; liver regeneration following partial hepatectomy[368]; and on the refeeding of starved *P. polycephalum*[38] and *Tetrahymena*.[369-371] Electrophoretic analysis has revealed that in many cases changes in the total amount of the nonhistone chromosomal proteins are due to changes in the levels of a few specific proteins.[38,367,372-375] The increases in specific nonhistone chromosomal proteins which occur when cells are stimulated to divide precede increases in RNA and DNA synthesis, and thus, it is reasonable to postulate that these proteins are involved in the control of gene transcription at the onset of cell proliferation. However, the levels of some nonhistone proteins decrease when cells are stimulated to divide, and these may be involved in the maintenance of the quiescent state.

2. Changes in Nonhistone Chromosomal Proteins During Development and Differentiation

During the course of development and differentiation, batteries of genes are activated and others are repressed; thus, developing and differentiating systems provide good opportunities to study the molecules involved in controlling selective gene expression. Quantitative and qualitative developmental stage-specific changes in the nonhistone chromosomal proteins have been observed in sea urchin embryos,[18,155,188,376,377] *Xenopus laevis* tadpoles,[378] Oncopeltus (milkweed bug) embryos,[379] and during the development of chick oviduct[165] and embryonic red blood cells.[380] These changes in the amount of nonhistone proteins paralleled changes in transcriptional activity[165,377,379,380] and structure[377] of chromatin.

Changes have also been observed in the complement of nonhistone chromosomal proteins during the differentiation of pollen from *Hippeastrum belladonna*,[381] during the conversion of lymphoid spleen to an erythroid organ,[382] and in the dimethyl sulphoxide-stimulated erythroid differentiation of Friend cells.[213,383] Again, these changes parallel changes in the RNA synthetic capacity of the tissues. Further evidence for a link between the level of nonhistone chromosomal proteins in a cell and the RNA synthetic capacity of that cell is provided by the reduction in amount and the loss of specific nonhistone proteins observed during the condensation of chromatin and concomitant repression of RNA synthesis during spermatogenesis[384,385] and the maturation of erythroid cells.[19,386] However, in contrast to the above findings, some groups have found only minimal changes in the complement of nonhistone chromosomal proteins during prostaglandin and cAMP-induced differentiation of neuroblastoma cells,[387] during the normal or hydrocortisone-induced embryonic development of the neural retina,[388] and during the normal development of various brain tissues.[207,335,389]

3. Changes in Nonhistone Chromosomal Proteins Associated with Gene Activation by Hormones and Drugs

Several hormones activate the expression of specific genes in their target tissues, and increases in the synthesis and amount of nonhistone chromosomal proteins have been demonstrated to occur during gene activation by insulin,[390] aldosterone,[391] and phenobarbital.[392] The conclusion that these proteins are somehow involved in the hormonal control of gene expression is further supported by the evidence that the synthesis of specific nonhistone proteins is augmented at times of gene activation by cortisol,[159] estradiol,[393,394] estrogen,[395] testosterone,[384,396] and glucagon;[397] and specific proteins accumulate in the "puffed" regions of insect chromosomes after treatment with ecdysone.[398] These changes are steroid- and target-tissue-specific. The changes in nonhistone proteins that occurred in prostate gland in response to testosterone were negated when the antiandrogen, cyproterone acetate, was administered together with testosterone in vivo.[396]

4. Changes in Nonhistone Chromosomal Proteins Associated with Carcinogenesis and Cell Transformation

Another finding which supports the hypothesis that the nonhistone chromosomal proteins are involved in the control of gene expression is that they undergo quantitative and qualitative changes during carcinogenesis and transformation, and some of these changes are evident within hours of the treatment of normal tissues with carcinogens. Although no changes were found in the complement of rat liver nonhistone proteins 3 hr after administration of diethylnitrosamine, their rate of synthesis had increased by 50% 1 hr after the administration.[399] However, when rats were treated with thioacetamide, substantial changes were found in both the levels and rates of synthesis of specific liver nonhistone proteins.[185] Similar results have been obtained for cancer of the breast,[400] liver,[374,401,402] colon,[403,404] brain,[405,406] prostate,[407] and lymphocytes.[375] However, in some cases, such as the treatment of human diploid fibroblasts with UV radiation or N-acetoxy-2-acetylaminofluorene, no changes were observed in the nonhistone proteins.[408] In the above studies, differences between the nonhistone proteins of normal and neoplastic tissues were detected by one- or two-dimensional gel electrophoresis, but it has been confirmed, by immunological techniques,[328] that there are differences between the nonhistone proteins of normal and neoplastic tissues. A paticularly interesting observation by Busch's group was that a protein which appeared in lymphocytes only when they became leukemic corresponded to a protein detected in hepatomas but not in normal liver.[374,375] This protein may be involved in some general mechanism of carcinogenesis such as the perturbation of replicative control.

Nonhistone chromosomal proteins also seem to be involved in mediating viral-induced modifications in gene expression. It was shown, by immunological techniques, that the nonhistone proteins of SV40-transformed WI-38 human fibroblasts differed from those of untransformed cells.[326] Gel-electrophoretic and radioactive-labeling studies have also demonstrated differences in the levels and rates of synthesis of specific nonhistone proteins in SV40-transformed and untransformed WI-38 cells[409-414] and in Rous sarcoma virus-infected chick embryo fibroblasts.[415] Although Gonzalez and Rees[416] did not find significant differences between the nonhistones of SV40-transformed and normal 3T3 mouse embryo fibroblasts, Krause et al.[417] found differences which were similar to those observed between SV40-transformed and normal WI-38 cells, and the latter group proposed that these changes may be a specific feature of SV40-mediated cell transformation. The possible involvement of nonhistone chromosomal proteins as mediators of aberrant gene expression in neoplastic cells has recently been reviewed.[459]

F. Phosphorylation of Nonhistone Chromosomal Proteins and the Control of Gene Expression

One aspect of nonhistone chromosomal protein metabolism that may play an important role in the control of gene expression is their rapid phosphorylation and dephosphorylation. The postsynthetic phosphorylation of proteins may well be a general method of physiological control.[418-420] Because a large proportion of the nonhistone chromosomal proteins are phosphoproteins, the evidence, discussed above, concerning the involement of these proteins in the regulation of gene expression also applies to their phosphoprotein component.

1. Tissue Specificity of Nonhistone Chromosomal Phosphoproteins

SDS-polyacrylamide gel electrophoresis of ^{32}P-labeled nonhistone chromosomal proteins has shown that most, but not all, of the bands contain phosphorylated proteins; and the phosphorylation patterns, although exhibiting major similarities, are tissue-specific.[114,115,161,211,319,338]

2. Localization of Nonhistone Chromosomal Phosphoproteins in Chromatin

There is a correlation between the level of phosphorylation of nonhistone chromosomal phosphoproteins and the RNA synthetic capacity of a tissue.[107,421] Phosphoproteins were found to be preferentially localized in the euchromatin,[150] and this was confirmed by direct autoradiographic observation of ^{32}P-labeled phosphoproteins.[111]

3. Phosphorylation and Dephosphorylation of Nonhistone Chromosomal Phosphoproteins During the Cell Cycle of Continuously Dividing Cells

Platz et al.,[187] working with synchronized HeLa cells, found that the rate of phosphate incorporation into the nonhistone chromosomal proteins was high in S and G1 but maximal in G2. They also found that one protein was specifically phosphorylated in G1. The enhanced ^{32}P incorporation in vivo during G2 corresponded to an enhanced level of in vitro cAMP-independent nuclear protein kinase activity[135] at this time during the cell cycle. LeStourgeon and Rusch,[38] working with *P. polycephalum,* also found that maximal phosphorylation occurred during G2. However, Allfrey and co-workers[47,230] found that in HeLa cells, the rate of phosphorylation of nonhistone proteins was maximal in early S and early G1, and depressed in late S, G2, and M. These periods of active phosphorylation were not due to changes in the specific activity of the cellular ATP pools, and they correspond to the cell cycle peaks in RNA synthesis,[422-424] the intracellular cAMP concentration,[425] and the cAMP-dependent protein kinase activity.[47] Although the total phosphate present in the nonhistone proteins remains constant throughout the cell cycle, the phosphate groups turn over rapidly. This turnover is independent of protein turnover and differs for individual proteins with half-life ($t_{1/2}$) values ranging from 5.5 to 12 hr.[47]

4. Changes in Nonhistone Chromosomal Protein Phosphorylation Following Stimulation of Cell Proliferation

An increase in the rate of phosphorylation of nonhistone chromosomal proteins occurs after human lymphocytes have been stimulated to proliferate with phytohemagglutinin or concanavalin A.[365,426,427] This increased rate of phosphorylation precedes the increase in RNA synthesis (and is accompanied by an eight- to tenfold stimulation of nuclear phosphoprotein kinase activity[428]). Similar increases in the rate of phosphorylation were observed in starved *P. polycephalum* stimulated to divide by refeeding;[38] in Yoshida ascites sarcoma cells moving from the exponential to the stationary growth phase;[421] in rat salivary glands stimulated by isoproterenol;[429,430] in Chinese hamster (K$_{12}$) cells;[431] in hamster kidney (BHK$_{21}$ C$_{13}$) cells;[432] and in WI-38 human fibroblasts stimulated to divide by fresh medium.[433] The pattern of phosphorylation of the nonhistones, and the phosphate turnover rates of specific proteins, differed between nondividing and dividing cells.[433] Similar changes were also observed during early kidney regeneration following folic acid treatment[434] and rat liver regeneration.[435]

5. Changes in Nonhistone Chromosomal Protein Phosphorylation During Differentiation and Development

Changes in the levels of phosphorylation of the nonhistone chromosomal proteins during development and differentiation correspond to the variations that take place in the amount of these proteins and in the RNA synthetic activity of the chromatin. Thus, the level of nonhistone chromosomal protein phosphorylation decreases during spermatogenesis[384] and red blood cell maturation[343] and increases rapidly during the early development of sea urchin, with significant increases being associated with the fertilization and hatching processes.[188,385] Changes in phosphorylation have also been found to occur during muscle differentiation in vitro.[436] It is interesting to note that even though no changes in the synthesis of the nonhistone chromosomal proteins were observed during the differentiation of neuroblastoma cells[387] or the development of neural retina,[388] distinct differences were found in their phosphorylation.

6. Changes in Nonhistone Chromosomal Protein Phosphorylation Associated with Gene Activation by Hormones and Drugs

In addition to increasing the synthesis and amount of nonhistone chromosomal proteins and the rate of RNA synthesis, several hormones and drugs also increase the phosphorylation of these proteins. The systems in which this increase has been found include: the stimulation of mammary epithelial cells by insulin and prolactin;[437] liver cells by glucagon[438] or cortisol and corticosterone;[386,439-441] prostate cells by testosterone;[112,442-444] rat testis by pituitary gonadotropic hormones and epididymis by testosterone;[400] kidney cells by aldosterone;[445] uterus by estradiol;[446] ovary by chorionic gonadotropin;[447] liver by triiodothyronine;[448] and glial cells by norepinephrine.[449] Similar results were found when liver was treated with phenobarbital.[450] In many of the above studies, the increase in nonhistone protein phosphorylation was mediated by an increase in the activity of the nonhistone chromosomal protein kinases.[438,443]

7. Nonhistone Chromosomal Protein Phosphorylation During Carcinogenesis and Cell Transformation

During carcinogenesis or cell transformation, increases in the level of phosphorylation of specific molecular weight classes of nonhistone chromosomal polypeptides have been observed. These findings have been reported in breast carcinoma;[400] carcinogen-induced carcinogenesis in liver;[451-454] and in SV40 transformation of WI-38 human fibroblasts.[412,455] Changes in the activities of nuclear protein kinases have also been found during carcinogenesis.[126,456]

8. Effects of Histones on Nonhistone Chromosomal Protein Phosphorylation

In addition to hormones, drugs, and cAMP, the presence of histones also influences the phosphorylation of the nonhistone chromosomal proteins. The addition of histones stimulated the phosphorylation of a nonhistone chromosomal protein fraction by endogenous protein kinase.[457] At a histone to nonhistone protein ratio of 15, histones H2A, H4, and H1 were potent stimulators of nonhistone protein phosphorylation, whereas H2B and H3 were less effective. Under optimal conditions, H1 increased the rate and extent of phosphorylation by a factor of ten. The increase in phosphorylation was uniform throughout the spectrum of nonhistone proteins, and the histones themselves were not phosphorylated. This phenomenon was found to be specific for histones, and other small basic proteins such as cytochrome c had no effect on nonhistone protein phosphorylation.[457] The most probable mechanism for this is that the binding of histones by nonhistone proteins promotes an increase in the number of accessible phosphate-acceptor sites.

The effects of histones on nonhistone chromosomal protein phosphorylation have also been examined by the addition of highly purified histones to intact isolated nuclei.[458] These workers found that the histones quantitatively entered the nucleus and bound to the chromatin. The various histones had specific differential effects on nonhistone protein phosphorylation. H4 enhanced the phosphorylation of a low molecular weight (22,000 daltons) nonhistone protein by 70%, whereas H1 had a similar effect on proteins in the molecular weight range 30,000 to 60,000 daltons, and both these histones completely inhibited the phosphorylation of a polypeptide of 7,000 daltons. Histones H2A, H2B, and H3 had no significant effects on nonhistone protein phosphorylation. One nonhistone chromosomal protein which bound to the acetylated histones H1 and H4 was a histone deacetylase,[272] and this prompted the speculation[458] that there may be an interlocking control between nonhistone chromosomal protein phosphorylation and histone deacetylation.

9. Control of Gene Expression Through Phosphorylation of RNA Polymerases

A possible mechanism whereby nonhistone chromosomal proteins could control transcription is through direct interaction with the RNA polymerase molecules leading to a modification of their activity. There is evidence which suggests that one such modification is the phosphorylation of the RNA polymerases. The phosphorylation of bacterial RNA polymerases, with a concomitant increase in RNA synthesis, has been reported.[460,461] The first suggestion that a similar mechanism existed in eukaryotes were reports by several groups of the cAMP-dependent and -independent protein kinase-mediated activation of eukaryotic RNA polymerases I and II.[131,462-464] The stimulation of RNA polymerase activity may not have been due to the phosphorylation of the polymerases themselves but instead to the phosphorylation of another nonhistone chromosomal protein and the subsequent interaction of this phosphorylated protein with the polymerases. However, studies with purified polymerases have shown that several subunits of RNA polymerases from yeast[465,466] and rat liver[467] are phosphorylated in vitro and in vivo, and the phosphorylation of rat liver RNA polymerase I seems to be mediated by a cAMP-dependent protein kinase which was found to be closely associated with the polymerase.[468] The phosphorylation of the 24,000-dalton subunit of yeast RNA polymerase I was found to be essential for polymerase activity[469] and Kranias and co-workers have shown that the in vitro phosphorylation of calf thymus RNA poymerase II by both a homologous cAMP-dependent[470] and -independent protein kinase[471] increased the polymerase activity. However, it has not yet been demonstrated that this phosphorylation-mediated stimulation occurs in vivo. Phosphorylation may also be involved in the activation of DNA polymerases. A protein has been found which interacts with avian myeloblastosis virus DNA polymerase; in its dephosphorylated form, it had no effect on enzyme activity, but in its phosphorylated form, it increased the rate of DNA synthesis as much as tenfold.[472]

G. The Involvement of Nonhistone Chromosomal Proteins in Steroid Hormone Action

In addition to the findings that steroid hormones increase the rate of synthesis and phosphorylation of specific nonhistone chromosomal proteins, there is a large body of evidence which suggests that components of the nonhistone proteins mediate some of the primary actions of steroid hormones.[473-475]

After steroid hormones enter the cell, they form a complex with a "receptor" protein. The hormone-receptor complex then enters the nucleus and binds to the chromatin. The nature of the specific chromatin-binding sites has been extensively studied in vitro with both the isolated progesterone-receptor complex and oviduct nuclei. The hormone-receptor complex bound more extensively to chromatin than did the free hormone,[476] and these workers also found that the bound hormone could be reextracted from the chromatin as a hormone-receptor complex. This result suggested that the cytoplasmic receptor is itself, at some stage, a nonhistone chromosomal protein and is an example of the movement of some of these proteins between the cytoplasm, nucleoplasm, and chromatin. The hormone-receptor complex bound more extensively to oviduct chromatin than to chromatin of "nontarget" tissues,[476] suggesting that the chromatin of target tissue contained specific "acceptor sites" for the hormone-receptor complex.

The use of chromatin reconstitution techniques showed that the nonhistone chromosomal proteins, and not the histones, are involved in the tissue-specific binding of the hormone-receptor complex.[152,476] Therefore, both the receptor and acceptor molecules for progesterone may be considerd nonhistone chromosomal proteins. A heterogeneous fraction of nonhistone proteins which contained the acceptor sites was isolated[165] and was shown by immunological techniques[325] to be tissue-specific. Similar results were obtained for the chromatin binding of several steroid hormones including corticosterone and estradiol,[477] thyroid hormone,[478] and testosterone.[479]

Multiple binding sites for the progesterone-receptor complex have been found,[480,481] and these binding sites have different binding affinities for the hormone-receptor complex. Most of the high-affinity, tissue-specific binding sites were masked by nonhistone chromosomal proteins.[480,482] This was also found to be the case for testosterone-binding sites.[479] Chromatin acceptor sites for the progesterone-receptor complex seem to be present in "nontarget" as well as "target" tissues; however, in the nontarget tissues, they are completely masked by nonhistone chromosomal proteins.[475,483] In the developing oviduct, marked changes in the extent of availability of acceptor sites have been observed.[483,484] The receptor-progesterone complex seems to be associated with particular DNA sites in the genome.[475,485] These sites may represent specific sequences of DNA to which the acceptor proteins are selectively bound. Thus, nonhistone chromosomal proteins may constitute part of the acceptor sites for steroid hormones, define the segment of the genome to which the hormone is bound, and regulate the availability of the acceptor sites. Since, in their target tissues, steroid hormones increase the number of sites available for transcription[486] and activate the transcription of defined messenger RNA sequences such as ovalbumin[487] mRNA, the mediation of their action by nonhistone chromosomal proteins is strong evidence supporting the role of these proteins in selective gene expression.

H. DNA Binding of Nonhistone Chromosomal Proteins

Selective gene expression implies the restriction of some genetic loci and the specific activation of others, and there is evidence supporting the hypothesis that nonhistone chromosomal proteins play a role in these processes. If this is, indeed, the case, it is reasonable to postulate that the mechanisms through which transcriptional control is achieved will depend, in part, on associations between these proteins and DNA. In prokaryotes, there are several examples of DNA-binding proteins that regulate RNA synthesis, for example, the lac repressor[1,3] which inhibits transcription of the lac operon, and the cAMP receptor protein which selectively facilitates initiation of lac and gal mRNAs.[488,489]

Specific DNA-binding nonhistone proteins have been isolated by several groups of workers, and the techniques used, together with their associated problems, were described in the section on fractionating the nonhistone chromosomal proteins by DNA affinity techniques. In this section, we will discuss some of the properties of these DNA-binding proteins which may have a bearing on their postulated role in the control of gene expression.

Only a small proportion of the total nonhistone chromosomal proteins binds specifically to homologous DNA,[168] and many of these proteins are phosphoproteins.[225] Some groups have found that these proteins are highly heterogeneous,[161,225] whereas others suggest that they are composed of only a small number of low molecular weight proteins.[168,223,226] Although most groups have reported that nonhistone proteins bind selectively to homologous DNA,[161,168,224,330] Jost et al.[334] found little, if any, species-specific binding and argued that, similar to the case of histones, interaction with DNA has severely restricted the evolutionary diversity of these proteins. The HMG proteins appear to be a subset of the nonhistone DNA-binding proteins.[221,332,333] These proteins are present in a wide variety of species and have little species specificity.[23] Thus, the HMG proteins (analogously to the histones) may be involved in some general interaction with DNA, whereas other, species-specific, DNA-binding proteins may play a role in more selective DNA interactions of the type expected in transcriptional control, for example, by binding a specific nucleotide sequence as does the lac repressor in *Escherichia coli*.[3] However, this type of repressor-DNA interaction would be complicated in eukaryotes by the existence of repetitive DNA sequences.[490] Some nonhistone proteins bind preferentially to repetitive sequences and others to unique sequences.[229,231,233] Preferential binding to single- or double-stranded DNA is also exhibited by these proteins.[227,229,231,232] The preferential binding of nonhistone chromosomal proteins to unique or repetitive DNA sequences may be of consequence in postulating mechanisms of gene control and chromatin structure.

Eukaryotic DNA-unwinding proteins have been isolated which unwind DNA helices and stabilize the resulting single strands.[227,262,491,492] These proteins bind preferentially to A-T-rich regions[227,491] and stimulate homologous DNA polymerase-α.[492] A protein which binds preferentially to A-T-rich regions of DNA has been isolated from rat liver and found to decrease in amount during growth.[208]

While undoubtedly DNA binding represents a powerful tool for isolation of subsets of the chromosomal proteins, caution must be exercised in assuming that the types of protein-DNA interactions which are observed by these affinity methods are biologically meaningful and are those which occur in the nuclei of intact cells.

VII. DIRECT EVIDENCE FOR NONHISTONE CHROMOSOMAL PROTEINS AS REGULATORY MOLECULES

A. Effects of Nonhistone Chromosomal Proteins on Chromatin Template Activity

The evidence already discussed indicates that there is a correlation between the amount and type of nonhistone chromosomal proteins and the RNA synthetic capacity of a tissue. More direct evidence for the involvement of these proteins in the control of gene transcription comes from experiments in which the effects of these proteins on chromatin template activity were studied by the incorporation of radioactively labeled nucleotides into RNA in the presence of bacterial or homologous RNA polymerase. Wang[493] and Kamiyama and Wang[494] found that a fraction of nonhistone chromosomal proteins stimulated RNA synthesis from rat liver chromatin. This activation was later shown to be specific to the tissue of origin of the nonhistone proteins.[320,495,496] Nonhistone chromosomal proteins were also found to stimulate the template activity of pure DNA using bacterial[161,497] or homologous RNA polymerase.[498] Transcription was only stimulated by homologous nonhistone proteins and was due to an increase in the number of RNA chains initiated. The protein fractions that stimulated transcription were rich in phosphoproteins, and there was a correlation between their level of protein kinase activity and their degree of activation of RNA synthesis.[113,499,500] Dephosphorylating the nonhistone proteins abolished their stimulatory effect.[498] These results support correlations, discussed previously, between the degree of nonhistone chromosomal protein phosphorylation and the transcriptional activity of a tissue.

A loosely bound, phosphate-rich nonhistone chromosomal protein fraction which stimulated the template capacity of homologous DNA in the presence of homologous RNA polymerase II was isolated from Ehrlich ascites tumor.[192] No stimulation was observed when a bacterial polymerase was used, indicating that the activation process may involve some form of specific interaction between the nonhistone proteins and the polymerase. In addition to proteins which stimulate transcriptional activity, a tightly bound nonhistone chromosomal phosphoprotein which inhibits transcription has also been isolated from Ehrlich ascites cells.[501] The inhibitory effect of this protein was not altered by the addition of excess RNA polymerase but was reduced by increasing the amount of DNA, indicating that the inhibitory reaction involved the template and not the enzyme. The transcription stimulator bound selectively to unique sequences of DNA and activated their transcription,[502] whereas the inhibitor protein bound to, and inhibited the transcription of, only reiterated DNA sequences.[503] The same group of workers isolated a nonhistone protein from calf thymus which had a similar inhibitory effect on transcription. However, the calf thymus and Ehrlich ascites inhibitors differed in molecular weight and subunit composition and only inhibited transcription from homologous DNA.[504] Thus, both the stimulatory and inhibitory proteins act in a tissue-specific manner which suggests that they are capable of recognizing and binding to specific tissue-specific DNA sequences. Several other groups have also isolated nonhistone chromosomal proteins which stimulate eukaryotic RNA polymerase II[505-509] or I.[236,507,510] In one case, a protein factor which enhances the formation of initiation complexes[509] was found to be active only when another "helper" protein was bound to the polymerase.[511]

While these results are, indeed, consistent with a regulatory role for components of the complex and heterogeneous nonhistone chromosomal proteins, caution must be exercised in interpretation of data from these experiments. Direct addition of nonhistone chromosomal proteins to protein-DNA complexes may result in nonspecific aggregation. Additionally, results from such experiments do not provide definitive answers with respect to regulation of specific genetic sequences.

B. Nonhistone Chromosomal Proteins and Transcription of Specific Genetic Sequences

The techniques of chromatin reconstitution and in vitro transcription and the availability of complementary DNA probes for specific genetic sequences have facilitated assessment of the involvement of nonhistone chromosomal proteins in the transcription of several genes; the globin, ovalbumin, and histone genes have been studied most extensively. Globin gene expression is discussed in the chapter by Gilmour in Volume I, and O'Malley et al. have recently reviewed the work from his laboratory on regulation of ovalbumin gene expression.[513] In this chapter, we will focus on studies carried out in this laboratory directed toward understanding the role of nonhistone chromosomal proteins in the transcription of histone genes from chromatin during the cell cycle.

1. Evidence for Cell Cycle Stage-Specific Histone Gene Transcription

Several lines of evidence suggest that transcription of histone mRNA sequences is restricted to the S phase of the cell cycle. Early evidence which was interpreted to support synthesis of histone mRNA only during S phase in continuously dividing HeLa cells came from pulse-labeling experiments in which ^{3}H-uridine-labeled 7-9S RNAs were isolated from the polysomes of S phase cells but not from the polysomes of G_1 cells.[514] This observation is consistent with the possibility of transcriptional control of gene expression, an interpretation which is further supported by in vitro translation[515,516] and nucleic acid hybridization[517] data suggesting the presence of histone mRNA sequences on the polysomes, in the postpolysomal cytoplasmic fraction, and in the nuclei of S phase, but not G_1 phase, HeLa cells. Other data suggesting that control of histone gene expression may be mediated transcriptionally come from experiments which show that nuclei[215,518] and chromatin[519] of S phase, but not G_1, HeLa cells transcribe RNAs which hybridize with a ^{3}H-labeled DNA complementary to the mRNAs for the five principal histones. Similar results were obtained following stimulation of nondividing human diploid fibroblasts to proliferate.[520]

While taken together these results seem to support control of histone gene readout residing at least in part at the transcriptional level, caution must be exercised in interpreting the in vitro translation and transcription experiments. The limits of detection of histones synthesized in vitro when very small quantities of RNA template are available leave something to be desired. Interpretation of data from in vitro nuclear transcription experiments is complicated by an inability to establish definitively the initiation of RNA chains in vitro and by the presence of endogenous nuclear histone mRNA sequences. Results from in vitro chromatin transcription experiments can be misleading since trancription is carried out with bacterial RNA polymerase, and endogenous chromatin-associated RNA sequences can also interfere with evaluation of nucleic acid hybridization. It must also be pointed out that because, in the experiments just described, hybridization was carried out in RNA excess using unlabeled RNA and a ^{3}H-labeled histone DNA complementary to the mRNAs for the five histones, the presence of rapidly turning over histone mRNA sequences in the nuclear RNA or in the nuclear or chromatin transcripts of G_1 cells might not have been detected. In fact, Melli et al.[521] have detected the presence of histone mRNA sequences in the nucleus throughout the cell cycle of HeLa cells by hybridizing ^{3}H-labeled RNA with excess sea urchin histone DNA. However, there are some reservations concerning the experiments of Melli et al.[521] (1) The method utilized for cell synchronization was double thymidine block, a procedure which results in at least 20% of the G_1 and G_2 cells actually being S phase cells (as measured by ^{3}H-thymidine labeling and autoradiography). This is in contrast to experiments in which the HeLa cDNA probe was used and in which G_1 cells were obtained by mitotic selective detachment, a procedure which yields a population of G_1 cells containing less than 0.1% S phase cells. (2) Hybridization analysis of HeLa cell RNAs was carried out with sea urchin DNA and there appears to be only 10 to 15% sequence homology between human and sea urchin histone sequences.[556]

Determination of the presence or absence of histone mRNA sequence in G_2 HeLa cells is complex. By nucleic acid hybridization analysis, we have observed a limited representation of histone mRNA sequences in the polysomal, postpolysomal cyto-plasmic, and nuclear RNA fractions of G_2 cells.[522] The rate of hybridization of these subcellular RNA fractions from G_2 cells with histone cDNA is approximately 20% of that observed with similar RNA fractions of S phase cells. However, thymidine label-ing followed by autoradiography indicates that at least 20% of the G_2 population (ob-tained by double thymidine block or mitotic selective detachment) consists of cells which are undergoing DNA replication.[28] Because effective methodologies are not available for obtaining a pure population of G_2 phase HeLa cells, it is difficult to determine unequivocally whether or not G_2 cells contain histone mRNA sequences.

2. Chromosomal Proteins and Regulation of Histone Gene Expression

If control of histone gene expression is mediated at the transcriptional level, it be-comes important to identify and characterize the nuclear and chromatin components (chromosomal proteins and/or RNAs) which render histone sequences transcribable. If control of histone gene expression is at a posttranscriptional level and the synthesis of histone mRNA sequences occurs throughout the cell cycle, it is still important to determine the mechanism by which the genes are rendered transcribable and main-tained in a transcriptionally active structural configuration. Posttranscriptional regu-lation of histone gene expression during the cell cycle also raises a broad spectrum of questions relevant to posttranscriptonal mechanisms: Are there variations in the rate of turnover of histone mRNA sequences in various intracellular compartments during the cell cycle? Are there cell cycle stage-specific changes in the abilities of histone mRNA sequences to be translated in vitro? Are there differences in proteins associated with histone mRNA sequences during the cell cycle? Are there variations in the pres-ence or activity of enzymes involved in the processing and/or degradation of histone mRNA sequences during the cell cycle? Are there changes in the binding of histone mRNAs to ribosomes during the cell cycle, resulting from alterations in histone mRNAs and/or the properties of the ribosomes? Unfortunately, to date, little is under-stood regarding processes associated with posttranscriptional regulation of the expres-sion of protein-coding genes in eukaryotes, and most of these questions are beyond the scope of this chapter.

a. Nonhistone Chromosomal Proteins and Histone Gene Transcription in Continu-ously Dividing Cells

A role for nonhistone chromosomal proteins in the regulation of gene expression during the cell cycle has been suggested by several lines of evidence. Variations ob-served in the composition and metabolism of the nonhistone chromosomal proteins during G_1, G_2, S, and mitosis and their correlation with changes in transcription are consistent with a regulatory function for these proteins (reviewed in references 473 and 523). Further evidence that nonhistone chromosomal proteins may be responsible for specific transcription at various stages of the cell cycle comes from a series of chro-matin reconstitution studies which indicate that nonhistone chromosomal proteins are involved in determining the quantitative differences in availability of DNA as template for RNA synthesis during the cell cycle of continuously dividing cells,[525] as well as after stimulation of nondividing cells to proliferate.[526]

To examine the involvement of nonhistone chromosomal proteins in rendering hi-stone genes available for transcription in vitro from chromatin during the cell cycle, we have pursued the following approach. Chromatin isolated from G_1 and S phase cells was dissociated in 3 M NaCl, 5 M urea, and each chromatin preparation was fractionated into DNA, histones, and nonhistone chromosomal proteins. Chromatin preparations were then reconstituted by the gradient dialysis procedure of Bekhor et al.[173] utilizing DNA and histones pooled from G_1 and S phase cells and either G_1 or S phase nonhistone chromosomal proteins. Essentially DNA, histones, and nonhistone chromosomal proteins were combined in high-salt-urea, and the salt was progressively removed by stepwise dialysis, followed by removal of the urea. In vitro RNA transcripts from chromatin reconstituted with G_1 nonhistone chromosomal proteins and from chromatin reconstituted with S phase nonhistone chromosomal proteins were annealed with histone cDNA. RNA transcripts from chromatin reconstituted with S phase nonhistone chromosomal proteins hybridized with histone cDNA while those from chromatin reconstituted with G_1 nonhistone chromosomal proteins did not exhibit a significant degree of hybrid formation. It should be emphasized that the kinetics of hybridization with the cDNA were the same for transcripts of native S phase chromatin and transcripts of chromatin reconstituted with S phase nonhistone chromosomal protein (Cr_o $t_{1/2} = 2 \times 10^{-1}$). Furthermore, the amount of RNA transcribed and the recoveries during isolation of these transcripts from native and reconstituted preparations were essentially identical. These results[519] suggest the possibility that nonhistone chromosomal proteins may be involved in determining the availability of histone sequences for transcription from chromatin during the cell cycle. Such a regulatory role for nonhistone chromosomal proteins is in agreement with results from several laboratories which have pointed to these proteins as potentially important for tissue-specific transcription of globin genes.[527-529]

i. Fidelity of Chromatin Reconstitution and Transcription

Several lines of evidence have previously suggested similarity of native and reconstituted chromatin.[173,525,526,530-533] However, because chromatin reconstitution has been extensively used in our studies, considerable effort over the past several years has been devoted to assessing the validity of the procedure. Native and reconstituted chromatin from HeLa cells were compared with respect to the following parameters and found to be indistinguishable:[534] (1) the banding patterns of histones and nonhistone chromosomal proteins when fractionated electrophoretically according to charge and molecular weight on polyacrylamide gels; (2) the binding of histones and nonhistone chromosomal proteins in chromatin when assayed by extractibility with dilute mineral acid and ionic detergents; (3) the extent of γ-ray-induced thymine damage in the DNA; (4) the availability of sites for binding of "reporter molecules" which exhibit specificity for intercalation in the major or minor grooves of the DNA helix; (5) the circular dichroism spectra; and (6) the in vitro transcription under conditions which prohibit reinitiation. Additional evidence for fidelity of chromatin reconstitution is that Cr_o $t_{1/2}$ values for the hybridization of histone cDNA with RNA transcripts from native and reconstituted S phase chromatin do not differ significantly (2×10^{-1} in both cases).[519] This result suggests that histone genes are transcribed to the same extent from native and reconstituted chromatin. In other systems, reconstituted chromatin has been reported to transcribe, with fidelity, globin[527-529] and ovalbumin[487,535] genes as well as total poly(A)$^+$ mRNA species.[557] However, at least with respect to globin gene transcription, the possibility has recently been raised that bona fide transcription of these genes does not occur in vitro — from native or reconstituted chromatin.[536,537]

It must also be emphasized that absolute criteria for fidelity of chromatin reconstitution have not been established and that numerous parameters of native and reconstituted chromatin have not been compared. Yet still, it seems rather naive to assume that native and reconstituted chromatin are structurally and functionally identical in every respect. It is quite clear, however, that chromatin reconstitution provides a potentially important approach for further defining the roles of chromosomal proteins in the structural and transcriptional properties of chromatin, particularly with defined

DNA sequences, thus necessitating critical evaluation of the technique and its applications. It should also be pointed out that although the structure and function of chromatin are interrelated, it has not yet been resolved which components of chromatin structure must be preserved during reconstitution to retain integrity of function. For example, Woodcock[538] has reported that the method we have been using for chromatin reconstitution does not efficiently reconstruct the "beads on a string" type structures seen by electron microsopy; but this does not necessarily indicate that the nuclease digest pattern generated by nucleosomes or transcriptional fidelity have been lost.

Extreme caution must also be exercised with regard to in vitro chromatin transcription and interpretation of results from such experiments. Meeting the following criteria should be considered minimal to justify chromatin as a bona fide in vitro system which reflects, with complete in vivo fidelity, the transcription of histone mRNA sequences:

1. The probe used to identify histone mRNA sequences should be homologous and should accurately reflect the complete mRNA. Eventually it will be desirable for the probe to represent all the nucleotide sequences of the primary gene transcript. Specific probes should be available so that hybridization analysis of histone gene transcripts can be carried out in RNA as well as in DNA excess.
2. Conditions for RNA transcription, isolation of transcripts, and hybridization analysis should be such that endogenous, chromatin-associated RNAs do not interfere with quantitation of histone gene transcripts.
3. Precautions must be taken to eliminate or account for RNA-dependent RNA synthesis when transcription is carried out with *Escherichia coli* RNA polymerase. Eventually it will be desirable to transcribe chromatin with the appropriate homologous RNA polymerase — in which case it would be necessary to demonstrate that *only* the enzyme responsible for transcription of histone genes in vivo is operative in the in vitro system.
4. It should be established that initiation of RNA synthesis is taking place in vitro, not merely elongaion of RNA molecules initiated in vivo.
5. It would be desirable to establish that initiation and termination of transcription in vitro from chromatin are at the sites on the DNA molecule at which they occur in vivo.
6. It should be shown that the degree of symmetric or asymmetric transcription of histone genes from chromatin is the same as that which takes place in intact cells.
7. In addition to establishing fidelity of histone gene transcription from chromatin in vitro, it is necessary to show that the availability *and* lack of availability of other genetic sequences for in vitro transcription from chromatin reflect transcription in intact cells.

Not all of the above criteria need to be met for in vitro chromatin transcription to be a useful model system for examining regulation of histone gene expression. In fact, failure to meet certain of these criteria may provide information regarding structural and functional properties of chromatin. However, in order to consider in vitro chromatin transcription justifiable for studying the regulation of histone gene expression, it must be unambiguously shown that histone mRNA sequences are transcribed in vitro only from chromatin derived from cells in which the genes are transcribed in vivo.

ii. In Vitro Transcription of Histone mRNA Sequences from DNA and DNA-Chromosomal Protein Complexes

To elucidate further the manner in which histones and nonhistone chromosomal proteins interact to render histone genes transcribable in HeLa S$_3$ cells, we have examined in vitro transcription of histone mRNA sequences from DNA as well as from several DNA-chromosomal protein complexes.[539] Our results suggest that DNA is an effective template for transcription of histone mRNA sequences and that histones by themselves inhibit transcription from DNA, including transcription of histone genes, in a dose-dependent, nonspecific manner. When complexed to DNA alone, nonhistone chromosomal proteins from either G_1 or S phase cells do not affect the transcription of histone mRNA sequences. However, when associated with DNA in the presence of histones, nonhistone chromosomal proteins from S phase seem to render histone genes transcribable selectively. A possible role for nonhistone chromosomal proteins in mediating the interaction of histones with DNA to render histone genes transcribable is, therefore, indicated and is consistent with a histone displacement model.[540,541]

iii. G_1 vs. S phase Nonhistone Chromosomal Proteins as Mediators of In Vitro Histone Gene Transcription

We have attempted to address the question of whether the difference in the in vitro transcription of histone genes from G_1 and S phase chromatin is due to a component of the S phase nonhistone chromosomal proteins which renders histone genes transcribable or, alternatively, to a specific component of the G_1 nonhistone chromosomal proteins which inhibits histone gene transcription.[542,543] If the difference in histone gene activity of G_1 and S phase chromatin were due to a component which is present or operative only in S phase, one would anticipate that the dissociation of G_1 chromatin with high-salt and urea followed by reconstitution in the presence of S phase nonhistone chromosomal proteins would result in an increase in the availability of histone genes for transcription. One would not anticipate any major effect on in vitro histone gene transcription if S phase chromatin were reconstituted in the presence of G_1 nonhistone chromosomal proteins. In contrast, if the difference in in vitro histone gene transcription of G_1 and S phase chromatin can be accounted for by a component of the nonhistone chromosomal proteins which is associated with chromatin during the G_1 phase of the cell cycle, one would anticipate that dissociation of S phase chromatin followed by reconstitution in the presence of increasing amounts of G_1 nonhistone chromosomal proteins would result in a progressive decrease in the availability of histone genes for transcription. If the latter alternative prevails, the presence of S phase chromosomal proteins during reconstitution would not be expected to affect significantly the in vitro transcription of histone genes from G_1 chromatin. If the regulation of in vitro histone gene transcription from chromatin involves G_1 and S phase proteins acting in an antagonistic manner, one would anticipate a more complex, intermediate result.

We observed that when G_1 chromatin was dissociated and then reconstituted in the presence of increasing amounts of S phase nonhistone chromosomal proteins, hybridization between in vitro transcripts of these chromatins and histone cDNA was seen at progressively lower $C_r{}_ot_{1/2}$ values, indicating that the presence of S phase nonhistone chromosomal proteins resulted in a dose-dependent increase in availability of histone genes for transcription from G_1 chromatin. By comparing the kinetics of the hybridization of histone cDNA and in vitro transcripts from S phase chromatin ($C_{r_o}t_{1/2} = 2 \times 10^{-1}$) with the kinetics of the hybridization of histone cDNA and in vitro transcripts from G_1 chromatin reconstituted with a 1:1 ratio of S phase nonhistone chromosomal protein to DNA ($C_{r_o}t_{1/2} = 3 \times 10^{-1}$), it can be determined that histone genes from G_1 chromatin can be rendered transcribable to approximately the same degree as in native S phase chromatin. A dose-dependent increase in the availability of histone genes for in vitro transcription was also observed when G_1 chromatin was dissociated and reconstituted with increasing amounts of total chromosomal proteins from S phase HeLa cells. The fidelity of the hybrids formed between the transcripts and histone cDNA as well as the validity of comparing $C_r{}_ot_{1/2}$ values is suggested by the fact that the melting temperature (T_m) of the hybrids in all cases is the same as the T_m of the hybrids formed between histone mRNA and histone ^{3}H-cDNA. Also, the maximal hybridization as estimated by a double reciprocal plot is equal, in all cases, to that of the histone mRNA-cDNA hybridization reaction. In contrast, when G_1 chromatin was dissociated and then reconstituted in the presence of S phase histones, even at a 1:1 ratio of S phase histone to DNA, a significant stimulation of the in vitro transcription of histone genes was not observed. It should be noted that there were no significant differences among the various chromatin preparations in the yield or recovery of RNA during isolation, even though the presence of S phase nonhistone chromosomal proteins during reconstitution caused a greater than 1000-fold stimulation in the amount of histone sequences transcribed from G_1 chromatin. Therefore, the observed increase in the representation of histone mRNA sequences cannot be attributed to nonspecific alteration of template activity. Stimulation of in vitro histone gene transcription was not observed when G_1 chromatin was dissociated and then reconstituted in the presence of additional G_1 chromosomal proteins — even at a 1:1 ratio of additional protein to DNA. The latter result suggests the possibility that specific chromosomal proteins are required to render histone sequences transcribable.

To address the possibility that the small amount of nucleic acid present in the S phase chromosomal proteins is responsible for the observed hybridization with histone ^{3}H-cDNA, either by containing histone sequences or by having the ability to render histone genes transcribable, the residual nucleic acid was removed from the S phase chromosomal proteins by buoyant density centrifugation in CsCl-urea.[543] There was no significant difference in the kinetics of hybridization with histone cDNA of transcripts of G_1 chromatin reconstituted with equal amounts of either CsCl-treated S phase chromosomal proteins or untreated S phase chromosomal proteins — the hybridization reactions in both cases had $Cr_0t_{1/2}$ values of 2×10^{-1}. Total chromosomal proteins, as well as fractions of S phase nonhistone chromosomal proteins, were assayed by this procedure. These results suggest that it is a protein component of the S phase chromatin and not a nucleic acid which is responsible for rendering histone sequences transcribable. Of course, the possibility of nucleic acid covalently bound to an S phase nonhistone chromosomal protein cannot be totally dismissed. However, results from chromatin reconstitution experiments with nuclease-treated S phase nonhistone chromosomal proteins are inconsistent with the latter alternative.[215,216] In the nuclease experiments, 3.4 μg/mℓ of nonhistone chromosomal proteins in 2 M urea-0.1 M Tris-1 mM CaCl$_2$ (pH 8.3) were digested for 30 min at 37°C with 0.06 μg/mℓ of micrococcal nuclease (a quantity of micrococcal nuclease sufficient to degrade at least 50 μg/mℓ of single- and double-stranded nucleic acids under these conditions). The nuclease reaction, which is calcium-dependent, was stopped by the addition of [ethylene-bis(oxyethylenenitrile)]tetraacetic acid (EGTA) to a final concentration of 5 mM. Control and nuclease-digested nonhistone chromosomal protein preparations were compared for ability to render histone sequences in G_1 chromatin transcribable by the reconstitution-transcription assay described above. Nuclease treatment did not decrease the ability of the nonhistone chromosomal proteins to render histone genes transcribable. However, when S phase nonhistone chromosomal proteins were treated with agarose-immobilized chymotrypsin, their abiity to render histone genes transcribable was lost.[215,216] These nuclease and protease experiments seem to support the involvement of a protein or proteins in regulation of in vitro histone gene transcription from chromatin. However, the possibility cannot be overlooked that nucleic acid tightly complexed with protein (such that it is resistant to micrococcal nuclease) is necessary for the protein to be active in the reconstitution-transcription system.

To investigate whether G_1 chromatin contains an inhibitor of histone gene transcription which is degraded or inactivated as cells progress from the G_1 to the S phase of the cell cycle, chromatin from S phase cells was dissociated and then reconstituted in the presence of total chomosomal proteins from G_1 phase cells.[543] The ability of transcripts from this reconstituted chromatin preparation to hybridize with histone cDNA was determined. The presence of G_1 total chromosomal protein — even at a 1:1 ratio of G_1 total chromosomal protein to DNA — did not significantly inhibit histone gene transcription from S phase chromatin. This is not to say that there is nothing in G_1 chromosomal proteins which can inhibit histone gene transciption. We have observed that histones inhibit transcription of histone genes from naked DNA to the same degree which they inhibit total RNA synthesis. However, it appears that there is nothing in G_1 chromosomal proteins which can inhibit in vitro histone gene transcription in the presence of S phase chromosomal proteins. This would suggest that any additional specific repressor of histone gene transcription is lost during isolation, dissociation, fractionation, or reconstitution, or that any inhibition of histone gene transcription by G_1 chromosomal proteins can be overridden by S phase chromosomal proteins. Similar results were obtained when S phase chromatin was dissociated and then reconstituted in the presence of G_1 phase nonhistone chromosomal proteins. Again, the T_m of the hybrids formed and the maximal hybridization were the same as seen with the histone mRNA-cDNA reaction.

These results provide support for the contention that the difference in the in vitro transcription of histone sequences from G_1 and S phase chromatin is due to the nonhistone chromosomal protein portion of the genome. Furthermore, this difference may be accounted for by a component (or components) of the S phase nonhistone chromosomal protein which has the ability to render histone genes of G_1 phase chromatin available for transcription in a dose-dependent fashion. These results do not indicate which component (or components) on the S phase nonhistone chromosomal proteins is responsible or by what mechanism it may act, but they do provide an assay which we are currently using to monitor fractionation and characterization of nonhistone chromosomal proteins which possess the ability to render histone genes transcribable in vitro from chromatin. We want to emphasize that there may exist in intact cells an additional level of regulation which does not function, or is not recognized, in the in vitro reconstitution-transcription system, perhaps involving homologous eukaryotic polymerases.

b. Regulation of Histone Gene Expression in Human Diploid Cells Stimulated to Proliferate

The control of histone gene expression was similarly studied in nondividing human diploid fibroblasts following stimulation to proliferate.[520] Hybridization analysis of RNAs isolated from various intracellular compartments suggests the presence of histone mRNAs only in cells undergoing DNA synthesis and transcription of histone mRNA sequences only from chromatin of S phase cells. Chromatin reconstitution experiments provide evidence for a role for the nonhistone chromosomal proteins in the regulation of histone gene transcription.

c. Fractionation of Nonhistone Chromosomal Proteins

In order to isolate macromolecules involved in the regulation of specific genes, it is necessary to determine not only whether a given fraction has activity but also how much activity is present. If activity is found only in one fraction, without the ability to quantitate one cannot tell whether the activity has been destroyed in the other fractions, whether all the components of the activity are present only in that fraction, or whether the activity has actually been fractionated. Our laboratory has used the techniques of chromatin reconstitution and in vitro transcription in an attempt to assay and quantitate the activity of nonhistone protein fractions and their involvement in determining the availability of histone genes for transcription in vitro from chromatin.[215,544] The approach which has been used to assay protein fractions for ability to render histone genes transcribable is as follows. G_1 chromatin, which does not serve as a template for in vitro histone gene transcription, was dissociated in 3 M NaCl-5 M urea and reconstituted in the presence of added S phase nonhistone chromosomal protein fractions. Reconstituted chromatin preparations were then transcribed in a cell-free system with *E. coli* RNA polymerase, and transcripts were assayed for their ability to hybridize with histone cDNA. When G_1 chromatin was dissociated and then reconstituted in the presence of increasing amounts (10, 100, and 1000 μg) of S phase nonhistone chromosomal proteins per milligram of G_1 DNA (as chromatin), a progressive and dose-dependent increase in the representation of histone mRNA sequences in the RNA transcripts from these preparations (as shown in Figure 1) was observed. This increase is indicated by progressively lower $Cr_ot_{1/2}$ values for the hybridization reactions of chromatin transcripts and histone cDNA, suggesting that histone genes are being made available for transcription. Such enhancement of histone gene transcription was not seen when G_1 chromatin was reconstituted in the presence of additional G_1 chromosomal proteins. Since this system responds to additional S phase nonhistone chromosomal proteins by rendering histone genes transcribable in a somewhat dose-dependent manner, it appears that we have a method for monitoring nonhistone chromosomal protein fractionation.

We have recently been able to achieve approximately a 100-fold purification of S phase HeLa cell nonhistone chromosomal proteins which exhibit ability to render histone mRNA sequences transcribable from chromatin. This fractionation of S phase HeLa cell nonhistone chromosomal proteins has been accomplished by ion-exchange chromatography and then gel-filtration chromatography.[215,216,544]

Ion-exchange chromatography of S phase HeLa cell chromosomal proteins on QAE-Sephadex® was carried out as follows: Chromosomal proteins from which nucleic acids had been removed by ultracentrifugation were dialyzed against 5 M urea-10 mM Tris (pH 8.3) and were loaded on the column of QAE-Sephadex® A-25, previously equilibrated with the same buffer. The proteins were then eluted with two column volumes each of 5 M urea-10 mM Tris (pH 8.3) containing 0, 0.1, 0.25, 0.5, and 3.0 M NaCl. As shown in Figure 2, the histones and approximately 10% of the nonhistone chromosomal proteins were not bound and were eluted in the void volume, whereas a complex but electrophoretically distinct class of nonhistone chromosomal proteins was eluted by each salt concentration (as shown in Figure 3). The total recovery of protein from the column was approximately 85%. In order to determine the ability of each of the QAE fractions to render histone genes available for transcription, 3 mg of chromatin from G_1 phase cells (containing approximately 1 mg of DNA) were dissociated with 3 M NaCl-5 M urea-10 mM Tris (pH 8.3) and were reconstituted in the presence of 100 μg of each of the QAE fractions. The reconstituted chromatin was then transcribed in vitro with *E. coli* RNA polymerase, and the isolated transcripts were assayed for histone mRNA sequences by hybridization to histone cDNA. As shown in Figure 4, the transcripts from G_1 chromatin reconstituted in the presence of the unbound fraction or in the presence of material eluted with 0.1, 0.25, or 3 M NaCl did not show significant hybrid formation with histone cDNA — the same results observed with transcripts from native G_1 chromatin. In contrast, even though the total amount of RNA was similar, transcripts from G_1 chromatin reconstituted in the presence of the 0.5 M NaCl fraction hybridized efficiently with histone cDNA ($Cr_o t_{1/2} = 4 \times 10^{-1}$).

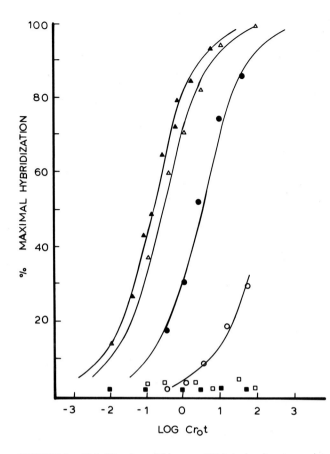

FIGURE 1. Hybridization of histone cDNA to in vitro transcripts from G_1 phase HeLa chromatin reconstituted in the presence of various amounts of S phase HeLa nonhistone chromosomal proteins. cDNA was annealed to RNA transcripts from G_1 chromatin reconstituted in the presence of 0.01 (○), 0.10 (●), or 1.00 (△) mg of S phase nonhistone chromosomal protein or 1.0 mg of S phase histones (□) per milligram of G_1 DNA as chromatin. cDNA was also annealed to RNA transcripts from G_1 chromatin reconstituted in the presence of 1.0 mg of G_1 total chromosomal protein per milligram of G_1 DNA as chromatin (■) and to RNA transcripts from native chromatin of S (▲) phase cells.

As discussed previously, when G_1 chromatin was reconstituted in the presence of various amounts of S phase chromosomal proteins, there was a dose-dependent increase in histone gene transcription. Specifically, transcripts from G_1 chromatin reconstituted in the presence of 1000 μg of S phase chromosomal proteins per milligram of G_1 chromatin DNA contained approximately ten times more histone mRNA sequences than transcripts from the same amount of G_1 chromatin reconstituted in the presence of 100 μg of these proteins. Since the 0.5 M NaCl fraction contained only approximately 10% of the total chromosomal protein, one would anticipate that 100 μg of the 0.5 M NaCl fraction should render histone genes transcribable from G_1 chromatin to the same degree as 1000 μg of the total S phase HeLa chromosomal proteins. As can be seen in Figure 4, there are no significant differences in the kinetics of hybrid formation with histone cDNA between transcripts from G_1 phase chromatin reconstituted in the presence of 100 μg of the 0.5 M NaCl fraction and 1000 μg of the total

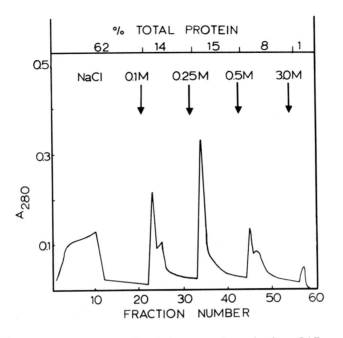

FIGURE 2.   Elution profile of chromosomal proteins from QAE-Sephadex®. Proteins were loaded in 5 *M* urea-10 m*M* Tris-HCl (pH 8.3), and were eluted with this buffer containing 0.10 *M*, 0.25 *M*, and 3.0 *M* NaCl. The percentage of protein eluted in each peak is shown in the upper panel.

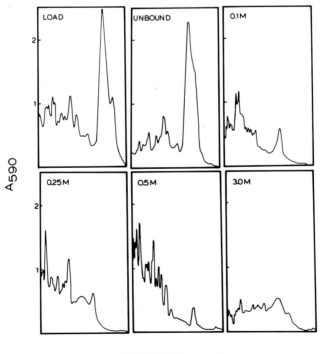

FIGURE 3.   SDS polyacrylamide gel electrophoretic profiles of chromosomal proteins fractionated with QAE-Sephadex®.

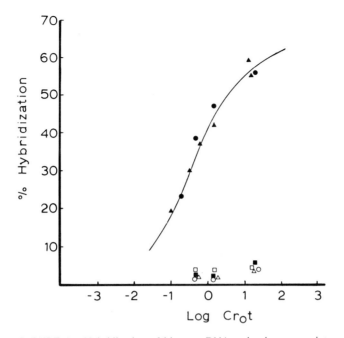

FIGURE 4. Hybridization of histone cDNA to in vitro transcripts from G_1 HeLa chromatin reconstituted in the presence of S phase HeLa cell chromosomal protein fractions. Transcripts from 1 mg of G_1 DNA as chromatin reconstituted in the presence of 100 μg of S phase chromosomal proteins eluted from QAE-Sephadex® A-25 by 5 M urea-10 mM Tris (pH 8.3) containing 0 M (□), 0.1 M (■), 0.25 M (○), 0.5 M (•) and 3.0 M (△) NaCl or in the presence of 1000 μg of S phase total chromosomal proteins (▲).

HeLa chromosomal proteins per milligram of G_1 chromatin DNA, suggesting that at least a tenfold purification of the S phase nonhistone chromosomal protein or proteins involved in transcription of histone genes has been achieved.

An additional eightfold purification of the S phase nonhistone chromosoal proteins involved with transcription of histone genes was obtained by chromatography of the 0.5 M NaCl QAE-Sephadex fraction on SP-Sephadex®. The SP-Sephadex® column was equilibrated against 5 M urea-10 mM sodium acetate-0.1 M NaCl (pH 5.2) and the chromosomal proteins were eluted with the same buffer containing 0.15, 0.2, 0.3, 0.4, 0.6, and 3 M NaCl and 3 M NaCl at pH 8.3. The fractions shown in Figure 5 were assayed for ability to render histone genes transcribable in chromatin from G_1 HeLa cells. Greater than 96% of such activity was recovered in the fraction which was eluted with 0.4 M NaCl. It should be noted that 1 μg of the 0.4 M SP fraction was as effective as 10 μg of the same fraction in rendering the maximal level of histone sequences available for transcription form G_1 chromatin (the same level as observed from native S phase chromatin). It therefore appears that the extent to which histone genes can be rendered transcribable by the SP fraction is *saturable*. This result would not be expected if endogenous histone mRNA sequences were present in the SP fraction and were responsible for the observed hybridization of histone cDNA.

Preliminary results suggest that further purification of the S phase nonhistone chromosomal protein fraction can be achieved by gel-filtration chromatography, since the proteins which have the ability to render histone genes transcribable were recovered in the 40,000- to 60,000-dalton fraction of the column. The bulk of the nonhistone chromosomal proteins, which did not appear to influence transcription of histone genes,

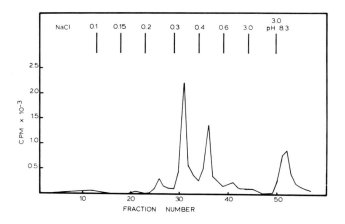

FIGURE 5.   Elution profile of chromosomal proteins from SP-Seph-adex®. NaCl concentrations used for elution of proteins are indicated.

were of higher molecular weights. The fraction from the SP-Sephadex® column which has the property of influencing histone gene transcription has been characterized by SDS-polyacrylamide gel electrophoresis and is still quite heterogeneous, although obviously less complex than the total nonhistone proteins. We have determined by CsCl equilibrium centrifugation and nuclease digestion that this protein fraction is not appreciably contaminated with nucleic acid.

We have also approached the problem of nonhistone chromosomal protein fractionation by extracting proteins from chromatin with progressively increasing concentrations of NaCl in the presence of 5 *M* urea-10 m*M* Tris (pH 8.0). The proteins solubilized by each concentration of NaCl were assayed for ability to render histone genes transcribable in the reconstitution assay described above. The proteins which remained bound to the chromatin were dissociated with 3 *M* NaCl-5 *M* urea-10 m*M* Tris (pH 8.3), the DNA was pelleted by centrifugation, and the proteins in the supernatant were assayed. While proteins capable of rendering histone genes transcribable were extracted from chromatin with 0.4 *M* NaCl, significant amounts of proteins with such activity remained associated with chromatin and were not removed from total chromatin which was subjected to extraction with NaCl at concentrations of 0.8 *M* and higher. These results raise the possibility that all proteins involved with the regulation of histone gene readout may not be associated with chromatin in a similar manner. If one postulates that a single species dictates the availability of histone genes for transcription, then the present data can be interpreted to reflect this protein being "loosely" as well as "tenaciously" bound to chromatin. Such differences in binding may indicate variations in the functional state of the protein-chromatin interactions, i.e., interactions with histone genes which result in transcription of histone sequences and nonspecific interactions which do not influence histone gene readout. Alternatively, differential extractability may mean that more than one species of nonhistone chromosomal protein can affect availability of histone genes for transcription.

While results discussed thus far suggest an important role for nonhistone chromosomal proteins in the regulation of histone gene transcription in both continuously dividing HeLa S₃ cells and contact-inhibited WI-38 cells, it is not known whether the mechanism by which histone gene transcription is regulated is the same in different tissues and species. It is of particular interest to determine whether a highly transformed continuously dividing cell, such as HeLa, contains components necessary to render histone genes transcribable from chromatin of other cells which have greater degrees of growth control. To examine these questions, chromatins from both contact-inhibited WI-38 human diploid fibroblasts and adult mouse liver (both nonproliferating) were dissociated and then reconstituted in the presence of added chromosomal proteins from S phase HeLa cells. Reconstituted chromatin was transcribed in vitro, and transcripts were assayed for histone mRNA sequences by hybridization with histone cDNA. The results of these studies suggest that S phase HeLa chromosomal proteins can render histone genes from chromatin of contact-inhibited WI-38 cells or from nondividing mouse liver available for transcription.[544] Specifically, these studies suggest that when the S phase HeLa chromosomal proteins are fractionated on QAE-Sephadex® in the presence of 5 M urea, only the fractions eluted by 0.5 M NaCl can render histone genes transcribable from chromatin of G_1 phase HeLa cells, contact-inhibited WI-38 fibroblasts, or mouse liver — indicating that transcription of histone sequences from these heterologous chromatins is not an effect elicited by S phase nonhistone chromosomal proteins in general. Several lines of evidence also suggest that in vitro histone gene transcription from mouse liver chromatin after addition of S phase HeLa cell nonhistone chromosomal proteins is not a random phenomenon. Addition of the HeLa cell proteins to mouse liver does not modify chromatin template activity, and, more specifically, the HeLa cell chromosomal proteins do not render mouse globin sequences transcribable (assayed by hybridization of chromatin transcripts with mouse globin ^{3}H-cDNA).[544]

Results from a number of laboratories indicate that histone proteins are similar in different mammalian species and in different cell types of the same species. Our data would seem to suggest that the involvement of the nonhistone chromosomal proteins in the in vitro transcription of histone genes from chromatin of HeLa cells, WI-38 cells, and mouse liver may be the same or similar. This raises the possibility that the DNA sequences with which certain nonhistone chromosomal proteins interact, perhaps regulatory sequences, are conserved between mouse and human. Alternatively, the DNA sequences involved with determining the availability of histone genes for transcription may differ between mouse and human, but both types of sequences may be recognized by the HeLa nonhistone chromosomal proteins. However, our results suggest that a highly transformed, continuously dividing cervical carcinoma cell, such as HeLa, may contain components necessary to make the histone genes of contact-inhibited tissue culture cells or nondividing cells from an intact organism available for transcription by E. coli RNA polymerase.

It should be noted that these results must be cautiously interpreted. The QAE fraction of S phase nonhistone chromosomal proteins is a very heterogeneous class of proteins. It is not known which component(s) is involved in determining the availability of histone genes for transcription or what the mechanism may be. It cannot be ruled out that regulatory molecules have been lost or inactivated in the course of elution, fractionation, and reconstitution of chromatin; it is also quite possible that in vitro transcription is different from that seen in vivo. These studies were performed using E. coli polymerase; one might anticipate that there may be other, perhaps more subtle, factors regulating histone gene transcription that interact only with the homologous RNA polymerase or that act in the intact cell. Also, caution must be exercised in assuming that the mode of histone gene control is the same in all biological situations; the primary level of regulation of histone gene expression may very likely vary from one system to another.

The data presently available do not permit us to determine if proteins involved in rendering histone sequences transcribable from S phase chromatin become associated with chromatin during the transition from the G_1 to the S phase of the cell cycle or, alternatively, if proteins involved with the control of histone gene transcription are associated with chromatin throughout the cell cycle and are modified during the G_1-S phase transition. Within this context, we have obtained two lines of evidence which suggest that the phosphate groups added posttranslationally to serine and threonine residues of nonhistone chromosomal proteins may play an important role in the regulation of in vitro histone gene transcription from chromatin. Not only are the proteins which appear to be involved in the control of histone gene transcription found in the fraction of the nonhistone chromosomal proteins which are highly phosphorylated,[545] but additionally, enzymatic dephosphorylation of S phase nonhistone chromosomal proteins significantly reduces the ability of these proteins to render histone genes transcribable.[140] While it is tempting to postulate positive control of histone gene transcription, the possibility should not be eliminated that a G_1 repressor is modified and thereby inactivated during the transition from the G_1 to the S phase of the cell cycle.

VIII. NONHISTONE CHROMOSOMAL PROTEINS AND CHROMATIN STRUCTURE: NONHISTONE PROTEINS ASSOCIATED WITH DNase I-SENSITIVE (ACTIVE) REGIONS OF THE GENOME

All DNA sequences, whether or not they are being transcribed, are associated with nucleosomes.[546-548] Thus, the positive control of gene expression cannot take place via a simple mechanism such as the complete removal of histones from a particular sequence by nonhistone chromosomal proteins. DNase I digestion studies indicate that sequences which are in an "active" configuration are preferentially digested by the nuclease.[549-553] This preferential nuclease sensitivity is not a consequence of the transcription process itself, since sequences being transcribed at different rates[552] and those which are no longer being transcribed all have equal sensitivities.[549] These results suggest that there is a structural difference between the chromatin of active and inactive regions of the genome and that the structure of active regions is necessary, but not sufficient, for transcription. There is evidence which suggests that the maintenance of the active structure of chromatin may be mediated by nonhistone chromosomal proteins associated with the nucleosomes. Using immunofluorescence techniques, a subfraction of nonhistone chromosomal proteins was shown to be specifically located at the active (puffed) regions of *Drosophila* polytene chromosomes.[304] Heat shock treatment resulted in the appearance of new transcriptionally active sites (puffs), and immunofluorescence showed that the nonhistone proteins associated with puffed regions were present at the new puffs.[304] Additional evidence supporting the hypothesis that nonhistone proteins are responsible for the active configuration of chromatin comes from the finding that, during nuclease digestion of active genes, a subset of nonhistone proteins was preferentially released from chromatin.[294,296,554] These proteins may be associated with the DNase I-sensitive loci in vivo, and some of the major proteins in this fraction were related to the HMG proteins which have been shown to interact with nucleosomes[23,293,296] One of the proteins was shown, by immunofluorescence, to be specifically associated with puffed (active) regions of *Drosophila* chromatin.[554] Thus, one way in which nonhistone chromosomal proteins could control selective gene expression is by interacting with nucleosomes in such a way as to change their structure into an "active" configuration. Other nonhistone proteins could possibly be responsible for maintaining the structure of nucleosomes in repressed (inactive) regions.

IX. NONHISTONE CHROMOSOMAL PROTEINS AS REGULATORY MOLECULES

In this chapter, we have attempted to review progress which has been made during the past several years toward elucidating the role of chromosomal proteins in determining the structural and functional properties of the genome. However, we are only at the threshold of understanding the nature of eukaryotic regulatory macromolecules and their mode of action. With regard to the regulation of gene expression, histones appear to act as nonspecific repressors of DNA-dependent RNA synthesis. In contrast, amongst the complex and heterogeneous nonhistone chromosomal proteins are components which appear to regulate the transcription of specific genetic sequences. Yet, many perplexing problems concerning the nonhistone chromosomal proteins remain to be resolved.

The specific nonhistone chromosomal proteins responsible for rendering particular genetic sequences transcribable must be identified. This is an especially difficult problem since, to date, the nature of the regulatory proteins is an enigma. It is generally assumed that specific regulatory proteins comprise only a very small percentage of the nonhistone chromosomal proteins. However, experimental evidence to support this assumption is lacking. It is also reasonable to construct a viable model for gene regulation in which multiple copies of regulatory proteins are associatd with the genome, with only a limited number of these proteins existing in a "functonal interaction". An important concept which should be considered is that a single protein may regulate several genes — particularly in situations where cellular events are functionally interrelated or coupled. For example, one may envision several genes involved with genome replication being controlled by a single regulatory protein. A similar situation may exist with hormone-stimulated processes. It is not clear whether regulatory proteins should comprise a subset of the nonhistone chromosomal proteins with common characteristics such as molecular weight, charge, or structure. In this regard, it will be interesting to establish whether similar types of proteins control "single-copy genes", such as globin genes, as opposed to "reiterated genes", such as histone and ribosomal genes.

A basic question to be answered is whether activation of genes is brought about by newly synthesized nonhistone chromosomal proteins or by modifications of preexisting genome-associated nonhistone chromosomal proteins. Alternatively, proteins residing in the cytoplasm or in the nucleoplasm may be modified in such a manner that they become associated with the genome and thereby render genes transcribable. Johnson and co-workers have observed that activation of lymphocytes by mitogenic agents results in accumulation of preexisting cytoplasmic proteins in the nucleus.[365] A nucleoplasmic pool of nonhistone chromosomal proteins has also been reported.[147] These latter two observations are consistent with the possibility that alterations in gene readout involve recruitment of proteins from the cytoplasm or nucleoplasm and their subsequent association with the genome. However, other studies suggest that protein synthesis is required for activation of transcription in human diploid fibroblasts following stimulation to proliferate.[555] In addition to numerous correlations between posttranslational modifications of nonhistone chromosomal proteins and changes in gene readout, recent studies suggest that the phosphate groups on nonhistone chromosomal proteins are important in rendering histone genes transcribable.[140,545]

Elucidating the manner in which nonhistone chromosomal proteins are associated with other genome components should significantly enhance our understanding of the mechanisms by which regulatory proteins interact with defined regions of the genome to render specific genes transcribable. While tenaciously bound as well as readily dissociable nonhistone chromosomal proteins have been purported to be the subclass of nonhistone chromosomal proteins which contains regulatory macromolecules, direct experimental evidence to distinguish between these two alternatives is, at present, limited. It is also presently unclear if nonhistone chromosomal proteins interact directly with DNA or with histone-DNA complexes.

In addition to understanding the mechanism by which nonhistone chromosomal proteins activate transcription of specific genes, the mechanism by which transcription is "turned off" must also be accounted for. One may envision inactivation of a gene or set of genes via degradation of the activator protein or proteins. Proteases which may utilized nonhistone chromosomal proteins as substrates have been shown to be associated with chromatin. An alternative mechanism for inactivation of regulatory proteins may involve acetate and/or phosphate groups added posttranslationally to nonhistone chromosomal proteins. One can speculate that repression of genetic sequences may be brought about by removal of such moieties from nonhistone chromosomal protein molecules. Deacetylases as well as phosphatases have been identified within the nucleus, lending credence to such speculation.

As fractionation and characterization of the nonhistone chromosomal proteins progress and as preparative scale quantities of cloned eukaryotic DNA sequences become available, the functional properties of eukaryotic gene regulators may become more apparent.

ADDENDUM

The regulation of histone gene expression during the cell cycle of HeLa S₃ cells was recently reassessed by Stein's laboratory using homologous H4 histone cDNA as a probe for detection of histone mRNA sequences.[557] S phase cells were obtained by double thymidine block and G1 cells were obtained by double thymidine block or mitotic selective detachment. Nuclear and cytoplasmic RNAs from S phase cells hybridized with H4 histone cDNA as did nuclear and cytoplasmic RNAs from G1 cells synchronized by double thymidine block. In contrast, significant levels of hybridization were not observed between H4 histone cDNA and nuclear, polysomal, or postpolysomal cytoplasmic RNAs of G1 cells synchronized by mitotic selective detachment. Double thymidine block yields a G1 cell population containing 20 to 25% S phase cells while G1 cells obtained by mitotic selective detachment contained less than 0.1% S phase cells. The ability of H4 histone cDNA to hybridize with RNAs from G1 cells obtained following release from double thymidine block as reported by Melli et al.[558] can therefore be explained by the presence of S phase cells in such a G1 population — an artifact of the synchronization procedure. These results are consistent with previous results[518,562,563] which indicate the presence of H4 histone mRNA sequences during the S but not G1 phase of the cell cycle in continuously dividing HeLa S₃ cells. Recently Marzluff and co-workers (personal communication) assayed pulse-labeled RNAs isolated from G1 and S phase mouse myeloma cells synchronized by the isoleucine deprivation method for the presence of histone mRNA sequences by hybridization to cloned sea urchin histone DNA. Consistent with transcriptional level control of histone gene expression during the cell cycle of continuously dividing cells, they found that synthesis of H3 and H4 histone mRNAs were prominent only during S phase. Parker and Fitschen (manuscript submitted) have also observed a difference (greater than 500-fold) in the representation of histone mRNA sequences in G1 and S phase mouse 3T6 cells. In the latter experiments, histone mRNA sequences were identified by hybridization of nuclear and cytoplasmic RNAs to homologous histone cDNA.

The control of gene expression by nonhistone chromosomal proteins may be mediated partially through alterations of chromatin structure. An acidic protein that assembles nucleosomes by first binding histones and then transferring them to DNA has been isolated from *Xenopus laevis* eggs.[559] Proteins that are able to alter the structure of nucleosomes after assembly may also exist. Recently, a subclass of nonhistone chromosomal proteins responsible for conferring a DNase I-sensitive structure on "active" globin genes has been isolated.[560] This fraction of proteins was enriched in HMG proteins 14 and 17.

Sequence analysis of cloned eukaryotic genomic DNA has revealed the existence, in the 5'-noncoding sequences of several genes, of an AT-rich region similar to a prokaryotic promoter site and of other regions with partial two-fold symmetry that are analogous to those found in prokaryotic operators.[561] These regions may provide interaction sites for nonhistone chromosomal proteins involved in the control of gene expression. In the near future, it should be possible to study the role of these proteins in selective gene expression through the use of in vitro systems containing cloned complete genes, histones, purified eukaryotic RNA polymerases and various nonhistone chromosomal proteins (possibly selected by affinity chromatographs to specific DNA sequences).

ACKNOWLEDGMENTS

We are indebted to Carlyn Ebert for her expert editorial assistance. Studies from this laboratory which are described in the chapter were supported by the following research grants: GM20535 from National Institutes of Health and PCM 77-15947 from the National Science Foundation.

REFERENCES

1. **Gilbert, W. and Mueller-Hill, B.,** Isolation of the *lac* repressor, *Proc. Natl. Acad. Sci. U.S.A.*, 56, 1891, 1966.
2. **Ptashne, M.,** Isolation of the λ-phage repressor, *Proc. Natl. Acad. Sci. U.S.A.*, 57, 306, 1967.
3. **Adler, K., Beyreuther, K., Fanning, E., Geisler, N., Gronenborn, B., Klemm, A., Mueller-Hill, B., Pfahl, M., and Schmitz, A.,** How *lac* repressor binds to DNA, *Nature (London)*, 237, 322, 1972.
4. **Jobe, A. and Bourgeois, S.,** *Lac* repressor-operator interaction. VI. The natural inducer of the *lac* operon, *J. Mol. Biol.*, 69, 397, 1972.
5. **Beckwith, J. R. and Zipser, D., Eds.,** *The Lactose Operon*, Cold Spring Harbor Laboratory, Cold Spring Harbor, New York, 1970.
6. **Hershey, A. D. and Dove, W.,** Introduction to lambda, in *The Bacteriophage Lambda*, Hershey, A. D., Ed., Cold Spring Harbor Laboratory, Cold Spring Harbor, New York, 1971, 3.
7. **Breathnach, R., Mandel, J. L., and Chambon, P.,** Ovalbumin gene is split in chicken DNA, *Nature (London)*, 270, 314, 1977.
8. **Jeffreys, A. J. and Flavell, R. A.,** The rabbit β-globin gene contains a large insert in the coding sequence, *Cell*, 12, 1097, 1977.
9. **Kornberg, R. D.,** Structure of chromatin, *Annu. Rev. Biochem.*, 46, 931, 1977.
10. **Felsenfeld, G., Chromatin,** *Nature (London)*, 271, 115, 1978.
11. **Benjamin, W. B. and Gelhorn, A.,** Acidic proteins of mammalian nuclei: isolation and characterization, *Proc. Natl. Acad. Sci. U.S.A.*, 59, 262, 1968.
12. **Marushige, K., Brutlag, D., and Bonner, J.,** Properties of chromosomal nonhistone protein of rat liver, *Biochemistry*, 7, 3149, 1968.
13. **MacGillivray, A. J., Cameron, A., Krauze, R. J., Rickwood, D., and Paul, J.,** The non-histone proteins of chromatin. Their isolaion and composition in a number of tissues, *Biochim. Biophys. Acta*, 277, 384, 1972.
14. **LeStourgeon, W. M. and Wray, W.,** Extraction and characterization of phenol-soluble acidic nuclear proteins, in *Acidic Proteins of the Nucleus*, Cameron, I. L. and Jeter, J. R., Jr., Eds., Academic Press, New York, 1974, 59.
15. **Shaw, L. M. J. and Huang, R. C.** A description of two procedures which avoid the use of extreme pH conditions for the resolution of components isolated from chromatins prepared from pig cerebellar and pituitary nuclei, *Biochemistry*, 9, 4530, 1970.

16. **Stein, G. and Baserga, R.,** The synthesis of acidic nuclear proteins in the prereplicative phase of the isoproterenol-stimulated salivary gland, *J. Biol. Chem.,* 245, 6097, 1970.

17. **Graziano, S. L. and Huang, R. C. C.,** Chromatographic separation of chick brain chromatin proteins using a SP-Sephadex column, *Biochemistry,* 10, 4770, 1971.

18. **Hill, R. J., Poccia, D. L., and Doty, P.,** Towards a total macromolecular analysis of sea urchin embryo chromatin, *J. Mol. Biol.,* 61, 445, 1971.

19. **Shelton, K. R. and Neelin, J. M.,** Nuclear residual proteins from goose erythroid cells and liver, *Biochemistry,* 10, 2342, 1971.

20. **Busch, H.,** *Histones and Other Nuclear Proteins,* Academic Press, New York, 1965, 200.

21. **Walker, J. M., Shooter, K. V., Goodwin, G. H., and Johns, E. W.,** The isolation of two peptides from a non-histone chromosomal protein showing irregular charge distributon within the molecule, *Biochem. Biophys. Res. Commun.,* 70, 88, 1976.

22. **Walker, J. M., Hastings, J. R. B., and Johns, E. W.,** The primary structure of a non-histone chromosomal protein, *Eur. J. Biochem.,* 76, 461, 1977.

23. **Goodwin, G. H., Walker, J. M., and Johns, E. W.,** The high mobility group (HMG) non-histone chromosomal proteins, in *The Cell Nucleus,* Vol. 6, Busch, H., Ed., Academic Press, New York, 1978, 181.

24. **Mamrack, M. D., Olson, M. O. J., and Busch, H.,** Acidic sequences containing phosphorylated sites in nucleolar nonhistone protein C23 of Novikoff hepatoma ascites cells, *Fed. Proc.,* 37, 1786, 1978.

25. **Stein, G. and Baserga, R.,** Cytoplasmic synthesis of acidic chromosomal proteins, *Biochem. Biophys. Res. Commun.,* 44, 218, 1971.

26. **Stein, G. S. and Baserga, R.,** Continued synthesis of non-histone chromosomal proteins during mitosis, *Biochem. Biophys. Res. Commun.,* 41, 715, 1970.

27. **Baserga, R. and Stein, G. S.,** Nuclear acidic proteins and cell proliferation, *Fed. Proc.,* 30, 1752, 1971.

28. **Stein, G. S. and Borun, T. W.,** The synthesis of acidic chromosomal proteins during the cell cycle of HeLa S-3 cells. I. The accelerated accumulation of acidic residual nuclear protein before the initiation of DNA replication, *J. Cell Biol.,* 52, 292, 1972.

29. **Borun, T. W. and Stein, G. S.,** The synthesis of acidic chromosomal proteins during the cell cycle of HeLa S-3 cells. II. The kinetics of residual protein synthesis and transport, *J. Cell Biol.,* 52, 308, 1972.

30. **Stein, G. S. and Matthews, D. E.,** Nonhistone chromosomal protein synthesis: utilization of preexisting and newly transcribed messenger RNAs, *Science,* 181, 71, 1973.

31. **Rovera, G. and Baserga, R.,** Early changes in the synthesis of acidic nuclear proteins in human diploid fibroblasts stimulated to synthesize DNA by changing the medium, *J. Cell Physiol.,* 77, 201, 1971.

32. **Tsuboi, A. and Baserga, R.,** Synthesis of nuclear acidic proteins in density-inhibited fibroblasts stimulated to proliferate, *J. Cell Physiol.,* 80, 107, 1972.

33. **Levy, R., Levy, S., Rosenberg, S. A., and Simpson, R. T.,** Selective stimulation of nonhistone chromatin protein synthesis in lymphoid cells by phytohemagglutinin, *Biochemistry,* 12, 224, 1973.

34. **Stein, G. S. and Thrall, C. L.,** Uncoupling of nonhistone chromosomal protein synthesis and DNA replication in human diploid WI-38 fibroblasts, *FEBS Letts.,* 34, 35, 1973.

35. **Gerner, E. W. and Humphrey, R. M.,** The cell-cycle phase synthesis of non-histone proteins in mammalian cells, *Biochim. Biophys. Acta,* 331, 117, 1973.

36. **Bhorjee, J. S. and Pederson, T.,** Nonhistone chromosomal proteins in synchronized HeLa cells, *Proc. Natl. Acad. Sci. U.S.A.,* 69, 3345, 1972.

37. **Bhorjee, J. S. and Pederson, T.,** Chromatin: its isolation from cultured mammalian cells with particular reference to contamination by nuclear ribonucleoprotein particles, *Biochemistry,* 12, 2766, 1973.

38. **LeStourgeon, W. M. and Rusch, H. P.,** Nuclear acid protein changes during differentiation in *Physarum polycephalum, Science,* 174, 1233, 1971.

39. **Becker, H. and Staners, C. P.,** Control of macromolecular synthesis in proliferating and resting Syrian hamster cells in monolayer culture. III. Electrophoretic patterns of newly synthesized proteins in synchronized proliferating cells and resting cells, *J. Cell Physiol.,* 80, 51, 1972.

40. **Daly, M. M., Allfrey, V. G., and Mirsky, A. E.,** Uptake of glycine-N[15] by components of cell nuclei, *J. Gen. Physiol.,* 36, 173, 1952.

41. **Allfrey, V. G., Daly, M. M., and Mirsky, A. E.,** Some observations on protein metabolism in chromosomes of non-dividing cells, *J. Gen. Physiol.,* 38, 415, 1955.

42. **Byvoet, P.,** Metabolic integrity of deoxyribonucleohistones, *J. Mol. Biol.,* 17, 311, 1966.

43. **Holoubek, V., and Crocker, T. T.,** DNA-associated acidic proteins, *Biochim. Biophys. Acta,* 157, 352, 1968.

44. **Hancock, R.,** Conservation of histones in chromatin during growth and mitosis in vitro, *J. Mol. Biol.,* 40, 457, 1969.

45. **Bondy, S. C.,** The synthesis and decay of histone fractions and of deoxyribonucleic acid in the developing avian brain, *Biochem. J.,* 123, 465, 1971.

46. **Dice, J. F. and Schimke, R. T.,** Turnover of chromosomal proteins from rat liver, *Arch. Biochem. Biophys.,* 158, 97, 1973.

47. **Karn, G., Johnson, E. M., Vidali, G., and Allfrey, V. G.,** Differential phosphorylation and turnover of nuclear acidic proteins during the cell cycle of synchronized HeLa cells, *J. Biol. Chem.,* 249, 667, 1974.

48. **Vidali, G., Karn, G., and Allfrey, V. G.,** Selective effects of inhibitors of protein synthesis on metabolism of nuclear and cytoplasmic proteins: evidence for coordinate synthesis of non-histone chromosomal proteins, *Proc. Nal. Acad. Sci. U.S.A.,* 72, 4450, 1975.

49. **Wilhelm, J. A., Groves, C. M., and Hnilica, L. S.,** Nucleolar and extranucleolar chromatin of rat Novikoff hepatoma cells. A comparison of histone and nonhistone protein acetylation, *Biochim. Biophys. Acta,* 238, 295, 1971.

50. **Libby, P. R.,** Histone acetylation and hormone action. Early effects of oestradiol-17β on histone acetylation in rat uterus, *Biochem. J.,* 130, 663, 1972.

51. **Suria, D. and Liew, C. C.,** Isolation of nuclear proteins from rat tissues. Characterization of acetylated liver nuclear acidic proteins, *Biochem. J.,* 137, 355, 1974.

52. **Friedman, M., Shull, K. H., and Farber, E.,** Highly selective in vivo ethylation of rat liver nuclear protein, *Biochem. Biophys. Res. Commun.,* 34, 857, 1969.

53. **Borun, T. W., Pearson, D., and Paik, W. K.,** Studies of histone methylation during the HeLa S-3 cell cycle, *J. Biol. Chem.,* 247, 4288, 1972.

54. **Byvoet, P., Shepherd, G. R., Hardin, J. M., and Noland, B. J.,** The distribution and turnover of labeled methyl groups in histone fractions of cultured mammalian cells, *Arch. Biochem. Biophys.,* 148, 558, 1972.

55. **Doenecke, D., Beato, M., Congote, L. F., and Sekeris, C. E.,** Effect of cortisol on the thiol content of rat liver nuclear proteins, *Biochem. J.,* 126, 1171, 1972.

56. **Gronow, M. and Thackrah, T.,** The nonhistone nuclear proteins of some rat tissues, *Arch. Biochem. Biophys.,* 158, 377, 1973.

57. **Gronow, M. and Lewis, F. A.,** Thiols attached to rat liver non-histone nuclear proteins, *Exp. Cell Res.,* 93, 225, 1975.

58. **Kaji, H.,** Amino-terminal arginylation of chromosomal proteins by arginyl-tRNA, *Biochemistry,* 15, 5121, 1976.

59. **Ljiljana, S. and Koviljka, K.,** Demonstration of glycoproteins which are associated with chromatin nonhistone proteins, *Int. J. Biochem.,* 4, 345, 1973.

60. **Stein G. S., Roberts, R. M., Davis, J. L., Head, W. J., Stein, J. L., Thrall, C. L., Van Veen, J., and Welch, D. W.,** Are glycoproteins and glycosaminoglycans components of the eukaryotic genome?, *Nature (London),* 258, 639, 1975.

61. **Jackson, R. C.,** On the identity of nuclear membrane and non-histone nuclear proteins, *Biochemistry,* 15, 5652, 1976.

62. **Rizzo, W. B. and Bustin, M.,** Lectins as probes of chromatin structure. Binding of concanavalin A to purified rat liver chromatin, *J. Biol. Chem.,* 252, 7062, 1977.

63. **Lu, C. Y. and Koenig, H.,** Isolation of acidic lipoproteins from brain chromatin — their relation to the acidic nonhistone proteins, *FEBS Letts.,* 34, 48, 1973.

64. **Manzoli, F. A., Cocco, L., Facchini, A., Casali, A. M., Maraldi, N. M., and Grossi, C. E.,** Phospholipids bound to acidic nuclear proteins in human B and T lymphocytes, *Mol. Cell. Biochem.,* 12, 67, 1976.

65. **Tata, J. R., Hamilton, M. J., and Cole, R. D.,** Membrane phospholipids associated with nuclei and chromatin. Melting profile, template activity and stability of chromatin, *J. Mol. Biol.,* 67, 231, 1972.

66. **Haussler, M. R., Thomson, W. W., and Norman, A. W.** The isolation of purified nuclear and chromatin fractions from chick intestinal mucosa, *Exp. Cell Res.,* 58, 234, 1969.

67. **Harlow, R., Tolstoshev, P., and Wells, J. R. E.,** Membrane. Major source of chromatin-associated RNA and non-histone proteins in avian erythroid cells, *Cell Differ.,* 1, 341, 1972.

68. **Huang, R. C. C. and Huang, P. C.,** Effect of protein-bound RNA associated with chick embryo chromatin on template specificity of the chromatin, *J. Mol. Biol.,* 39, 365, 1969.

69. **Bhorjee, J. S. and Pederson, T.,** Chromosomal proteins: tightly bound nucleic acids and its bearing on the measurement of nonhistone protein phosphorylation, *Anal. Biochem.,* 71, 393, 1976.

70. **MacGillivray, A. J. and Rickwood, D.,** Role of chromosomal proteins as gene regulators, in *Biochemistry of Differentiation and Development,* MTP Int. Rev. Sci.: Biochem. Ser. 1, Vol. 9, Paul, J., Ed., Butterworth, London, 1974, 301.

71. **Chambon, P., Weill, J. D., Doly, J., Strosser, M. T., and Mandel, P.,** On the formation of a novel adenylic compound by enzymatic extracts of liver nuclei, *Biochem. Biophys. Res. Commun.,* 25, 638, 1966.

72. **Nishizuka, Y., Ueda, K., Nakazawa, K., and Hayaishi, O.,** Studies on the polymer of adenosine diphosphate ribose. I. Enzymic formation from nicotinamide adenine dinucleotide in mammalian nuclei, *J. Biol. Chem.,* 242, 3164, 1967.

73. **Sugimura, T., Fujimura, S., Hasegawa, S., and Kawamura, Y.,** Polymerization of the adenosine 5'-diphosphate ribose moiety of NAD by rat liver nuclear enzyme, *Biochim. Biophys. Acta,* 138, 438, 1967.

74. **Nishizuka, Y., Ueda, K., Honjo, T., and Hayaishi, O.,** Enzymic adenosine diphosphate ribosylation of histone and poly adenosine diphosphate ribose synthesis in rat liver nuclei, *J. Biol. Chem.,* 243, 3765, 1968.

75. **Otake, H., Miwa, M., Fujimura, S., and Sugimura, T.,** Binding of ADP-ribose polymer with histone, *J. Biochem.,* 65, 145, 1969.

76. **Adamietz, P. and Hilz, H.,** Covalent linkage of poly(adenosine diphosphate ribose) to nuclear proteins of rat liver by two types of bonds, *Biochem. Soc. Trans.,* 3, 1118, 1975.

77. **Adameitz, P. and Hilz, H.,** Poly(adenosine diphosphate ribose) is covalently linked to nuclear proteins by two types of bonds, *Hoppe-Seyler's Z. Physiol. Chem.,* 357, 527, 1976.

78. **Rickwood, D., MacGillivray, A. J., and Whish, W. J. D.,** The modification of nuclear proteins by ADP-ribosylation, *Eur. J. Biochem.,* 79, 589, 1977.

79. **Nishizuka, Y., Ueda, K., Yoshihara, K., Yamamura, H., Takeda, M., and Hayaishi, O.,** Enzymic adenosine diphosphoribosylation of nuclear proteins, *Cold Spring Harbor Symp. Quant. Biol.,* 34, 781, 1969.

80. **Ueda, K., Omachi, A., Kawaichi, M., and Hayaishi, O.,** Natural occurrence of poly(ADP-ribosyl) histones in rat liver, *Proc. Natl. Acad. Sci. U.S.A.,* 72, 205, 1975.

81. **Smith, J. A. and Stocken, L. A.,** Chemical and metabolic properties of adenosine diphosphate ribose derivatives of nuclear proteins, *Biochem. J.,* 147, 523, 1975.

82. **Yoshihara, K., Tanigawa, Y., Burzio, L., and Koide, S. S.,** Evidence for adenosine diphosphate ribosylation of Ca^{2+}, Mg^{2+}-dependent endonuclease, *Proc. Natl. Acad. Sci. U.S.A.,* 72, 289, 1975.

83. **Okayama, H., Ueda, K., and Hayaishi, O.,** Purification of ADP-ribosylated nuclear proteins by covalent chromatography on dihydroxyboryl polyacrylamide beads and their characterization, *Proc. Natl. Acad. Sci. U.S.A.,* 75, 1111, 1978.

84. **Mullins, D. W., Jr., Giri, C. P., and Smulson, M.,** Poly(ADP) polymerase: the distribution of a chromosome-associated enzyme within the chromatin substructure, *Biochemistry,* 16, 506, 1977.

85. **Yukioka, M., Okai, Y., Hasuma, T., and Inoue, A.,** Non-preferential localization of poly(ADP-ribose) polymerase activity in transcriptionally active chromatin, *FEBS Lett.,* 86, 85, 1978.

86. **Okayama, H., Edson, C. M., Fukushima, M., Ueda, K., and Hayaishi, O.,** Purification and properties of poly(adenosine diphosphate ribose) synthetase. Role of histone in poly(ADP-ribose) synthesis, *J. Biol. Chem.,* 252, 7000, 1977.

87. **Miyakawa, N., Ueda, K., and Hayaishi, O.,** Association of poly ADP-ribose glycohydrolase with liver chromatin, *Biochem. Biophys. Res. Commun.,* 49, 239, 1972.

88. **Burzio, L. and Koide, S. S.,** A functional role of poly ADPR in DNA synthesis, *Biochem. Biophys. Res. Commun.,* 40, 1013, 1970.

89. **Hilz, H. and Kittler, M.,** Lack of correlation between poly ADP-ribose formation and DNA synthesis, *Hoppe-Seyler's Z. Physiol. Chem.,* 352, 1693, 1971.

90. **Brightwell, M. and Shall, S.,** Poly(adenosine diphosphate ribose) polymerase in *Physarum polycephalum* nuclei, *Biochem. J.,* 125, 67p, 1971.

91. **Burzio, L. and Koide, S. S.,** In vitro effect of NAD on DNA synthesis in isolated nuclei from regenerating rat liver and Novikoff hepatoma, *FEBS Lett.,* 20, 29, 1972.

92. **Roberts J. H., Stark, P., and Smulson, M.,** Poly(ADP-ribose): release of template restriction in HeLa cells, *Proc. Natl. Acad. Sci. U.S.A.,* 71, 3212, 1974.

93. **Smulson, M. E., Stark, P., Gazzoli, M., and Roberts, J. H.,** Release of template restriction for DNA synthesis by poly ADP(ribose) polymerase during the HeLa cell cycle, *Exp. Cell Res.,* 90, 175, 1975.

94. **Leiber, U., Kittler, M., and Hilz, H.,** Enzymes of poly(ADPR) metabolism in proliferating and nonproliferating liver tissues, *Hoppe-Seyler's Z. Physiol. Chem.,* 354, 1347, 1973.

95. **Lehman, A. R., Kirk-Bell, S., Shall, S., and Whish, W. J. D.,** The relationship between cell growth, macromolecular synthesis and poly ADP-ribose polymerase in lymphoid cells, *Exp. Cell Res.,* 83, 63, 1974.

96. **Müller, W. E. G., Totsuka, A., Nusser, I., Obermeier, J., Rhode, H. J., and Zahn, R. K.,** Poly(adenosine diphosphate-ribose) polymerase in quail oviduct. Changes during estrogen and progesterone induction, *Nucleic Acids Res.,* 1, 1317, 1974.

97. **Burzio, L., Reich, L., and Koide, S. S.,** Poly(adenosine diphosphoribose) synthetase activity of isolated nuclei and leukemic leukocytes, *Proc. Soc. Exp. Biol. Med.,* 149, 933, 1975.

98. **Kidwell, W. R. and Mage, M. G.,** Changes in poly(adenosine diphosphate-ribose) and poly(adnosine diphosphate-ribose) polymerase in synchronous HeLa cells, *Biochemistry,* 15, 1213, 1976.

99. **Shall, S., Goodwin, P., Halldorsson, H., Khan, G., Skidmore, C., and Tsopanakis, C.,** Post-synthetic modifications of nuclear macromolecules, *Biochem. Soc. Symp.,* 42, 103, 1977.

100. **Lorimer, W. S., III, Stone, P. R., and Kidwell, W. R.,** Adenosine diphosphate ribosylation of basic nuclear proteins, *Fed. Proc.,* 35, 1624, 1976.

101. **Goff, C. G.,** Chemical structure of a modification of the *Escherichia coli* ribonucleic acid polymerase α polypeptides induced by bacteriophage T₄ infection, *J. Biol. Chem.,* 249, 6181, 1974.

102. **Rohrer, H., Zillig, W., and Mailhammer, R.,** ADP-ribosyation of DNA-dependent RNA polymerase of *Escherichia coli* by an NAD⁺: protein ADP-ribosyltransferase from bacteriophage T₄, *Eur. J. Biochem.,* 60, 227, 1975.

103. **Davidson, J. N., Frazer, S. C., and Hutchinson, H. C.,** Phosphorus compounds in the cell. I. Protein-bound phosphorus fractions studied with the aid of radioactive phosphorus, *Biochem. J.,* 49, 311, 1951.

104. **Johnson, R. M. and Albert, S.,** Incorporation of phosphorus³² into the phosphoprotein fraction of mammalian tissue, *J. Biol. Chem.,* 200, 335, 1953.

105. **Langan, T. A.,** A phosphoprotein preparation from liver nuclei and its effect on the inhibition of RNA synthesis by histones, in *Regulation of Nucleic Acid and Protein Biosynthesis,* Koningsberger, V. V. and Bosch, L., Eds., Elsevier, Amsterdam, 1967, 233.

106. **Kleinsmith, L. J., Allfrey, V. G., and Mirsky, A. E,** Phosphoprotein metabolism in isolated lymphocyte nuclei, *Proc. Natl. Acad. Sci. U.S.A.,* 55, 1182, 1966.

107. **Kleinsmith, L. J. and Allfrey, V. G,** Nuclear phosphoproteins. I. Isolation and characterization of a phosphoprotein fraction from calf thymus nuclei, *Biochim. Biophys. Acta,* 175, 123, 1969.

108. **Schiltz, E. and Sekeris, C. E.,** Enzymatic phosphorylation of nuclear proteins by [γ-³²P]ATP in isolated rat liver nuclei, *Hoppe-Seyler's Z. Physiol. Chem.,* 350, 317, 1969.

109. **Chen, C., Smith, D. L., Bruegger, B. B., Halpern, R. M., and Smith, R. A.,** Occurrence and distribution of acid-labile histone phosphates in regenerating rat liver, *Biochemistry,* 13, 3785, 1974.

110. **Schiltz E. and Sekeris, C. E.,** Enzymatic phosphorylation of proteins of rat liver chromatin by (γ-³²P) ATP in vitro, *Experientia,* 27, 30, 1971.

111. **Benjamin, W. and Goodman, R. M.,** Phosphorylation of dipteran chromosomes and rat liver nuclei, *Science,* 166, 629, 1969.

112. **Ahmed, K.,** Studies of nuclear phosphoproteins of rat ventral prostate: incorporation of ³²P from [γ-³²P]ATP, *Biochim. Biophys. Acta,* 243, 38, 1971.

113. **Kamiyama, M. and Dastugue, B.,** Rat liver non-histone proteins: correlation between protein kinase activity and activation of RNA synthesis, *Biochim. Biophys. Res. Commun.,* 44, 29, 1971.

114. **Rickwood, D., Riches, P. G., and MacGillivray, A. J.,** Studies of the in vitro phosphorylation of chromatin non-histone proteins in isolated nuclei, *Biochim. Biophys. Acta,* 299, 162, 1973.

115. **Phillips, I. R. and Mathias, A. P.,** Tissue specificity and phosphorylation of nonhistone chromosomal proteins studied by two-dimensional gel electrophoresis, submitted for publication.

116. **Kleinsmith, L. J. and Allfrey, V. G.,** Nuclear phosphoproteins. II. Metabolism of exogenous phosphoprotein by intact nuclei, *Biochim. Biophys. Acta,* 175, 136, 1969.

117. **Ruddon, R. W. and Anderson, S. L.,** Presence of multiple protein kinase activities in rat liver nuclei, *Biochem. Biophys. Res. Commun.,* 46, 1499, 1972.

118. **Desjardins, P. R., Lue, P. F., Liew, C. C., and Gornall, A. G.,** Purification and properties of rat liver nuclear protein kinases, *Can. J. Biochem.,* 50, 1249, 1972.

119. **Desjardins, P. R., Liew, C. C., and Gornall, A. G.,** Rat liver nuclear protein kinases, *Can. J. Biochem.,* 53, 354, 1975.

120. **Desjardins, P. R., Mendelson, I. M., and Anderson, K. M.,** Relationship between RNA polymerase and protein kinase, *Can. J. Biochem.,* 53, 591, 1975.

121. **Rikans, L. E. and Ruddon, R. W.,** Role of 3', 5'-cyclic AMP in the control of nuclear protein kinase activity, *Biochem. Biophys. Res. Commun.,* 54, 387, 1973.

122. **Rikans, L. E. and Ruddon, R. W.,** Partial purification and properties of a chromatin-associated phosphoprotein kinase from rat liver nuclei, *Biochim. Biophys. Acta,* 422, 73, 1976.

123. **Dastugue, B., Tichonicky, L., and Kruh, J.,** Multiple forms of protein kinase in liver cell. II. Nuclear kinase and cytosol phosvitin kinase, *Biochimie,* 56, 490, 1974.

124. **Takeda, M., Matsumura, S., and Nakaya, Y.,** Nuclear phosphoprotein kinases from rat liver, *J. Biochem.,* 75, 743, 1974.

125. **Gamo, S. and Lindell, T. J.,** Presence of two protein kinases in highly purified rat liver nucleoli, *Life Sci.,* 15, 2179, 1974.

126. **Thomson, J. A., Chiu, J.-F., and Hnilica, L. S.,** Nuclear phosphoprotein kinase activities in normal and neoplastic tissues, *Biochim. Biophys. Acta,* 407, 114, 1975.

127. **Farron-Furstenthal, F. and Lightholder, J. R.,** The regulation of nuclear protein kinases, in *Onco-Developmental Gene Expression,* Fishman, W. H. and Sell, S., Eds., Academic Press, New York, 1976, 57.

128. **Kish, V. M. and Kleinsmith, L. J.**, Nuclear protein kinases. Evidence for their heterogeneity, tissue specificity, substrate specificities, and differential responses to cyclic adenoside 3′-5′-monophosphate, *J. Biol. Chem.*, 249, 750, 1974.

129. **Kemp, B. E., Froscio, M., Rogers, A., and Murray, A. W.**, Multiple protein kinases from human lymphocytes. Identification of enzymes phosphorylating exogenous histone and casein, *Biochem. J.*, 145, 241, 1975.

130. **Johnson, E. M., Hadden, J. W., Inoue, A., and Allfrey, V. G.**, DNA binding by cyclic adenosine 3′,5′-monophosphate dependent protein kinase from calf thymus nuclei, *Biochemistry*, 14, 3873, 1975.

131. **Jungmann, R. A. and Kranias, E. G.**, Cyclic AMP-mediated protein kinase activation and its regulatory effect on mammalian RNA polymerase, in *Advances in Biochemical Psychopharmacology*, Vol. 15, Costa, E., Giacobini, E., and Paoletti, R., Eds., Raven Press, New York, 1976, 413.

132. **Keller, R. K., Chandra, T., Schrader, W. T., and O' Malley, B. W.**, Protein kinases of the chick oviduct: a study of the cytoplasmic and nuclear enzymes, *Biochemistry*, 15, 1958, 1976.

133. **Spielvogel, A. M., Mednicks, M. I., Eppenberger, U., and Jungmann, R. A.**, Evidence for the identity of nuclear and cytoplasmic adenosine-3′-5′-monophosphate-dependent protein kinase from porcine ovaries and nuclear translocation of the cytoplasmic proteins, *Eur. J. Biochem.*, 73, 199, 1977.

134. **Thomson, J. A., Mon, M. J., Stein, J. L., DuVal, K. A., Kleinsmith, L. J., and Stein, G. S.**, Partial fractionation and characterization of nuclear protein kinases of HeLa S₃ cells, *Cell Differ.*, 8, 305, 1979.

135. **Phillips, I. R., Shephard, E. A., Stein, J. L., Kleinsmith, L. J., and Stein, G. S.**, Nuclear protein kinases during the cell cycle of HeLa S₃ cells, *Biochim. Biophys. Acta*, 565, 326, 1979.

136. **Keely, S. L., Corbin, J. D., and Park, C. R.**, On the question of translocation of heart cAMP-dependent protein kinase, *Proc. Natl. Acad. Sci. U.S.A.*, 72, 1501, 1975.

137. **Jungmann, R. A., Hiestand, P. C., and Schweppe, J. S**, Mechanism of action of gonadotropin. IV. Cyclic adenosine monophosphate-dependent translocation of ovarian cytoplasmic cyclic adenosine monophosphate-binding protein and protein kinase to nuclear acceptor sites, *Endocrinology*, 94, 168, 1974.

138. **Jungmann, R. A., Lee, S.-G., and DeAngelo, A. B.**, Translocation of cytoplasmic protein kinase and cyclic adenosine monophosphate-binding protein to intracellular acceptor sites, in *Advances in Cyclic Nucleotide Research*, Vol. 5, Drummond, G. I., Greengard, P., and Robison, G. A., Eds., Raven Press, New York, 1975, 281.

139. **Kleinsmith, L. J.**, Do phosphorylated proteins regulate gene activity?, in *Chromosomal Proteins and their Role in the Regulation of Gene Expression*, Stein, G. S. and Kleinsmith, L. J., Eds., Academic Press, New York, 1975, 45.

140. **Kleinsmith, L. J., Stein, J., and Stein, G.**, Dephosphorylation of nonhistone proteins specifically alters the pattern of gene transcription in reconstituted chromatin, *Proc. Natl. Acad. Sci. U.S.A.*, 73, 1174, 1976.

141. **Wilhelm, J. A. Groves, C. M., and Hnilica, L. S.**, Lack of major cytoplasmic protein contamination of rat liver nuclear chromatin, *Experientia*, 28, 514, 1972.

142. **Johns, E. W. and Forrester, S.**, Studies on nuclear proteins. The binding of extra acidic proteins to deoxyribonucleoprotein during the preparation of nuclear proteins, *Eur. J. Biochem.*, 8, 547, 1969.

143. **Lin, P. P-C., Wilson, R. F., and Bonner, J.**, Isolation and properties of nonhistone chromosomal proteins from pea chromatin, *Mol. Cell Biochem.*, 1, 197, 1973.

144. **O'Malley, B. W., Toft, D. O., and Sherman, M. R.**, Progesterone-binding components of chick oviduct. II. Nuclear components, *J. Biol. Chem.*, 246, 1117, 1971.

145. **Carlsson, S.-A., Moore, G. P. M., and Ringertz, N. R.**, Nucleo-cytoplasmic protein migration during the activation of chick erythrocyte nuclei in heterokaryons, *Exp. Cell Res.*, 76, 234, 1973.

146. **Kirsh, W. M., Leitner, J. W., Gairney, M., Schultz, D., Lasher, R., and Nakone, P.**, Bulk isolation in nonaqueous media of nuclei from lyophilized cells, *Science*, 168, 1592, 1970.

147. **Stein, G. S. and Thrall, C. L.**, Evidence for the presence of non-histone chromosomal proteins in the nucleoplasm of HeLa S₃ cells, *FEBS Lett.*, 32, 41, 1973.

148. **Frenster, J. H., Allfrey, V. G., and Mirsky, A. E.**, Repressed and active chromatin isolated from interphase lymphocytes, *Proc. Natl. Acad. Sci. U.S.A.*, 50, 1026, 1963.

149. **Dingman, W. C. and Sporn, M. B.**, Studies on chromatin. I. Isolation and characterization of nuclear complexes of deoxyribonucleic acid, ribonucleic acid, and protein from embryonic and adult tissues of the chicken, *J. Biol. Chem.*, 239, 3483, 1964.

150. **Frenster, J. H.**, Nuclear polyanions as de-repressors of synthesis of ribonucleic acid, *Nature (London)*, 206, 680, 1965.

151. **Chonda, S. X. and Cherion, M. G.**, Isolation and partial characterization of a mercury-binding nonhistone protein component from rat kidney nuclei, *Biochem. Biophys. Res. Commun.*, 50, 1013, 1973.

152. **Spelsberg, T. C., Steggles, A. W., Chytil, F., and O'Malley, B. W.,** Progesterone-binding components of chick oviduct. V. Exchange of progesterone-binding capacity from target to nontarget tissue chromatins, *J. Biol. Chem.*, 247, 1368, 1972.

153. **Jungmann, R. A. and Schweppe, J. S.,** Binding of chemical carcinogens to nuclear proteins of rat liver, *Cancer Res.*, 32, 952, 1972.

154. **Elgin, S. C. R. and Bonner, J.,** Limited heterogeneity of the major nonhistone chromosomal proteins, *Biochemistry*, 9, 4440, 1970.

155. **Seale, R. L. and Aronson, A. I.,** Chromatin-associated proteins of the developing sea urchin embryo. I. Kinetics of synthesis and characterization of non-histone proteins, *J. Mol. Biol.*, 75, 633, 1973.

156. **Wilson, E. M. and Spelsberg, T. C.,** Rapid isolation of total acidic proteins from chromatin of various chick tissues, *Biochim. Biophys. Acta*, 322, 145, 1973.

157. **Yeoman, L. C., Taylor, C. W., Jordan, J. J., and Busch, H.,** Two-dimensional polyacrylamide gel electrophoresis of chromatin proteins of normal rat liver and Novikoff hepatoma ascites cells, *Biochem. Biophys. Res. Commun.*, 53, 1067, 1973.

158. **Steele, W. J. and Busch, H.,** Acidic nuclear proteins of the Walker tumor and liver, *Cancer Res.*, 23, 1153, 1963.

159. **Shelton, K. R. and Allfrey, V. G.,** Selective synthesis of a nuclear acidic protein in liver cells stimulated by cortisol, *Nature (London)*, 228, 132, 1970.

160. **Teng, C. T., Teng, C. S., and Allfrey, V. G.,** Species-specific interactions between nuclear phosphoproteins and DNA, *Biochem. Biophys. Res. Commun.*, 41, 690, 1970.

161. **Teng, C. S., Teng, C. T., and Allfrey, V. G.,** Studies of nuclear acidic proteins. Evidence for their phosphorylation, tissue specificity, selective binding to deoxyribonucleic acid, and stimulatory effects on transcription, *J. Biol. Chem.*, 246, 3597, 1971.

162. **Shelton, K. R., Seligy, V. L., and Neelin, J. M.,** Phosphate incorporation into "nuclear" residual proteins of goose erythrocytes, *Arch. Biochem. Biophys.*, 153, 375, 1972.

163. **Shelton, K. R.,** Plasma membrane and nuclear proteins of the goose erythrocyte, *Can. J. Biochem.*, 51, 1442, 1973.

164. **LeStourgeon, W. M. and Rusch, H. P.,** Localization of nucleolar and chromatin residual acidic protein changes during differentiation in *Physarum polycephalum*, *Arch. Biochem. Biophys.*, 155, 144, 1973.

165. **Spelsberg, T. C., Mitchell, W. M., Chytil, F., Wilson, E. M., and O'Malley, B. W.,** Chromatin of the developing chick oviduct: changes in the acidic proteins, *Biochim. Biophys. Acta*, 312, 765, 1973.

166. **Patel, G. and Wang, T. Y.,** Chromatography and electrophoresis of nuclear soluble proteins, *Exp. Cell Res.*, 34, 120, 1964.

167. **Wang, T. Y.,** The isolation, properties, and possible functions of chromatin acidic proteins, *J. Biol. Chem.*, 242, 1220, 1967.

168. **van den Broek, H. W. J., Nooden, L. D., Sevall, J. S., and Bonner, J.,** Isolation, purification, and fractionation of nonhistone chromosomal proteins, *Biochemistry*, 12, 229, 1973.

169. **Tuan, D., Smith, S., Folkman, J., and Merler, E.,** Isolation of the nonhistone proteins of rat Walker carcinoma 256. Their association with tumor angiogenesis, *Biochemistry*, 12, 3159, 1973.

170. **Arnold, E. A. and Young, K. E.,** Isolation and partial electrophoretic characterization of total protein from non-sheared rat liver chromatin, *Biochim. Biophys. Acta*, 257, 482, 1972.

171. **Levy, S., Simpson, R. T., and Sober, H. H.,** Fractionation of chromatin components, *Biochemistry*, 11, 1547, 1972.

172. **Augenlicht, L. H. and Baserga, R.,** Preparation and partial fractionation of nonhistone chromosomal proteins from human diploid fibroblasts, *Arch. Biochem. Biophys.*, 158, 89, 1973.

173. **Bekhor, I., Kung, G. M., and Bonner, J.,** Sequence-specific interaction of DNA and chromosomal protein, *J. Mol. Biol.*, 39, 351, 1969.

174. **Umanskii, S. R., Tokarskaya, V. I., Zotova, R. N., and Migushina, V. L.,** Isolation and heterogeneity of nonhistone proteins of the rat liver chromatin, *Mol. Biol. (Moscow)*, 5, 215, 1971.

175. **Richter, K. H. and Sekeris, C. E.,** Isolation and partial purification of non-histone chromosomal proteins from rat liver, thymus and kidney, *Arch. Biochem. Biophys.*, 148, 44, 1972.

176. **Chaudhuri, S.,** Fractionation of chromatin nonhistone proteins, *Biochim. Biophys. Acta*, 322, 155, 1973.

177. **Monahan, J. J. and Hall, R. H.,** Fractionation of chromatin components, *Can. J. Biochem.*, 51, 709, 1973.

178. **Yoshida, M. and Shimura, K.,** Isolation of nonhistone chromosomal protein from calf thymus *Biochim. Biophys. Acta*, 263, 690, 1972.

179. **MacGillivray, A. J., Carroll, D., and Paul, J.,** The heterogeneity of the non-histone chromatin proteins from mouse tissues, *FEBS Lett.*, 13, 204, 1971.

180. **Rickwood, D. and Macillivray, A. J.,** Improved techniques for the fractionation of non-histone proteins of chromatin on hydroxyapatite, *Eur. J. Biochem.*, 51, 593, 1975.

181. **Shirey, T. and Huang, R. C. C.**, Use of sodium dodecyl sulphate, alone, to separate chromatin proteins from deoxyribonucleoprotein of *Arabacia punctulata* sperm chromatin, *Biochemistry*, 8, 4138, 1969.

182. **Elgin, S. C. R. and Bonner, J.**, Partial fractionation and chemical characterization of the major nonhistone chromosomal proteins, *Biochemistry*, 11, 722, 1972.

183. **Gronow, M.**, Solubilization and partial fractionation of the sulphur-containing nuclear proteins of hepatoma 233 ascites cells, *Eur. J. Cancer*, 5, 497, 1969.

184. **Gronow, M. and Griffiths, G.**, Rapid isolation and separation of the nonhistone proteins of rat liver nuclei, *FEBS Lett.*, 15, 340, 1971.

185. **Gonzalez-Mujica, F. and Mathias, A. P.**, Proteins from different classes of liver nuclei in normal and thioacetamide-treated rats, *Biochem. J.*, 133, 441, 1973.

186. **Gershey, E. L. and Kleinsmith, L. J.**, Phosphoproteins from calf-thymus nuclei: studies on the method of isolation, *Biochim. Biophys. Acta*, 194, 331, 1969.

187. **Platz, R D., Stein, G. S., and Kleinsmith, L. J.**, Changes in the phosphorylation of non-histone chromatin proteins during the cell cycle of HeLa S₃ cells, *Biochem. Biophys. Res. Commun.*, 51, 735, 1973.

188. **Platz, R. D. and Hnilica, L. S.**, Phosphorylation of nonhistone chromatin proteins during sea urchin development, *Biochem. Biophys. Res. Commun.*, 54, 222, 1973.

189. **Fujitani, H. and Holoubek, V.**, Similarity of the 0.35 *M* NaCl soluble nuclear proteins and the nonhistone chromosomal proteins, *Biochem. Biophys. Res. Commun.*, 54, 1300, 1973.

190. **Fujitani, H. and Holoubek, V.**, Fractionation of nuclear proteins by extraction with solutions of different ionic strength, *Int. J. Biochem.*, 6, 547, 1975.

191. **Comings, D. E. and Tack, L. O.**, Non-histone proteins. The effect of nuclear washes and comparison of metaphase and interphase chromatin, *Exp. Cell Res.*, 82, 175, 1973.

192. **Kostraba, N. C., Montagna, R. A., and Wang, T. Y.**, Study of the loosely bound non-histone chromatin proteins. Stimulation of deoxyribonucleic acid-templated ribonucleic acid synthesis by a specific deoxyribonucleic acid-binding phosphoprotein fraction, *J. Biol. Chem.*, 250, 1548, 1975.

193. **Prestayko, A. W., Crane, P. M., and Busch, H.**, Phosphorylation and DNA binding of nuclear rat liver proteins soluble at low ionic strength, *Biochemistry*, 15, 414, 1976.

194. **Comings, D. E. and Harris, D. C.**, Nuclear proteins. II. Similarity of nonhistone proteins in nuclear sap and chromatin, and essential absence of contractile proteins from mouse liver nuclei, *J. Cell Biol.*, 70, 440, 1976.

195. **Bekhor, I., Lapeyre, J. -N., and Kim, J.**, Fractionation of nonhistone chromosomal proteins isolated from rabbit liver and submandibular salivary gland, *Arch. Biochem. Biophys.*, 161, 1, 1974.

196. **Murphy, R. F. and Bonner, J.**, Alkaline extraction of non-histone proteins from rat liver chromatin, *Biochim. Biophys. Acta*, 405, 62, 1975.

197. **Russev, G., Anachkova, B., and Tsanev, R.**, Fractionation of rat liver chromatin nonhistone proteins into two groups with different metabolic rates, *Eur. J. Biochem.*, 58, 253, 1975.

198. **Wang, T. Y. and Johns, E. W.**, Study of the chromatin acidic proteins of rat liver: heterogeneity and complex formation with histones, *Arch. Biochem. Biophys.*, 124, 176, 1968.

199. **Patel, G., Patel, V., Wang, T. Y. and Zobel, C. R.**, Studies of the nuclear residual proteins, *Arch. Biochem. Biophys.*, 128, 654, 1968.

200. **Loeb, J. and Creuzet, C.**, Electrophoretic comparison of acidic proteins of chromatin from different animal tissues, *FEBS Lett.*, 5, 37, 1969.

201. **Kostraba, N. C. and Wang, T. Y.**, Tissue variations of acidic nuclear proteins and their biosynthesis during liver regeneration, *Int. J. Biochem.*, 1, 327, 1970.

202. **Shapiro, A. L., Viñuela, E., and Maizel, J. A., Jr.**, Molecular weight estimation of polypeptide chains by electrophoresis in SDS-polyacrylamide gels, *Biochem. Biophys. Res. Commun.*, 28, 815, 1967.

203. **Laemmli, U. K.**, Cleavage of structural proteins during the assembly of the head of bacteriophage T4, *Nature (London)*, 227, 680, 1970.

204. **Wu, F. C., Elgin, S. C. R., and Hood, L. E.**, Nonhistone chromosomal proteins of rat tissues. A comparative study by gel electrophoresis, *Biochemistry*, 12, 2792, 1973.

205. **Elgin, S. C. R., Boyd, J. B., Hood, L. E., Wray, W., and Wu, F. C.**, A prologue to the study of the nonhistone chromosomal proteins, *Cold Spring Harb. Symp. Quant. Biol.*, 38, 821, 1974.

206. **Sevaljevic, L. and Stamenkovic, M.**, Separation of chromatin proteins by an isoelectric focusing method, *Int. J. Biochem.*, 3, 525, 1972.

207. **Tsitilou, S. G., Cox, D., Mathias, A. P., and Ridge, D.**, The characterization of the non-histone chromosomal proteins of the main classes of nuclei from rat brain fractionated by zonal centrifugation, *Biochem. J.*, 177, 331, 1979.

208. **Catino, J J., Yeoman, L. C., Mandel, M., and Busch, H.**, Characterization of a DNA binding protein from rat liver chromatin which decreases during growth, *Biochemistry*, 17, 983, 1978.

209. **Taylor, C. W., Yeoman, L. C., and Busch, H.,** The isolation of nuclei with citric acid and the analysis of proteins by two-dimensional polyacrylamide gel electrophoresis, in *Methods in Cell Biology,* Vol. 9, Prescott, D. M., Ed., Academic Press, New York, 1975, 349.

210. **Barrett, T. and Gould, H. J.,** Tissue and species specificity of non-histone chromatin proteins, *Biochim. Biophys. Acta,* 294, 165, 1973.

211. **MacGillivray, A. J. and Rickwood, D.,** The heterogeneity of mouse-chromatin nonhistone proteins as evidenced by two-dimensional polyacrylamide gel electrophoresis and ion-exchange chromatography, *Eur. J. Biochem.,* 41, 181, 1974.

212. **Peterson, J. L. and McConkey, E. H.,** Non-histone chromosomal proteins from HeLa cells. A survey by high resolution, two-dimensional electrophoresis, *J. Biol. Chem.,* 251, 548, 1976.

213. **Peterson, J. L. and McConkey, E. H.,** Proteins of Friend leukemia cells. Comparison of hemoglobin-synthesizing and noninduced populations, *J. Biol. Chem.,* 251, 555, 1976.

214. **O'Farrell, P. H.,** High resolution two-dimensional electrophoresis of proteins, *J. Biol. Chem.,* 250, 4007, 1975.

215. **Stein, G. S., Stein, J. L., Park, W. D., Detke, S., Lichtler, A. C., Shephard, E. A., Jansing, R. L., and Phillips, I. R.,** Regulation of gene expression in HeLa S_3 cells, *Cold Spring Harb. Symp. Quant. Biol.,* 42, 1107, 1977.

216. **Park, W. D., Stein, G. S., and Stein, J. L.,** Fractionation and partial characterization of S phase HeLa cell nonhistone chromosomal proteins involved with histone gene transcription, manuscript submitted.

217. **Wang, T. Y.,** Restoration of histone-inhibited DNA-dependent RNA synthesis by acidic chromatin proteins, *Exp. Cell Res.,* 53, 288, 1968.

218. **Gilmour, R. S. and Paul, J.,** RNA transcribed from reconstituted nucleoprotein is similar to natural RNA, *J. Mol. Biol.,* 40, 137, 1969.

219. **MacGillivray, A. J. and Rickwood, D.,** Further characterization of the chromatin non-histone proteins by ion-exchange chromatography and two-dimensional gel electrophoresis, *Biochem. Soc. Trans.,* 1, 686, 1973.

220. **Park, W., Jansing, R., Stein, J., and Stein, G.,** Activation of histone gene transcription in quiescent WI-38 cells or mouse liver by a nonhistone chromosomal fraction from HeLa S_3 cells, *Biochemistry,* 16, 3713, 1977.

221. **Goodwin, G. H., Shooter, K. V., and Johns, E. W.,** Interaction of a non-histone chromatin protein (high-mobility group protein 2) with DNA, *Eur. J. Biochem.,* 54, 427, 1975.

222. **Chaudhuri, S., Stein, G., and Baserga, R.,** Binding of chromosomal acidic proteins to DNA and chromatin, *Proc. Soc. Exp. Biol. Med.,* 139, 1363, 1972.

223. **Patel, G. L. and Thomas, T. L.,** Some binding parameters of chromatin acidic proteins with high affinity for deoxyribonucleic acid, *Proc. Natl. Acad. Sci. U.S.A.,* 70, 2524, 1973.

224. **Kleinsmith, L. J., Heidema, J., and Carroll, A.,** Specific binding of rat liver nuclear proteins to DNA, *Nature (London),* 226, 1025, 1970.

225. **Kleinsmith, L. J.,** Specific binding of phosphorylated non-histone chromatin proteins to deoxyribonucleic acid, *J. Biol. Chem.,* 248, 5648, 1973.

226. **Wakabayashi, K., Wang, S., Hord, G., and Hnilica, L. S.,** Tissue-specific non-histone chromatin proteins with affinity for DNA, *FEBS Lett.,* 32, 46, 1973.

227. **Thomas, T. L. and Patel, G. L.,** DNA unwinding component of the non-histone chromatin proteins, *Proc. Natl. Acad. Sci. U.S.A.,* 73, 4364, 1976.

228. **Yamamoto, K. R. and Alberts, B. M.,** In vitro conversion of estradiol-receptor protein to its nuclear form: dependence on hormone and DNA, *Proc. Natl. Acad. Sci. U.S.A.,* 69, 2105, 1972.

229. **Allfrey, V. G.,** DNA-binding proteins and transcriptional control in prokaryotic and eukaryotic systems, in *Acidic Proteins of the Nucleus,* Cameron, I. L. and Jeter, J. R., Jr., Eds., Academic Press, New York, 1974, 1.

230. **Allfrey, V. G., Inoue, A., Karn, J., Johnson, E. M., and Vidali, G.,** Phosphorylation of DNA-binding nuclear acidic proteins and gene activation in the HeLa cell cycle, *Cold Spring Harb. Symp. Quant. Biol.,* 38, 785, 1974.

231. **Allfrey, V. G., Inoue, A., and Johnson, E. M.,** Use of DNA columns to separate and characterize nuclear non-histone proteins, in *Chromosomal Proteins and their Role in the Regulation of Gene Expression,* Stein, G. S. and Kleinsmith, L. J., Eds., Academic Press, New York, 1975, 265.

232. **Patel, G. L. and Thomas, T. L.,** Interactions of a subclass of nonhistone chromatin proteins with DNA, in *Chromosomal Proteins and their Role in the Regulation of Gene Expression,* Stein, G. S. and Kleinsmith, L. J., Eds., Academic Press, New York, 1975, 249.

233. **Sevall, J. S., Cockburn, A., Savage, M., and Bonner, J.,** DNA-protein interactions of the rat liver non-histone chromosomal protein, *Biochemistry,* 14, 782, 1975.

234. **Kikuchi, H. and Sato, S.,** Fractionation of nonhistone proteins on a column of daunomycin-CH-Sepharose 4B, *Biochim. Biophys. Acta,* 532, 113, 1978.

235. **Conner, B. J. and Comings, D. E.,** Nuclear proteins. V. Studies of histone-binding proteins from mouse liver by affinity chromatography, *Biochim. Biophys. Acta*, 532, 122, 1978.
236. **James, G. T., Yeoman, L. C., Matsui, S., Goldberg, A. H., and Busch, H.,** Isolation and characterization of nonhistone chromosomal protein C-14 which stimulates RNA synthesis, *Biochemistry*, 16, 2384, 1977.
237. **Patel, G., Howk, R., and Wang, T. Y.,** Partial purification of a DNA-polymerase from the nonhistone chromatin proteins of rat liver, *Nature (London)*, 215, 1488, 1967.
238. **Howk, R. and Wang, T. Y.,** DNA polymerase from rat liver chromosomal proteins. Alteration of template specificity and alkaline deoxyribonuclease activity, *Eur. J. Biochem.*, 13, 455, 1970.
239. **Loeb, L. A.,** Molecular association of DNA polymerase with chromatin in sea urchin embryos, *Nature (London)*, 226, 448, 1970.
240. **Chang, L. M. S.,** Low molecular weight deoxyribonucleic acid polymerase from calf thymus chromatin. I. Preparation of homogeneous enzyme, *J. Biol. Chem.*, 248, 3789, 1973.
241. **Tsuruo, T. and Ukita, T.,** Purification and further characterization of three DNA polymerases of rat ascites hepatoma cells, *Biochim. Biophys. Acta*, 353, 146, 1974.
242. **Weiss, S. B.,** Enzymic incorporation of ribonucleoside triphosphates into the interpolynucleotide linkages of ribonucleic acid, *Proc. Natl. Acad. Sci. U.S.A.*, 46, 1020, 1960.
243. **Tata, J. R. and Baker, B.,** Sub-nuclear fractionation. I. Procedure and characterization of fractions, *Exp. Cell Res.*, 83, 111, 1974.
244. **Tata, J. R. and Baker, B.,** Sub-nuclear fractionation. II. Intranuclear compartmentation of transcription in vivo and in vitro, *Exp. Cell Res.*, 83, 125, 1974.
245. **Lentfer, D. and Lezius, A. G.,** Mouse-myeloma RNA polymerase B. Template specificities and the role of a transcription-stimulating factor, *Eur. J. Biochem.*, 30, 278, 1972.
246. **Mondal, H., Ganguly, A., Das, A., Mandal, R. K., and Biswas, B. B.,** Ribonucleic acid polymerase from eukaryotic cells. Effects of factors and rifampicin on the activity of RNA polymerase from chromatin of coconut nuclei, *Eur. J. Biochem.*, 28, 143, 1972.
247. **Cox, R. F.,** Transcription of high-molecular-weight RNA from hen-oviduct chromatin by bacterial and endogenous form-B RNA polymerases, *Eur. J. Biochem.*, 39, 49, 1973.
248. **Ganguly, A., Das, A., Mondal, H., Mandal, R. K., and Biswas, B. B.,** Molecular weight and subunit structure of RNA polymerase I and initiation factor from chromatin of plant cell nuclei, *FEBS Lett.*, 34, 27, 1973.
249. **O'Connor, P. J.,** Alkaline deoxyribonuclease from rat liver nonhistone chromatin proteins, *Biochem. Biophys. Res. Commun.*, 35, 805, 1969.
250. **Swingle, K. F., Cole, L. J., and Bailey, J. S.,** Association of neutral deoxyribonuclease with chromatin isolated from mammalian cells, *Biochim. Biophys. Acta*, 149, 467, 1969.
251. **Urbanczyk, J. and Studzinski, G. P.,** Chromatin-associated DNA endonuclease activities in HeLa cells, *Biochem. Biophys. Res. Commun.*, 59, 616, 1974.
252. **Gaziev, A. I. and Kuzin, A. M.,** Localization of DNA ligase in the chromatin of animal cells, *Eur. J. Biochem.*, 37, 7, 1973.
253. **Wang, T. Y.,** Isolation of a terminal DNA-nucleotidyltransferase from calf thymus nonhistone chromatin proteins, *Arch. Biochem. Biophys.*, 127, 235, 1968.
254. **Srivastava, B. I. S.,** Association of terminal deoxynucleotidyl transferase activity with chromatin from plant tissue, *Biochem. Biophys. Res. Commun.*, 48, 270, 1972.
255. **Sasaki, K. and Tazawa, T.,** Polyriboadenylate synthesizing activity in chromatin of wheat seedlings, *Biochem. Biophys. Res. Commun.*, 52, 1440, 1973.
256. **Burdon, R. H.,** Enzymic modification of chromosomal macromolecules. I. DNA and protein methylation in mouse tumor cell chromatin, *Biochim. Biophys. Acta*, 232, 359, 1971.
257. **Hotta, Y. and Stern, H.,** A DNA-binding protein in meiotic cells of *Lilium*, *Dev. Biol.*, 26, 87, 1971.
258. **Hotta, Y. and Stern, H.,** Meiotic protein in spermatocytes of mammals, *Nature (London) New Biol.*, 234, 83, 1971.
259. **Champoux, J. J. and Dulbecco, R.,** An activity from mammalian cells that untwists superhelical DNA — a possible swivel for DNA replication, *Proc. Natl. Acad. Sci. U.S.A.*, 69, 143, 1972.
260. **Basse, W. A. and Wang, J. C.,** An ω protein from *Drosophila melanogaster*, *Biochemistry*, 13, 4299, 1974.
261. **Herrick, G. and Alberts, B.,** Purification and physical characterization of nucleic acid helix-unwinding proteins from calf thymus, *J. Biol. Chem.*, 251, 2124, 1976.
262. **Champoux, J. J. and McConaughy, B. L.,** Purification and characterization of the DNA untwisting enzyme from rat liver, *Biochemistry*, 15, 4638, 1976.
263. **Bina-Stein, M., Vogel, T., Singer, D. S., and Singer, M. F.,** H_5 histone and DNA-relaxing enzyme of chicken erythrocytes, *J. Biol. Chem.*, 251, 7363, 1976.
264. **Bartley, J. and Chalkley, R.,** Further studies of a thymus nucleohistone-associated protease, *J. Biol. Chem.*, 245, 4286, 1970.

265. **Garrels, J. I., Elgin, S. C. R., and Bonner, J.,** Histone protease of rat liver chromatin, *Biochem. Biophys. Res. Commun.,* 46, 545, 1972.

266. **Chong, M. T., Garrard, W. T., and Bonner, J.,** Purification and properties of a neutral protease from rat liver chromatin, *Biochemistry,* 13, 5128, 1974.

267. **Carter, D. B. and Chae, C.-B.,** Chromatin bound protease: degradation of chromosomal proteins under chromatin dissociation conditions, *Biochemistry,* 15, 180, 1976.

268. **Racey, L. A. and Byvoet, P.,** Histone acetyltransferase in chromatin. Evidence for in vitro enzymatic transfer of acetate from acetyl-coenzyme A to histones, *Exp. Cell Res.,* 64, 366, 1971.

269. **Racey, L. A. and Byvoet, P.,** Histone acetyltransferase in chromatin. Extraction of transferase activity from chromatin, *Exp. Cell Res.,* 73, 329, 1972.

270. **Gallwitz, D. and Sures, I.,** Histone acetylation. Purification and properties of three histone-specific acetyltransferases from rat thymus nuclei, *Biochim. Biophys. Acta,* 263, 315, 1972.

271. **Libby, P. R.,** Calf liver nuclear N-acetyltransferases. Purification and properties of two enzymes with both spermidine acetyltransferase and histone acetyltransferase activities, *J. Biol. Chem.,* 253, 233, 1978.

272. **Vidali, G., Boffa, L. C., and Allfrey, V. G.** Properties of an acidic histone-binding protein fraction from cell nuclei. Selective precipitation and deacetylation of histone F_{2a1} and F_3, *J. Biol. Chem.,* 247, 7365, 1972.

273. **Krieger, D. E., Levine, R., Merrifield, R. B., Vidali, G., and Allfrey, V. G.,** Chemical studies of histone acetylation, substrate specificity of a histone deacetylase from calf thymus nuclei, *J. Biol. Chem.,* 249, 332, 1974.

274. **Smith, D. L., Chen, C.-C., Bruegger, B. B., Holtz, S. L., Halpern, R. M., and Smith, R. A.,** Characterization of protein kinases forming acid-labile histone phosphates in Walker-256 carcinosarcoma cell nuclei, *Biochemistry,* 13, 3780, 1974.

275. **Comb, D. G., Sarker, N., and Pinzino, C. J.,** The methylation of lysine residues in protein, *J. Biol. Chem.,* 241, 1857, 1966.

276. **Byvoet, P. and Baxter, C. S.,** Histone methylation, a functional enigma, in *Chromosomal Proteins and their Role in the Regulation of Gene Expression,* Stein, G. and Kleinsmith, L., Eds., Academic Press, New York, 1975, 127.

277. **Yamada, M. and Sugimura, T.,** Effects of deoxyribonucleic acid and histone on the number and length of chains of poly(adenosine diphosphate-ribose), *Biochemistry,* 12, 3303, 1973.

278. **Jockusch, B. M., Becker, M., Hindennach, I., and Jockusch, H.,** Slime mould actin: homology to vertebrate actin and presence in the nucleus, *Exp. Cell Res.,* 89, 241, 1974.

279. **LeStourgeon, W. M., Forer, A., Yang, Y-Z., Bertram, J. S., and Rusch, H. P.,** Contractile proteins. Major components of nuclear and chromosome nonhistone proteins, *Biochim. Biophys. Acta,* 379, 529, 1975.

280. **Pederson, T.,** Isolation and characterization of chromatin from the cellular slime mold, *Dictyostelium discoideum, Biochemistry,* 16, 2771, 1977.

281. **Fukui, Y.,** Intranuclear actin bundles induced by dimethyl sulfoxide in interphase nucleus of *Dictyostelium, J. Cell Biol.,* 76, 146, 1978.

282. **Douvas, A. S., Harrington, C. A., and Bonner, J.,** Major nonhistone proteins of rat liver chromatin: preliminary identification of myosin, actin, tubulin and tropomyosin, *Proc. Natl. Acad. Sci. U.S.A.,* 72, 3902, 1975.

283. **Bertram, J. S., Libby, P. R., and LeStourgeon, W. M.,** Changes in nuclear actin levels with change in growth state of C3H/10T½ cells and the lack of response in malignantly transformed cells, *Cancer Res.,* 37, 4104, 1977.

284. **Goldstein, L., Rubin, R., and Ko, C.,** The presence of actin in nuclei: a critical appraisal, *Cell,* 12, 601, 1977.

285. **Lazarides, E. and Lindberg, U.,** Actin is the naturally occurring inhibitor of deoxyribonuclease I, *Proc. Natl. Acad. Sci. U. S.A.,* 71, 4742, 1974.

286. **Adolph, K. W., Cheng, S. M., and Laemmli, U. K.,** Role of nonhistone proteins in metaphase chromatin structure, *Cell,* 12, 805, 1977.

287. **Paulson, J. R. and Laemmli, U. K.,** The structure of histone-depleted metaphase chromosomes, *Cell,* 12, 817, 1977.

288. **Adolph, K. W., Cheng, S. M., Paulson, J. R., and Laemmli, U. K.,** Isolation of a protein scaffold from mitotic HeLa cell chromosomes, *Proc. Natl. Acad. Sci. U.S.A.,* 74, 4937, 1977.

289. **Laemmli, U. K., Cheng, S. M., Adolph, K. W., Paulson, J. R., Brown, J. A., and Baumbach, W. R.,** Metaphase chromosome structure: a study of the role of non-histone proteins, *Cold Spring Harbor Symp. Quant. Biol.,* 42, 351, 1977.

290. **Augenlicht, L. H. and Lipkin, M.,** Chromatin monomer: absence of non-histone proteins, *Biochem. Biophys. Res. Commun.,* 70, 540, 1976.

291. **Liew, C. C. and Chan, P. K.,** Identification of nonhistone chromatin proteins in chromatin subunits, *Proc. Natl. Acad. Sci. U.S.A.,* 73, 3458, 1976.

292. **Paul, J. and Malcolm, S.,** A class of chromatin particles associated with nonhistone proteins, *Biochemistry*, 15, 3510, 1976.
293. **Goodwin, G. H., Woodhead, L., and Johns, E. W.,** The presence of high mobility group non-histone chromatin proteins in isolated nucleosomes, *FEBS Lett.*, 73, 85, 1977.
294. **Vidali, G., Boffa, L. C., and Allfrey, V. G.,** Selective release of chromosomal proteins during limited DNase I digestion of avian erythrocyte chromatin, *Cell*, 12, 409, 1977.
295. **Goldknopf, I. L., French, M. F., Musso, R., and Busch, H.,** Presence of protein A24 in rat liver nucleosomes, *Proc. Natl. Acad. Sci. U.S.A.*, 74, 5492, 1977.
296. **Levy, W. B., Wong, N. C. W., and Dixon, G. H.,** Selective association of the trout-specific H6 protein with chromatin regions susceptible to DNase I and DNase II: possible location of HMG-T in the spacer region between core nucleosomes, *Proc. Natl. Acad. Sci. U.S.A.*, 74, 2810, 1977.
297. **Smerdon, M. J. and Isenberg, I.,** Interactions between the subfractions of calf thymus H1 and non-histone chromosomal proteins HMG1 and HMG2, *Biochemistry*, 15, 4242, 1976.
298. **Goldknopf, I. L. and Busch, H.,** Isopeptide linkage between nonhistone and histone 2A polypeptides of chromosomal conjugate-protein A24, *Proc. Natl. Acad. Sci. U.S.A.*, 74, 864, 1977.
299. **Hunt, L. T. and Dayhoff, M. O.,** Amino-terminal sequence identity of ubiquitin and the nonhistone component of nuclear protein A24, *Biochem. Biophys. Res. Commun.*, 74, 650, 1977.
300. **Birnie, G. D., Rickwood, D., and Hell, A.,** Buoyant densities and hydration of nucleic acids, proteins and nucleoprotein complexes in metrizamide, *Biochim. Biophys. Acta*, 331, 283, 1973.
301. **Scott, S. E. M. and Sommerville, J.,** Location of nuclear proteins on the chromosomes of the newt oocytes, *Nature (London)*, 250, 680, 1974.
302. **Alfageme, C.R., Rudkin, G. T., and Cohen, L. H.,** Locations of chromosomal proteins in polytene chromosomes, *Proc. Natl. Acad. Sci. U.S.A.*, 73, 2038, 1976.
303. **Silver, L. M. and Elgin, S. C. R.,** A method for determination of the *in situ* distribution of chromosomal proteins, *Proc. Natl. Acad. Sci. U.S.A.*, 73, 423, 1976.
304. **Silver, L. M. and Elgin, S. C. R.,** Distribution patterns of three subfractions of *Drosophila* nonhistone chromosomal proteins: possible correlations with gene activity, *Cell*, 11, 971, 1977.
305. **Miller, O. L., Jr., and Hamkalo, B. A.,** Visualization of RNA synthesis on chromosomes, *Int. Rev. Cytol.*, 33, 1, 1972.
306. **Augenlicht, L. H. and Lipkin, M.,** Appearance of rapidly labeled, high molecular weight RNA in nuclear ribonucleoprotein, *J. Biol. Chem.*, 251, 2592, 1976.
307. **Samarina, O. P., Lukanidin, E. M., Molnar, J., and Georgiev, G. P.,** Structural organization of nuclear complexes containing DNA-like RNA, *J. Mol. Biol.*, 33, 251, 1968.
308. **Kierszenbaum, A. L. and Tres, L. L.,** Transcription sites in spread meiotic prophase chromosomes from mouse spermatocytes, *J. Cell Biol.*, 63, 923, 1974.
309. **Mott, M. R. and Callan, H. G.,** An electron microscope study of the lamp brush chromosomes of the newt *Triturus cristatus*, *J. Cell Sci.*, 17, 241, 1975.
310. **Malcolm, D. B. and Sommerville, J.,** The strucure of nuclear ribonucleoprotein of amphibian oocytes, *J. Cell Sci.*, 24, 143, 1977.
311. **Kish, V. M. and Pederson, T.,** Heterogeneous nuclear RNA secondary structure: oligo(U) sequences base-paired with poly(A) and their possible role as binding sites for heterogeneous nuclear RNA-specific proteins, *Proc. Natl. Acad. Sci. U.S.A.*, 74, 1426, 1977.
312. **Beyer, A. L., Christensen, M. E., Walker, B W., and LeStourgeon, W. M.,** Identification and characterization of the packaging proteins of core 40S HnRNP particles, *Cell*, 11, 127, 1977.
313. **Karn, J., Vidali, G., Boffa, L. C., and Allfrey, V. G.,** Characterization of the non-histone nuclear proteins associated with rapidly labeled heterogeneous nuclear RNA, *J. Biol. Chem.*, 20, 7307, 1977.
314. **LeStourgeon, W. M., Beyer, A. L., Christensen, M. E., Walker, B. W., Poupore, S. M., and Daniels, L. P.,** The packaging proteins of core HnRNP particles and the maintenance of proliferative cell states, *Cold Spring Harbor Symp. Quant. Biol.*, 42, 885, 1977.
315. **Martin, T., Billings, P., Pullman, J., Stevens, B., and Kinniburgh, A.,** Substructure of nuclear ribonucleoprotein complexes, *Cold Spring Harbor Symp. Quant. Biol.*, 42, 899, 1977.
316. **Goodwin, G. H., Nicolas, R. H., and Johns, E. W.,** Microheterogeneity in a non-histone chromosomal protein, *FEBS Lett.*, 64, 412, 1976.
317. **Delange, R. J. and Smith, E. L.,** Histones: structure and function, *Annu. Rev. Biochem.*, 40, 279, 1971.
318. **Kruh, J., Tichonicky, L., and Wajcman, H.,** Action des proteines acides du noyau sur la synthese accelulaire de l'hemoglobine et sur les RNA, *Biochim. Biophys. Acta*, 196, 549, 1969.
319. **Platz, R. D., Kish, V M., and Kleinsmith, L. J.,** Tissue specificity of nonhistone chromatin phosphoproteins, *FEBS Lett.*, 12, 38, 1970.
320. **Wang, T. Y.,** Tissue specificity of non-histone chromosomal proteins, *Exp. Cell Res.*, 69, 217, 1971.
321. **Wilhelm, J. A., Ansevin, A. T., Johnson, A. W., and Hnilica, L. S.,** Proteins of chromatin in genetic restriction. IV. Comparison of histone and nonhistone proteins of rat liver nucleolar and extranucleolar chromatin, *Biochim. Biophs. Acta*, 272, 220, 1972.

322. **Bekhor, I., Anne, L., Kim, J., Lapeyre, J.-N., and Stambaugh, R.,** Organ discrimination through organ-specific nonhistone chromosomal proteins, *Arch. Biochem. Biophys.,* 161, 11, 1974.

323. **Davis, R. H., Wilson, R. B., and Ebadi, M. S.,** Tissue specificity of nuclear acidic proteins isolated from bovine brain and adrenal medulla, *Can. J. Biochem.,* 53, 101, 1975.

324. **Fujitani, H. and Holoubek, V.,** Presence of the same types of nonhistone chromosomal proteins of different tissues, *Experientia,* 30, 474, 1974.

325. **Chytil, F. and Spelsberg, T. C.,** Tissue differences in antigenic properties of non-histone protein-DNA complexes, *Nature (London) New Biol.,* 233, 215, 1971.

326. **Zardi, L., Lin, J.-C., and Baserga, R.,** Immunospecificity to non-histone chromosomal proteins of anti-chomatin antibodies, *Nature (London) New Biol.,* 245, 211, 1973.

327. **Wakabayashi, K., and Hnilica, L. S.,** The immunospecificity of nonhistone protein complexes with DNA, *Nature (London) New Biol.,* 242, 153, 1973.

328. **Chiu, J.-F., Craddock, C., Morris, H. P., and Hnilica, L. S.,** Immunospecificity of chromatin non-histone protein-DNA complexes in normal and neoplastic growth, *FEBS Lett.,* 42, 94, 1974.

329. **Wakabayashi, K., Wang, S., and Hnilica, L. S.,** Immunospecificity of non-histone proteins in chromatin, *Biochemistry,* 13, 1027, 1974.

330. **Wang, S., Chiu, J.-F., Klyszejko-Stefanowicz, L., Fujitani, H., Hnilica, L. S., and Ansevin, A. T.,** Tissue-specific chromosomal non-histone protein interactions with DNA, *J. Biol. Chem.,* 5, 1471, 1976.

331. **Wu, F. C., Elgin, S. C. R., and Hood, L. E.** The nonhistone chromosomal proteins of vertebrate liver and kidney: a comparative study by gel electrophoresis, *J. Mol. Evol.,* 5, 87, 1975.

332. **Shooter, K. V., Goodwin, G. H., and Johns, E. W.,** Interactions of a purified non-histone chromosomal protein with DNA and histone, *Eur. J. Biochem.,* 47, 263, 1974.

333. **Yu, S. S., Li, H. J., Goodwin, G. H., and Johns, E. W.,** Interaction of non-histone chromosomal proteins HMG1 and HMG2 with DNA, *Eur. J. Biochem.,* 78, 497, 1977.

334. **Jost, E., Lennox, R., and Harris, H.,** Affinity chromatography of DNA-binding proteins from human, murine and man-mouse hybrid cell lines, *J. Cell Sci.,* 18, 41, 1975.

335. **Fujitani, H. and Holoubek, V.,** Nonhistone nuclear proteins of rat brain, *J. Neurochem.,* 23, 1215, 1974.

336. **Olpe, H.-R., von Hahn, H. P., and Honegger, C. G.,** Differences in electrophoretic patterns of nonhistone proteins from large and small nuclei of rat brain, *Brain Res.,* 58, 453, 1973.

337. **Tashiro, T., Mizobe, F., and Kurokawa, M.,** Characteristics of cerebral non-histone chromatin proteins as revealed by polyacrylamide gel electrophoresis, *FEBS Lett.,* 38, 121, 1974.

338. **Fleischer-Lambropoulos, H., Sarkander, H. I., and Brade, W. P.,** Phosphorylation of nonhistone chromatin protein from neuronal and glial nuclei-enriched fractions of rat brain, *FEBS Lett.,* 45, 329, 1974.

339. **Mirsky, A. E. and Ris, H.,** The composition and structure of isolated chromosomes, *J. Gen. Physiol.,* 34, 475, 1951.

340. **Busch, H., Ballal, N. R., Olson, M. O. J., and Yeoman, L. C.,** Chromatin and its nonhistone proteins, in *Methods in Cancer Research,* Vol. 11, Busch, H., Ed., Academic Press, New York, 1975, 43.

341. **Ozaki, H.,** Developmental studies of sea urchin chromatin. Chromatin isolated from spermatozoa of the sea urchin, *Strongylocentrotus purpuratus, Dev. Biol.,* 26, 209, 1971.

342. **Mohberg, J. and Rusch, H. P.,** Nuclear histones in *Physarum polycephalum* during growth and differentiation, *Arch. Biochem. Biophys.,* 138, 418, 1970.

343. **Gershey, E. L. and Kleinsmith, L. J.,** Phosphorylation of nuclear proteins in avian erythrocytes, *Biochim. Biophys. Acta,* 194, 519, 1969.

344. **Marushige, K. and Dixon, G. H.,** Developmental changes in chromosomal composition and template activity during spermatogenesis in trout testis, *Dev. Biol.,* 19, 397, 1969.

345. **Marushige, K. and Ozaki, H.,** Properties of isolated chromatin from sea urchin embryo, *Dev. Biol.,* 16, 474, 1967.

346. **Dolbeare, F. and Koenig, H.,** Fractionation of rat liver chromatin: effects of cations, hepatectomy and actinomycin D, *Proc. Soc. Exp. Biol. Med.,* 135, 636, 1970.

347. **Marushige, K. and Bonner, J.,** Fractionation of liver chromatin, *Proc. Natl. Acad. Sci. U.S.A.,* 68, 2941, 1971.

348. **Reeck, G. R., Simpson, R. T., and Sober, H. A.,** Resolution of a spectrum of nucleoprotein species in sonicated chromatin, *Proc. Natl. Acad. Sci. U.S.A.,* 69, 2317, 1972.

349. **Berkowitz, E. M. and Doty, P.,** Chemical and physical properties of fractionated chromatin, *Proc. Natl. Acad. Sci. U.S.A.,* 72, 3328, 1975.

350. **Neelin, J. M., Mazen, A., and Champagne, M.,** The fractionation of active and inactive chromatins from erythroid cells of chicken, *FEBS Lett.,* 65, 309, 1976.

351. **Rodriguez, L. V. and Becker, F. F.**, Rat liver chromatin. Distribution of histones and nonhistone proteins in eu- and heterochromatin, *Arch. Biochem Biophys.*, 173, 438, 1976.

352. **Comings, D. E., Harris, D. C., Okada, T. A., and Holmquist, G.**, Nuclear proteins. IV. Deficiency of non-histone proteins in condensed cromatin of *Drosophila virilis* and mouse, *Exp. Cell Res.*, 105, 349, 1977.

353. **Simpson, R. T. and Reeck, G. R.**, A comparison of the proteins of condensed and extended chromatin fractions of rabbit liver and calf thymus, *Biochemistry*, 12, 3853, 1973.

354. **Murphy, E. C., Hall, S. H., Shepherd, J. H., and Weiser, R. S.**, Fractionation of mouse myeloma chromatin, *Biochemistry*, 12, 3843, 1973.

355. **Gottesfeld, J. M., Garrard, W. T., Bagi, G., Wilson, R. F., ad Bonner, J.**, Partial purification of the template-active fraction of chromatin: a preliminary report, *Proc. Natl. Acad. Sci. U.S.A.*, 71, 2193, 1974.

356. **Comings, D. E. and Harris, D. C.**, Nuclear proteins. I. Electrophoretic comparison of mouse nuceoli, heterochromatin, euchromatin and contractile proteins, *Exp. Cell Res.*, 96, 161, 1975.

357. **Musich, P. R., Brown, F. L., and Maio, J. J.**, Subunit structure of chromatin and the organization of eukaryotic highly repetitive mammalian DNA, *Proc. Natl. Acad. Sci. U.S.A.*, 74, 3297, 1977.

358. **Chiu, N., Baserga, R., and Furth, J. J.**, Composition and template activity of chromatin fractionated by isoelectric focusing, *Biochemistry*, 16, 4796, 1977.

359. **Zardi, L.**, Chicken antichromatin antibodies: specificity to different chromatin fractions, *Eur. J. Biochem.*, 55, 231, 1975.

360. **Keller, R. K., Socher, S. H., Krall, J. F., Chandra, T., and O'Malley, B. W.**, Fractionation of chick oviduct chromatin. IV. Association of protein kinase with transcriptionally active chromatin, *Biochem. Biophys. Res. Commun.*, 66, 453, 1975.

361. **Gottsfeld, J. M. and Partington, G. A.**, Distribution of messenger RNA-coding sequences in fractionated chromatin, *Cell*, 12, 953, 1977.

362. **Wallace, R. B., Dube, S. K., and Bonner, J.**, Localization of the globin gene in the template active fraction of chromatin of Friend leukemia cells, *Science*, 198, 1166, 1977.

363. **Krieg, P. and Wells, J. R. E.**, The distribution of active genes (globin) and inactive genes (keratin) in fractionated chicken erythroid chromatin, *Biochemistry*, 15, 4549, 1976.

364. **Rovera, G. and Baserga, R.**, Effect of nutritional changes on chromatin template activity and non-histone chromosomal protein synthesis in WI-38 and 3T6 cells, *Exp. Cell Res.*, 78, 118, 1973.

365. **Johnson, E. M., Karn, J., and Allfrey, V. G.**, Early nuclear events in the induction of lymphocyte proliferation by mitogens. Effects of concanavalin A on the phosphorylation and distributon of non-histone chromatin proteins, *J. Biol. Chem.*, 249, 4990, 1974.

366. **Decker, J. M. and Marchalonis, J. J.**, Molecular events in lymphocyte differentiation: stimulation of nonhistone nuclear protein synthesis in rabbit peripheral blood lymphocytes by anti-immunoglobulin, *Biochem. Biophys. Res. Commun.*, 74, 584, 1977.

367. **Hemminki, K.**, Synthesis of chromatin proteins in resting and stimulated human lymphocyte populations, *Exp. Cell Res.*, 93, 63, 1975.

368. **Garrard, W. T. and Bonner, J.**, Changes in chromatin proteins during liver regeneration, *J. Biol. Chem.*, 249, 5570, 1974.

369. **Cameron, I. L., Griffin, E. E., and Rudick, M. J.**, Macromolecular events following refeeding of starved *Tetrahymena, Exp. Cell Res.*, 65, 262, 1971.

370. **Rudick, M. J. and Cameron, I. L.**, Regulation of DNA synthesis and cell division in starved-refed synchronized *Tetrahymena pyriformis, Exp. Cell Res.*, 70, 411, 1972.

371. **Jeter, J. R., Jr., Pavlat, W. A., and Cameron, I. L.**, Changes in the nuclear acidic proteins and chromatin structure in starved and refed *Tetrahymena, Exp. Cell Res.*, 93, 79, 1975.

372. **Weisenthal, L. M. and Ruddon, R. W.**, Characterization of human leukemia and Burkitt lymphoma cells by their acidic nuclear protein profiles, *Cancer Res.*, 32, 1009, 1972.

373. **Zornetzer, M. S. and Stein, G. S.**, Gene expression in mouse neuroblastoma cells: properties of the genome, *Proc. Natl. Acad. Sci. U.S.A.*, 72, 3119, 1975.

374. **Yeoman, L. C., Taylor, C. W., Jordan, J. J., and Busch, H.**, Differences in chromatin proteins of growing and non-growing tissues, *Exp. Cell Res.*, 91, 207, 1975.

375. **Yeoman, L. C., Seeber, S., Taylor, C. W., Fernbach, D. J., Falletta, J. M, Jordan, J. J., and Busch, H.**, Differences in chromatin proteins of resting and growing human lymphocytes, *Exp. Cell Res.*, 100, 47, 1976.

376. **Ševaljević, L., Popović, Ž., and Konstantinović, M.**, Investigation on stage-related changes of sea urchin chromatin proteins by hydroxyapatite chromatography, *Int. J. Biochem.*, 6, 903, 1975.

377. **Ševaljević, L., Krtolica, K., and Konstantinović, M.**, Embryonic stage-related properties of sea urchin embryo chromatin, *Bochim. Biophys. Acta*, 425, 76, 1976.

378. **Theriault, J. and Landesman, R.**, An analysis of acidic nuclear proteins during the development of *Xenopus laevis, Cell Differ.*, 3, 249, 1974.

379. **Teng, C. S.,** Nuclear acidic protein of the developing *Oncopeltus* embryos, *Biochim. Biophys. Acta,* 366, 385, 1974.

380. **Vidali, G., Boffa, L. C., Littau, V. C., Allfrey, K. M., and Allfrey, V. G.,** Changes in nuclear acidic protein complement of red blood cells during embryonic development, *J. Biol. Chem.,* 248, 4065, 1973.

381. **Pipkin, J. L., Jr. and Larson, D. A.,** Changing patterns of nucleic acids, basic and acidic proteins in generative and vegetative nuclei during pollen germination and pollen tube growth in *Hippeastrum belladonna, Exp. Cell Res.,* 79, 28, 1973.

382. **Spivak, J. L.,** Chromosomal protein synthesis during erythropoiesis in the mouse spleen, *Exp. Cell Res.,* 91, 253, 1975.

383. **Keppel, F., Allet, B. and Eisen, H.,** Appearance of a chromatin protein during the erythroid differentiation of Friend virus-transformed cells, *Proc. Natl. Acad. Sci. U.S.A.,* 74, 653, 1977.

384. **Kadohama, N. and Turkington, R. W.,** Changes in acidic chromatin proteins during the hormone-dependent development of rat testis and epididymis, *J. Biol. Chem.,* 249, 6225, 1974.

385. **Platz, R. D., Grimes, S. R, Hord, G., Meistrich, M. L., and Hnilica, L. S.,** Changes in nuclear proteins during embryonic development and cellular differentiation, in *Chromosomal Proteins and their Role in the Regulation of Gene Expression,* Stein, G. S. and Kleinsmith, L. J., Eds., Academic Press, New York, 1975, 67.

386. **Allfrey, V. G., Johnson, E. M., Karn, J., and Vidali, G.,** Phosphorylation of nuclear proteins at times of gene activation, in *Protein Phosphorylation in Control Mechanisms,* Miami Winter Symp., Vol. 5, Huijing, F. and Lee, E. Y. C., Eds., Academic Press, New York, 1973, 217.

387. **Lazo, J. S., Prasad, K. N., and Ruddon, R. W.,** Synthesis and phosphorylation of chromatin-associated proteins in cAMP-induced "differentiated" neuroblastoma cells in culture, *Exp. Cell Res.,* 100, 41, 1976.

388. **Banks-Schlegel, S., Martin, T. E., and Moscona, A. A.,** Synthesis and phosphorylation of chromosomal nonhistone proteins during embryonic development of neural retina, *Dev. Biol.,* 50, 1, 1976.

389. **Burdman, J A.,** The relationship between DNA synthesis and the synthesis of nuclear proteins in rat brain during development, *J. Neurochem.,* 19, 1459, 1972.

390. **Buck, M. D. and Schauder, P.,** In vivo stimulation of ^{14}C-amino acid incorporation into nonhistone proteins in rat liver chromatin induced by insulin and cortisol, *Biochim. Biophys. Acta,* 224, 644, 1970.

391. **Swaneck, G. E. Chu, L., and Edelman, I.,** Stereospecific binding of aldosterone to renal chromatin, *J. Biol. Chem.,* 245, 5382, 1970.

392. **Ruddon, R.W. and Rainey, C. H.,** Stimulation of nuclear protein synthesis in rat liver after phenobarbital administration, *Biochem. Biophys. Res. Commun.,* 40, 152, 1970.

393. **Teng, C. S. and Hamilton, T. H.,** Regulation by estrogen of organ-specific synthesis of a nuclear acidic protein, *Biochem. Biophys. Res. Commun.,* 40, 1231, 1970.

394. **Cohen, M. E. and Hamilton, T. H.** Effect of estradiol-17 β on the synthesis of specific uterine nonhistone chromosomal proteins, *Proc. Natl. Acad. Sci. U.S.A.,* 72, 4346, 1975.

395. **Hemminki, K.,** Labelling of oviduct nuclear and nucleolar proteins during estrogen induced differentiation, *Mol. Cell Biochem.,* 11, 9, 1976.

396. **Mainwaring, W. I. P., Rennie, P. S., and Keen, J.,** The androgenic regulation of prostate proteins with a high affinity for deoxyribonuceic acid. Evidence for a prostate deoxyribonucleic acid-unwinding protein, *Biochem. J.,* 156, 253, 1976.

397. **Enea, V. and Allfrey, V. G.** Selective synthesis of liver nuclear acidic proteins following glucagon administration in vivo, *Nature (London),* 242, 265, 1973.

398. **Helmsing, P. and Berendes, H.,** Induced accumulation of nonhistone proteins in polytene nuclei of *Drosophila hydei, J. Cell Biol.,* 50, 893, 1971.

399. **Alonso, A. and Arnold, H. P.,** Simulation of amino acid incorporation into rat liver nonhistone chromatin proteins after treatment with diethylnitrosamine, *FEBS Lett.,* 41, 8, 1974.

400. **Kadohama, N. and Turkington, R. W.,** Altered populations of acidic chromatin proteins in breast cancer cells, *Cancer Res.,* 33, 1194, 1973.

401. **Orrick, L. R., Olson, M. O. J., and Busch, H.,** Comparison of nucleolar proteins of normal rat liver and Novikoff hepatoma ascites cells by two-dimensional polyacrylamide gel electrophoresis, *Proc. Natl. Acad. Sci. U.S.A.,* 70, 1316, 1973.

402. **Chae, C.-B., Smith, M. C., and Morris, H. P.,** Chromosomal nonhistone proteins of rat hepatomas and normal rat liver, *Biochem. Biophys. Res. Commun.,* 60, 1468, 1974.

403. **Boffa, L. C., Vidali, G., and Allfrey, V. G.,** Selective synthesis and accumulation of nuclear nonhistone proteins during carcinogensis of the colon induced by 1,2-dimethylhydrazine, *Cancer,* 36, 2356, 1975.

404. **Boffa, L. C., Vidali, G., and Allfrey, V. G.,** Changes in nuclear non-histone protein composition during normal differentiation and carcinogenesis of intestinal epithelial cells, *Exp. Cell Res.,* 98, 396, 1976.

405. **Biessman, H. and Rajewsky, M. F.,** Nuclear protein patterns in developing and adult brain and in ethylnitrosourea-induced neuroectodermal tumours of the rat, *J. Neurochem.,* 24, 387, 1975.

406. **Biessman, H. and Rajewsky, M. F.,** The synthesis of brain chromosomal proteins after a pulse of the nervous system-specific carcinogen *N*-ethyl-*N*-nitrosourea to the fetal rat, *J. Neurochem.,* 27, 927, 1976.

407. **Kadohama, N. and Anderson, K. M.,** Nuclear non-histone proteins from rat ventral prostate cells undergoing hypertrophy or hyperplasia, *Exp. Cell Res.,* 99,135, 1976.

408. **Stein, G. S., Park, W. D., Stein, J. L., and Lieberman, M. W.,** Synthesis of nuclear proteins during DNA repair synthesis in human diploid fibroblasts damaged with ultraviolet radiation or *N*-acetoxy-2-acetylaminofluorene, *Proc. Natl. Acad. Sci. U.S.A.,* 73, 1466, 1976.

409. **Rovera, G., Baserga, R., and Defendi, V.,** Early increase in nuclear acidic protein synthesis after SV-40 infection, *Nature (London) New Biol.,* 237, 240, 1972.

410. **Ledinko, L.,** Nuclear acidic protein changes in adenovirus-infected human embryo kidney cultures, *Virology,* 54, 294, 1973.

411. **Krause, M. O. and Stein, G. S.,** Modifications in the chromosomal proteins of SV-40 transformed WI-38 human diploid fibroblasts, *Biochem. Biophys. Res. Commun.,* 59, 796, 1974.

412. **Krause, M. O., Kleinsmith, L. J., and Stein, G. S.,** Properties of the genome in normal and SV40 transformed WI38 human diploid fibroblasts. I. Composition and metabolism of nonhistone chromosomal proteins, *Exp. Cell Res.,* 92, 164, 1975.

413. **Krause, M. O., Kleinsmith, L. J., and Stein, G. S.,** Properties of the genome in normal and SV-40 transformed WI-38 human diploid fibroblasts. III. Turnover of nonhistone chromosomal proteins and their phosphate groups, *Life Sci.,* 16, 1047, 1975.

414. **Iida, H. and Oda, K.,** Stimulation of nonhistone chromosomal protein synthesis in simian virus 40-infected simian cells, *J. Virol.,* 15, 471, 1975.

415. **Stein, G. S., Moscovici, G., Moscovici, C., and Mons, M.,** Acidic nuclear protein synthesis in Rous sarcoma virus infected chick embryo fibroblasts, *FEBS Lett.,* 38, 295, 1974.

416. **Gonzalez, C. A. and Rees, K. R.,** Non-histone chromosomal proteins from virus-transformed and untransformed 3T3 mouse fibroblasts, *Biochim. Biophys. Acta,* 395, 361, 1975.

417. **Krause, M. O., Noonan, K. D., Kleinsmith, L. J., and Stein, G. S.,** The effect of SV40 transformation on the chromosomal proteins of 3T3 mouse embryo fibroblasts, *Cell Differ.,* 5, 83, 1976.

418. **Krebs, E. G.,** Protein kinases, *Curr. Top. Cell. Regul.,* 5, 99, 1972.

419. **Segal, H. L.,** Enzymatic interconversion of active and inactive forms of enzymes, *Science,* 180, 25, 1973.

420. **Greengard, P.,** Phosphorylated proteins as physiological effectors, *Science,* 199, 146, 1978.

421. **Riches, P. G., Harrap, K. R., Sellwood, S. M., Rickwood, D., and MacGillivray, A. J.,** Phosphorylation of nuclear proteins in rodent tissues, *Biochem. Soc. Trans.,* 1, 684, 1973.

422. **Johnson, T. C. and Holland, J. J.,** Ribonucleic acid and protein synthesis in mitotic HeLa cells, *J. Cell Biol.,* 27, 565,1965.

423. **Pfeiffer, S. E. and Tolmach, L. J.,** RNA synthesis in synchronously growing populations of HeLa S3 cells. I. Rate of total RNA synthesis and its relationship to DNA synthesis, *J. Cell Physiol.,* 71, 77, 1968.

424. **Farber, J., Stein, G., and Baserga, R.,** The regulation of RNA synthesis during mitosis, *Biochem. Biophys. Res. Commun.,* 47, 790, 1972.

425. **Zeilig, C. E., Johnson, R. A., Friedman, D. L., and Sutherland, E. W.,** Cyclic AMP concentrations in synchronized HeLa cells, *J. Cell Biol.,* 55, 296a, 1972.

426. **Kleinsmith, L. J., Allfrey, V. G., and Mirsky, A. E.,** Phosphorylation of nuclear protein early in the course of gene activation in lymphocytes, *Science,* 154, 780, 1966.

427. **Pogo, B. G. T. and Katz, J. R.,** Early events in lymphocyte transformation by phytohaemagglutinin. II. Synthesis and phosphorylation of nuclear proteins, *Differentiation,* 2, 119, 1974.

428. **Horenstein, A., Piras, M. M., Mordoh, J., and Piras, R.,** Protein phosphokinase activities of resting and proliferating human lymphocytes, *Exp. Cell Res.,* 101, 260, 1976.

429. **Ishida, H. and Ahmed, K.,** Studies on phosphoproteins of submandibular gland nuclei isolated from isoproterenol treated rats, *Exp. Cell Res.,* 78, 31, 1973.

430. **Ishida, H. and Ahmed, K.,** Studies on chromatin protein phosphokinase of submandibular gland from isoproterenol treated rats, *Exp. Cell Res.,* 84, 127, 1974.

431. **Rieber, M. and Bacalao, J.,** Alterations in nuclear phosphoproteins of a temperature-sensitive Chinese hamster cell line exposed to non-permissive conditions, *Exp. Cell Res.,* 85, 334, 1974.

432. **Marty de Morales, M., Blat, C., and Harel, L.,** Changes in the phosphorylation of non-histone chromosomal proteins in relationship to DNA and RNA synthesis in $BHK_{21}C_{13}$ cells, *Exp. Cell Res.,* 86, 111, 1974.

433. **Pumo, D. E., Stein, G. S., and Kleinsmith, L. J.,** Phosphorylation of nonhistone chromosomal proteins early during the prereplicative phase of the cell cycle of WI-38 human diploid fibroblasts, *Cell Differ.*, 5, 45, 1976.

434. **Brade, W. P., Thomson, J. A., Chiu, J.-F., and Hnilica, L. S.,** Chromatin-bound kinase activity and phosphoryation of chromatin non-histone proteins during early kidney regeneration after folic acid, *Exp. Cell Res.*, 84, 183, 1974.

435. **Ezrailson, E. G., Olson, M. O. J., Guetzow, K. A., and Busch, H.,** Phosphorylation of non-histone chromatin proteins in normal and regenerating rat liver, Novikoff hepatoma and rat heart, *FEBS Lett.*, 62, 69, 1976.

436. **Mân, N. T., Morris, G. E., and Cole, R. J.,** Phosphorylation of nuclear proteins during muscle differentiation in vitro, *FEBS Lett.*, 42, 257, 1974.

437. **Turkington, R. W. and Riddle, M.,** Hormone-dependent phosphorylation of nuclear proteins during mammary gland differentiation in vitro, *J. Cell. Biol.*, 244, 6040, 1969.

438. **Palmer, W. K., Castagna, M., and Walsh, D. A.,** Nuclear protein kinase activity in glucagon-stimulated perfused rat livers, *Biochem. J.*, 143, 469, 1974.

439. **Bottoms, G. D. and Jungmann, R. A.,** Effect of corticosterone on phosphorylation of rat liver nuclear proteins in vitro, *Proc. Soc. Exp. Biol. Med.*, 144, 83, 1973.

440. **Trajkovic, D., Ribarac-Stepic, N., and Kanazir, D.,** The effect of cortisol on the phosphorylation of rat liver nuclear acidic proteins and the role of these proteins in biosynthesis of nuclear RNA, *Arch. Int. Physiol. Biochim.*, 82, 211, 1974.

441. **Schauder, P., Starman, B. J., and Williams, R. H.,** Effect of cortisol on phosphorylation of acidic proteins in liver nuclei from adrenalectomized rats, *Experientia*, 30, 1277, 1974.

442. **Ahmed, K. and Ishida, H.,** Effect of testosterone on nuclear phosphoproteins of rat ventral prostate, *Mol. Pharmacol.*, 7, 323, 1971.

443. **Ahmed, K. and Wilson, M. J.,** Chomatin-associatd protein phosphokinases of rat ventral prostate, *J. Biol. Chem.*, 250, 2370, 1975.

444. **Schauder, P., Starman, B. J., and Williams, R. H.,** Effect of testosterone of phenol-soluble nuclear acidic proteins of rat ventral prostate, *Proc. Soc. Exp. Biol. Med.*, 145, 331, 1974.

445. **Liew, C. C., Suria, D., and Gornall, A. G.,** Effects of aldosterone on acetylation and phosphorylation of chromosomal proteins, *Endocrinology*, 93, 1025, 1973.

446. **Cohen, M. E. and Kleinsmith, L. J.,** Effect of estradiol-17β on the phosphorylation of uterine nonhistone chromosomal proteins, *Fed. Proc.*, 34, 704, 1975.

447. **Jungmann, R. A. and Schweppe, J. S.,** Mechanism of action of gonadotropin. I. Evidence for gonadotropin-induced modifications of ovarian nuclear basic and acidic protein biosynthesis, phosphorylation, and acetylation, *J. Biol. Chem.*, 247, 5535, 1972.

448. **Kruh, J. and Tichonicky, L.,** Effect of triiodothyronine on rat liver chromatin protein kinase, *Eur. J. Biochem.*, 62, 109, 1976.

449. **Salem, R. and DeVellis, J.,** Protein kinase activity and cAMP-dependent protein phosphorylation in subcellular fractions after norepinephrine treatment of glial cells, *Fed. Proc.*, 35, 296, 1976.

450. **Blankenship, J. and Bresnick, E.,** Effects of phenobarbital on the phosphorylation of acidic nuclear proteins of rat liver, *Biochim. Biophys. Acta*, 340, 218, 1974.

451. **Chiu, J.-F., Craddock, C., Getz, S., and Hnilica, L. S.,** Nonhistone chromatin protein phosphorylation during azo-dye carcinogenesis, *FEBS Lett.*, 33, 247, 1973.

452. **Chiu, J.-F., Brade, W. P., Thomson, J., Tsai, Y. H., and Hnilica, L. S.,** Non-histone protein phosphorylation in normal and neoplastic rat liver chromatin, *Exp. Cell Res.*, 91, 200, 1975.

453. **Ahmed, K.,** Increased phosphorylation of nuclear phosphoproteins in precancerous liver, *Res. Commun. Chem. Pathol. Pharmacol.*, 9, 771, 1974.

454. **Brade, W. P., Chiu, J.-F., and Hnilica, L. S.,** Phosphorylation of rat liver nuclear acidic phosphoproteins after administration of α-1,2,3,4,5,6-hexachlorocyclohexane in vivo, *Mol. Pharmacol.*, 10, 398, 1974.

455. **Pumo, D. E., Stein, G. S., and Kleinsmith, L. J.,** Stimulated phosphorylation of non-histone phosphoproteins in SV-40 transformed WI-38 human diploid fibroblasts, *Biochim. Biophys. Acta*, 402, 125, 1975.

456. **Farron-Fursthenthal, F.,** Protein kinases in hepatoma, and adult and fetal liver of the rat. I. Subcellular distribution, *Biochem. Biophys. Res. Commun.*, 67, 307, 1975.

457. **Kaplowitz, P. B., Platz, R. D., and Kleinsmith, L. J.,** Nuclear phosphoproteins. III. Increase in phosphorylation during histone-phosphoprotein interaction, *Biochim. Biophys. Acta*, 229, 739, 1971.

458. **Johnson, E. M., Vidali, G., Littau, V. C., and Allfrey, V. G.,** Modulation by exogenous histones of phosphorylation of non-histone nuclear proteins in isolated rat liver nuclei, *J. Biol. Chem.*, 248, 7595, 1973.

459. **Stein, G. S., Stein, J. L., and Thomson, J. A.,** Chromosomal proteins in transformed and neoplastic cells: a review, *Cancer Res.*, 38, 1181, 1978.

460. **Martelo, O. J., Woo, S. L. C., Reimann, E. M., and Davie, E. W.,** Effect of protein kinase on ribonucleic acid polymerase, *Biochemistry,* 9, 4807, 1970.

461. **Zillig, W., Fujiki, H., Blum, W., Janekovic, D., Schweiger, M., Rahmsdorf, H.-J., Ponta, H., and Hirsch-Kauffmann, M.,** In vivo and in vitro phosphorylation of DNA-dependent RNA polymerase of *Escherichia coli* by bacteriophage-T$_7$-induced protein kinase, *Proc. Natl. Acad. Sci. U.S.A.,* 72, 2506, 1975.

462. **Martelo, O. J. and Hirsch, J.,** Effect of nuclear protein kinases on mammalian RNA synthesis, *Biochem. Biophys. Res. Commun.,* 58, 1008, 1974.

463. **Jungmann, R. A., Hiestrand, P. C., and Schweppe, J. S.,** Adenosine 3′:5′-monophosphate-dependent protein kinase and the stimulation of ovarian nuclear ribonucleic acid polymerase activities, *J. Biol. Chem.,* 249, 5444, 1974.

464. **Dahmus, M. E.,** Stimulation of ascites tumor RNA polymerase II by protein kinase, *Biochemistry,* 15, 1821, 1976.

465. **Bell, G. I., Valenzuela, P., and Rutter, W. J.,** Phosphorylation of yeast RNA polymerases, *Nature (London),* 261, 429, 1976.

466. **Bell, G. I., Valenzuela, P., and Rutter, W. J.,** Phosphorylation of yeast DNA-dependent RNA polymerases in vivo and in vitro, *J. Biol. Chem.,* 252, 3082, 1977.

467. **Hirsch, J. and Martelo, O. J.,** Phosphorylation of rat liver ribonucleic acid polymerase I by nuclear protein kinases, *J. Biol. Chem.,* 251, 5408, 1976.

468. **Hirsch, J. and Martelo, O. J.,** Purification and properties of a nuclear protein kinase associated with ribonucleic acid polymerase I, *Biochem. J.,* 169, 355, 1978.

469. **Valenzuela, P., Bell, G. I., and Rutter, W. J.,** The 24,000-dalton subunit and the activity of yeast RNA polymerases, *Biochem. Biophys. Res. Commun.,* 71, 26, 1976.

470. **Kranias, E. G., Schweppe, J. S., and Jungmann, R. A.,** Phosphorylative and functional modifications of nucleoplasmic RNA polymerase II by homologous adenosine 3′:5′-monophosphate-dependent protein kinase from calf thymus and by heterologous phosphatase, *J. Biol. Chem.,* 252, 6750, 1977.

471. **Kranias, E. G. and Jungmann, R. A.,** Phosphorylation of calf thymus RNA polymerase II by nuclear cyclic 3′,5′-AMP-independent potein kinase, *Biochim. Biophys. Acta,* 517, 439, 1978.

472. **Tsiapalis, C. M.,** Chemical modification of DNA polymerase phosphoprotein from avian myeloblastosis virus, *Nature (London),* 266, 27, 1977.

473. **Stein, G. S., Spelsberg, T. C., and Kleinsmith, L. J.,** Nonhistone chromosomal proteins and gene regulation, *Science,* 183, 817, 1974.

474. **Spelsberg, T. C.,** The role of nuclear acidic proteins in binding steroid hormones, in *Acidic Proteins of the Nucleus,* Cameron, I. L. and Jeter, J. R., Jr., Eds., Academic Press, New York, 1974, 247.

475. **Thrall, C. L., and Webster, R. A., and Spelsberg, T. C.,** Steroid receptor interaction with chromatin, in *The Cell Nucleus,* Busch, H., Ed., Academic Press, New York, 1979.

476. **Spelsberg, T. C., Steggles, A. W., and O'Malley, B. W.,** Progesterone-binding components of chick oviduct. III. Chromatin acceptor sites, *J. Biol. Chem.,* 246, 4188, 1971.

477. **Defer, M., Dastugue, B., and Kruh, J.,** Direct binding of corticosterone and estradiol to rat liver nuclear non-histone proteins, *Biochimie,* 56, 559, 1974.

478. **Charles, M. A., Ryffel, G. U., Obinata, M., McCarthy, B. J., and Baxter, J. D.,** Nuclear receptors for thyroid hormone: evidence for nonrandom distribution within chromatin, *Proc. Natl. Acad. Sci. U.S.A.,* 72, 1787, 1975.

479. **Klyzsejko-Stefanowicz, L., Chiu, J.-F., Tsai, Y.-H., and Hnilica, L. S.,** Acceptor proteins in rat and androgenic tissue chromatin, *Proc. Natl. Acad. Sci. U.S.A.,* 73, 1954, 1976.

480. **Spelsberg, T. C., Webster, R., and Pikler, G. M.,** Multiple binding sites for progesterone in the hen oviduct nucleus: evidence that acidic proteins represent the acceptors, in *Chromosomal Proteins and their Role in the Regulation of Gene Expression,* Stein, G. S. and Kleinsmith, L. J., Eds., Academic Press, New York, 1975, 153.

481. **Webster, R. A., Pikler, G. M., and Spelsberg, T. C.,** Nuclear binding of progesterone hen oviduct. Role of acidic chromatin proteins in high-affinity binding, *Biochem. J.,* 156, 409, 1976.

482. **Spelsberg, T. C., Webster, R. A., and Pikler, G. M.,** Chromosomal proteins regulate steroid binding to chromatin, *Nature (London),* 262, 65, 1976.

483. **Spelsberg, T. C., Webster, R., Pikler, G., Thrall, C., and Wells, D.,** Role of nuclear proteins as high affinity sites ("acceptors") for progesterone in the avian oviduct, *J. Steroid Biochem.,* 7, 1091, 1976.

484. **Spelsberg, T. C., Webster, R. A., Pikler, G. M., Thrall, C. L., and Wells, D. J.,** Nuclear binding sites ("acceptors") for progesterone in avian oviduct: characterization of the highest-affinity sites, *Ann. N.Y. Acad. Sci.,* 286, 43, 1977.

485. **Spelsberg, T. C., Thrall, C. L., Webster, R. A., and Pikler, G. M.,** Hormone regulation of growth: stimulatory and inhibitory influences of estrogens on DNA synthesis, *J. Toxicol. Environ. Health,* 3, 309, 1977.

486. **Schwartz, R. J., Kuhn, R. W., Buller, R. E., Schrader, W. T., and O'Malley, B. W.,** Progesterone-binding components of chick oviduct. In vitro effects of purified hormone receptor complexes on the initiation of RNA synthesis in chromatin, *J. Biol. Chem.,* 251, 5166, 1976.

487. **Tsai, S.-Y., Tsai, M.-J., Harris, S. E., and O'Malley, B. W.,** Effects of estrogen on gene expression in the chick oviduct. Control of ovalbumin gene expression by non-histone proteins, *J. Biol. Chem.,* 251, 6475, 1976.

488. **Zubay, G., Schwartz, D., and Beckwith, J.,** Mechanism of activation of catabolite-sensitive genes: a positive control system, *Proc. Natl. Acad. Sci. U.S.A.,* 66, 104, 1970.

489. **Anderson, W. B., Schneider, A. B., Emmer, M., Perlman, P. L., and Pastan, I.,** Purification of and properties of the cyclic adenosine 3′,5′-monophosphate receptor protein which mediates cyclic adenosine 3′,5′-monophosphate-dependent gene transcription in *Escherichia coli, J. Biol. Chem.,* 246, 5929, 1971.

490. **Britten, R. J. and Kohne, D. E.,** Repeated sequences in DNA, *Science,* 161, 529, 1968.

491. **Herrick, G. and Alberts, B.,** Nucleic acid helix-coil transitions mediated by helix-unwinding proteins from calf thymus, *J. Biol. Chem.,* 251, 2133, 1976.

492. **Herrick, G., Delius, H., and Alberts, B.,** Single-stranded DNA structure and DNA polymerase activity in the presence of nucleic acid helix-unwinding proteins from calf thymus, *J. Biol. Chem.,* 251, 2142, 1976.

493. **Wang, T. Y.,** Activation of transcription in vitro from chromatin by nonhistone proteins, *Exp. Cell Res.,* 61, 455, 1970.

494. **Kamiyama, M. and Wang, T. Y.,** Activated transcription from rat liver chromatin by non-histone proteins, *Biochim. Biophys. Acta,* 228, 563, 1971.

495. **Kostraba, N. C. and Wang, T. Y.,** Transcriptional transformation of Walker tumor chromatin by nonhistone proteins, *Cancer Res.,* 32, 2348, 1972.

496. **Kostraba, N. C. and Wang, T. Y.,** Differential activation of transcription of chromatin by non-histone proteins, *Biochim. Biophys. Acta,* 262, 169, 1972.

497. **Rickwood, D., Threlfall, G., MacGillivray, A. J., Paul, J., and Riches, P.,** Studies on the phosphorylation of chromatin non-histone proteins and their effect on deoxyribonucleic acid transcription, *Biochem. J.,* 129, 50p, 1972.

498. **Shea, M. and Kleinsmith, L. J.,** Template-specific stimulation of RNA synthesis by phosphorylated non-histone chromatin proteins, *Biochem. Biophys. Res. Commun.,* 50, 473, 1973.

499. **Kamiyama, M., Dastugue, B., and Kruh, J.,** Action of phosphoproteins and protein kinase from rat liver chromatin on RNA synthesis, *Biochem. Biophys. Res. Commun.,* 44, 1345, 1971.

500. **Kamiyama, M., Dastugue, B., Defer, N., and Kruh, J.,** Liver chromatin non-histone proteins. Partial fractionation and mechanism of action on RNA synthesis, *Biochim. Biophys. Acta,* 277, 576, 1972.

501. **Kostraba, N. C. and Wang, T. Y.,** Inhibition of transcription in vitro by a non-histone protein isolated from Ehrlich ascites tumor chromatin, *J. Biol. Chem.,* 250, 8938, 1975.

502. **Kostraba, N. C., Montagna, R. A., and Wang, T. Y.,** Mode of action of non-histone proteins in the stimulation of transcription from DNA, *Biochem. Biophys. Res. Commun.,* 72, 334, 1976.

503. **Kostraba, N. C., Newman, R. S., and Wang, T. Y.,** Selective inhibition of transcription by a nonhistone protein isolated from Ehrlich ascites tumor chromatin, *Arch. Biochem. Biphys.,* 179, 100, 1977.

504. **Kostraba, N. C., Loor, R. M., and Wang, T. Y.,** Tissue-specificity of the nonhistone protein that inhibits RNA synthesis in vitro, *Biochem. Biophys. Res. Commun.,* 79, 347, 1977.

505. **Seifart, K. H.,** A factor stimulating the transcription on double-stranded DNA by purified RNA polymerase from rat liver nuclei, *Cold Spring Harbor Symp. Quant. Biol.,* 35, 719, 1970.

506. **Stein, H. and Hausen, F.,** A factor from calf thymus stimulating DNA-dependent RNA polymerase isolated from this tissue, *Eur. J. Biochem.,* 14, 270, 1970.

507. **Di Mauro, E., Hollenberg, C. P., and Hall, B. D.,** Transcription in yeast: a factor that stimulates yeast RNA polymerases, *Proc. Natl. Acad. Sci. U.S.A.,* 69, 2818, 1972.

508. **Lee, S.-C., and Dahmus, M. E.,** Stimulation of eukaryotic DNA-dependent RNA polymerase by protein factors, *Proc. Natl. Acad. Sci. U.S.A.,* 70, 1383, 1973.

509. **Sekimizu, K., Kobayashi, N., Mizuno, D., and Natori, S.,** Purification of a factor from Ehrlich ascites tumor cells specifically stimulating RNA polymerase II, *Biochemistry,* 15, 5064, 1976.

510. **Higashinakagawa, T., Onishi, T., and Muramatsu, M.,** A factor stimulating the transcription by nucleolar RNA polymerase in the nucleolus of rat liver, *Biochem. Biophys. Res. Commun.,* 48, 937, 1972.

511. **Kuroiwa, A., Mizuno, D., and Natori, S.,** Protein which interacts with a stimulatory factor of RNA polymerase II of Ehrlich ascites tumor cells, *Biochemistry,* 16, 5687, 1977.

512. **Rickwood, D., Hell, A., and Birnie, G. D.,** Isopycnic centrifugation of sheared chromatin in metrizamide gradients, *FEBS Lett.,* 33, 221, 1973.

513. **O'Malley, B. W., Towle, H. C., and Schwartz, R. J.,** Regulation of gene expression in eucaryotes, *Annu. Rev. Genet.,* 11, 239, 1977.

514. **Borun, T. W., Scharf, M. D., and Robbins, E.,** Rapidly labeled, polyribosome-associated RNA having the properties of histone messenger, *Proc. Natl. Acad. Sci. U.S.A.,* 58, 1977, 1967.

515. **Jacobs-Lorena, M., Baglioni, C., and Borun, T. W.,** Translation of messenger RNA for histones from HeLa cells by a cell-free extract from mouse ascites tumor, *Proc. Natl. Acad. Sci. U.S.A.,* 69, 2095, 1972.

516. **Gallwitz, D. and Breindl, M.,** Synthesis of histones in a rabbit reticulocyte cell-free system directed by a polyribosomal RNA fraction from synchronized HeLa cells, *Biochem. Biophys. Res. Commun.,* 47, 1106, 1972.

517. **Stein, J. L., Thrall, C. L., Park, W. D., Mans, R. J., and Stein, G. S.,** Hybridization analysis of histone messenger RNA association with polyribosomes during the cell cycle, *Science,* 189, 557, 1975.

518. **Detke, S., Stein, J., and Stein, G.,** Synthesis of histone messenger RNAs by RNA polymerase II in nuclei from S phase HeLa S$_3$ cells, *Nucleic Acids Res.,* 5, 1515, 1978.

519. **Stein, G. S., Park, W. D., Thrall, C. L., Mans, R. J., and Stein, J. L.,** Regulation of histone gene transcription during the cell cycle by nonhistone chromosomal proteins, *Nature (London),* 257, 764, 1975.

520. **Jansing, R. L., Stein, J. L., and Stein, G. S.,** Activation of histone gene transcription by nonhistone chromosomal proteins in WI-38 human diploid fibroblasts, *Proc. Natl. Acad. Sci. U.S.A.,* 74, 173, 1977.

521. **Melli, M., Spinelli, G., and Arnold, E.,** Synthesis of histone messenger RNA of HeLa cells during the cell cycle, *Cell,* 12, 167, 1977.

522. **Stein, J. L., Stein, G. S., and McGuire, P. M.,** Histone mRNA from HeLa cells: evidence for modified 5' termini, *Biochemistry,* 16, 2207, 1977.

523. **Baserga, R.,** Non-histone chromosomal proteins in normal and abnormal growth, *Life Sci.,* 15, 1057, 1974.

524. **Stein, G. S., Stein, J. L., Laipis, P. J., Chattopadhyay, S. K., Lichtler, A. C., Detke, S., Thomson, J. A., Phillips, I. R., and Shephard, E. A.,** Regulation of gene expression in normal and neoplastic cells, in *Differentiation and Development,* Miami Winter Symp., Vol. 15, Ahmed, F., Russell, T. R., Schultz, J., and Werner, R., Eds., Academic Press, New York, 1978, 125.

525. **Stein, G. S. and Farber, J. L.,** The role of nonhistone chromosomal proteins in the restriction of mitotic chromatin template activity, *Proc. Natl. Acad. Sci. U.S.A.,* 69, 2918, 1972.

526. **Stein, G. S., Chaudhuri, S. K., and Baserga, R.,** Gene activation in WI-38 fibroblasts stimulated to proliferate: role of nonhistone chromosomal proteins, *J. Biol. Chem.,* 247, 3019, 1972.

527. **Paul, J., Gilmour, R. S., Affara, N., Birnie, G., Harrison, P., Hell, A., Humphries, S., Windass, J., and Young, B.,** The globin gene: structure and expression, *Cold Spring Harbor Symp. Quant. Biol.,* 38, 885, 1973.

528. **Barrett, T., Maryanka, D., Hamlyn, P., and Gould, H. J.,** Nonhistone proteins control gene expression in reconstituted chromatin, *Proc. Natl. Acad. Sci. U.S.A.,* 71, 5057, 1974.

529. **Chiu, J.-F., Tsai, Y.-H., Sakuma, K., and Hnilica, L. S.,** Regulation of in vitro mRNA transcription by a fraction of chromosomal proteins, *J. Biol. Chem.,* 250, 9431, 1975.

530. **Gilmour, R. S. and Paul, J.,** Role of non-histone components in determining organ specificity of rabbit chromatins, *FEBS Lett.,* 9, 242, 1970.

531. **Paul, J. and More, I.,** Properties of reconstituted chromatin and nucleohistone complexes, *Nature (London) New Biol.,* 239, 134, 1972.

532. **Kleiman, L. and Huang, R. C.,** Reconstitution of chromatin. The sequential binding of histones to DNA in the presence of salt and urea, *J. Mol. Biol.,* 64, 1, 1972.

533. **Roti-Roti, J. L., Stein, G. S., and Cerutti, P.,** Reactivity of thymine to gamma-rays in HeLa chromatin and nucleoprotein preparations, *Biochemistry,* 13, 2900, 1974.

534. **Stein, G. S., Mans, R. J., Gabbay, E. J., Stein, J. L., Davis, J. L., and Adawadkar, P. D.,** Evidence for fidelity of chromatin reconstitution, *Biochemistry,* 14, 1859, 1975.

535. **Tsai, S. Y., Harris, S. E., Tsai, M.-J., and O'Malley, B. W.,** Effects of estrogen on gene expression in chick oviduct. The role of chromatin proteins in regulating transcription of the ovalbumin gene, *J. Biol. Chem.,* 251, 4713, 1976.

536. **Zasloff, M. and Felsenfeld, G.,** Analysis of in vitro transcription of duck reticulocyte chromatin using mercury-substituted ribonucleotide triphosphates, *Biochemistry,* 16, 5135, 1977.

537. **Gould, H. J., Maryanka, D., Fey, S. J., Cowling, G. J., and Allen, J.,** The assay of globin gene transcription in reconstituted chromatin, in *Methods in Cell Biology,* Vol. 19, Stein, G. S., Stein, J. L., and Kleinsmith, L. J., Eds., Academic Press, New York, 1979, 387.

538. **Woodcock, C. L. F.,** Reconstitution of chromatin subunits, *Science,* 195, 1350, 1977.

539. **Stein, J. L., Reed, K., and Stein, G. S.,** Effect of histones and nonhistone chromosomal proteins on the transcription of histone genes from HeLa S$_3$ cell DNA, *Biochemistry,* 15, 3291, 1976.

540. **Stein, G. S., Hunter, G., and Lavie, L.,** Nonhistone chromosomal proteins: evidence for their role in mediating the binding of histones to DNA during the cell cycle, *Biochem. J.,* 139, 71, 1974.

541. **Stein, G. S., Stein, J. L., Kleinsmith, L. J., Jansing, R. L., Park, W. D., and Thomson, J. A.,** Nonhistone chromosomal proteins: their role in the regulation of histone-gene expression, *Biochem. Soc. Symp.,* 42, 137, 1977.

542. **Park, W. D., Thrall, C. L., Stein, J. L., and Stein, G. S.,** Activation of histone gene transcription from chromatin of G1 HeLa cells by S phase nonhistone chromosomal proteins, *FEBS Lett.,* 62, 226, 1976.

543. **Park, W. D., Stein, J. L., and Stein, G. S.,** Activation of in vitro histone gene transcription from HeLa S_3 chromatin by S phase nonhistone chromosomal proteins, *Biochemistry,* 15, 3296, 1976.

544. **Park, W. D., Jansing, R. L., Stein, J. L., and Stein, G. S.,** Activation of histone gene transcription in quiescent WI-38 cells or mouse liver by a nonhistone chromosomal fraction from HeLa S_3 cells, *Biochemistry,* 16, 3713, 1977.

545. **Thomson, J. A., Stein, J. L., Kleinsmith, L. J., and Stein, G. S.,** Activation of histone gene transcription by nonhistone chromosomal phosphoproteins, *Science,* 194, 428, 1976.

546. **Lacy, E. and Axel, R.,** Analysis of DNA of isolated chromatin subunits, *Proc. Natl. Acad. Sci. U.S.A.,* 72, 3978, 1975.

547. **Kuo M. T., Sahasrabuddhe, C. G., and Saunders, G. F.,** Presence of messenger specifying sequences in the DNA of chromatin subunits, *Proc. Natl. Acad. Sci. U.S.A.,* 73, 1572, 1976.

548. **Reeves, R.,** Ribosomal genes of *Xenopus laevis:* evidence of nucleosomes in transcriptionally active chromatin, *Science,* 194, 529, 1976.

549. **Weintraub, H. and Groudine, M.,** Chromosomal subunits in active genes have an altered conformation, *Science,* 193, 848, 1976.

550. **Garel, A. and Axel, R.,** Selective digestion of transcriptionally active ovalbumin genes from oviduct nuclei, *Proc. Natl. Acad. Sci. U.S.A.,* 73, 3966, 1976.

551. **Levy, W. B., and Dixon, G. H.,** Renaturation kinetics of cDNA complementary to cytoplasmic polyadenylated RNA from rainbow trout testis. Accessibility of transcribed genes to pancreatic DNase, *Nucleic Acids Res.,* 4, 883, 1977.

552. **Garel, A., Zolan, M., and Axel, R.,** Genes transcribed at diverse rates have a similar conformation in chromatin, *Proc. Natl. Acad. Sci. U.S.A.,* 74, 4867, 1977.

553. **Flint, S. J. and Weintraub, H. M.,** An altered subunit configuration associated with the actively transcribed DNA of integrated adenovirus genes, *Cell,* 12, 783, 1977.

554. **Mayfield, J. E., Serunian, L. A., Silver, L. M., and Elgin, S. C. R.,** A protein released by DNase I digestion of *Drosophila* nuclei is preferentially associated with puffs, *Cell,* 14, 539, 1978.

555. **Rovera, G., Farber, J. L., and Baserga, R.,** Gene activation in WI-38 fibroblasts stimulated to proliferate: requirement for protein synthesis, *Proc. Natl. Acad. Sci. U.S.A.,* 68, 1725, 1971.

556. **Gadski, R. A., and Chae, C.-B.,** Effect of proteolysis on transcriptional fidelity of reconstituted chromatin, *Biochemistry,* 16, 3465, 1977.

557. **Detke, S., Lichtler, A., Phillips, I., Stein, J., and Stein, G.,** Reassessment of histone gene expression during cell cycle in human cells by using homologous H4 histone cDNA, *Proc. Natl. Acad. Sci.,* 76, 4995, 1979.

558. **Melli, M., Spinelli, G., and Arnold, E.,** Synthesis of histone messenger RNA of HeLa cells during the cell cycle, *Cell,* 12, 167, 1977.

559. **Laskey, R. A., Honda, B. M., Mills, A. D., and Finch, J. T.,** Nucleosomes are assembled by an acidic protein which binds histones and transfers them to DNA, *Nature (London),* 275, 416, 1978.

560. **Weisbrod, S. and Weintraub, H.,** Isolation of a subclass of nuclear proteins responsible for conferring a DNase I-sensitive structure on globin chromatin, *Proc. Natl. Acad. Sci.,* 76, 630, 1979.

561. **Gannon, F., O'Hare, K., Perrin, F., LePennec, J. P., Benoist, C., Cochet, M., Breathnach, R., Royal, A., Garapin, A., Cami, B. and Chambon, P.,** Organisation and sequences at the 5′ end of a cloned complete ovalbumin gene, *Nature (London),* 278, 428, 1979.

562. **Stein, J. L.,** *Science,* 189, 557, 1975.

563. **Stein, G. S.,** *Nature (London),* 257, 764, 1975.

Chapter 4

HORMONAL REGULATION OF GENE TRANSCRIPTION

R. F. Cox

TABLE OF CONTENTS

I. INTRODUCTION

Currently, and perhaps temporarily, transcription is in vogue. Before the spearhead of activity in the field of hormone action shifts to an analysis of the effects of "processing-out" of intervening gene sequences in nuclear RNA transcripts (already the trend has been from translation to transcription and it may well continue to RNA processing and then back to translation and mRNA stability), it is timely to collate current data relevant to our understanding of the action of hormones, both on transcriptional events and on RNA metabolism in eukaryotic cells. Much of the discussion relates to sex steroid action, due to the comparative profusion of the literature on this topic and the author's predisposition to this field.

In particular, this chapter attempts to critically evaluate studies on endogenous and solubilized RNA polymerase activities in isolated nuclei, on transcription of chromatin templates by exogenous enzymes, and on the effects of hormone-receptor (H-R) complexes on RNA synthesis in vitro. Speculation abounds in all of these areas. Happily, the attendant confusion is offset by the contrasting clarity of the effects of hormones on the expression of specific genes, and on the latter topic, models are proposed to account for the apparent "fine" control and multihormonal control of these steroid-sensitive loci.

The biochemistry of steroid-receptors and nuclear "acceptor" sites for these complexes are not considered here. The reader is referred to the treatise of King and Mainwaring,[1] reviews by Baulieu et al.,[2] Gorski and co-workers,[3,4] Rousseau,[5] Yamamoto and co-workers,[6,7] and Buller and O'Malley,[8] and discussions by Milgrom and Atger,[9] Buller et al.,[10] Clark et al.,[11] Puca et al.,[12] Spelsberg et al.,[13] and Jackson and Chalkley,[14] particularly for differing viewpoints on the transport of H-R complexes to the nucleus and the nature of the nuclear "acceptor" site. Stumpf and Sar[15] have recently summarized their extensive autoradiographic evidence showing that steroids associate with nuclei in target cells. It is assumed then that H-R complexes for all steroids must bind to topologically propitious sites in the nucleus prior to eliciting their effect on transcription.

II. EARLY EFFECTS ON TARGET CELLS

It is the author's impression that early effects of sex steroids at the cell surface have been underestimated as mediators of subsequent changes in RNA synthesis. In rat uterus, the early work of Spaziani and Szego[16,17] showed that estrogens promote the release of histamine (probably from mast cells) which, in turn, promotes vasodilation, increased capillary permeability, and reactive hyperemia. Concomitant with the ensuing uptake of water by the uterus, there is increased transport of sugars, amino acids, metal ions, and nucleosides.[18] Although the first three events seem to be dependent on RNA or protein synthesis, metal ion and nucleoside transport do not. Androgens trigger a similar series of events in their target tissues.[18] These data leave little doubt that, in many cases, target cell metabolism is modulated via an increased blood supply, a destabilization of (or alteration in) the cell membrane, and an increased availability (and, in some cases, transport) of precursors and nutrients.

Evidence that these effects per se are the immediate stimulus for hypertrophy and cell division are circumstantial, but recently it has been shown that levels of amino acids and nucleic acid precursors can indeed control rates of rRNA synthesis.[19,20] *It is not inconceivable, then, that many anabolic events are the result of a direct action of the steroid at the cell periphery.* In this context, specific binding sites for estrogens on rat endometrial membranes have recently been found.[21] (A note of caution should be injected here. While evidence for a direct action of estradiol (E) on precursor uptake is good, it is by no means established for other classes of steroid, the action of gluco-corticoids on thymic lymphocytes being a case in point.[22] These steroids may indeed have the opposite effects since cortisol (C) stabilizes membranes and can antagonize estrogen-mediated precursor uptake in rat uterus.[23])

Thus, *the existence of at least two sites of action for some steroids in some cells is suspected: the cell periphery* (possibly the plasma membrane) *and the nucleus,* where hormones alter gene expression (see Section VI). A possible third site, which cannot be ignored in the light of recent evidence, is the lysosome. Szego[23,24] claims that steroids (and possibly ACTH) destabilize lysosomal membranes in their respective target tis-sues, causing a dramatic influx of nucleases, proteases, and phosphatases into cell nuclei (see Section III.D).

The very early effects of hormones on phosphorylation and acetylation of nuclear proteins is discussed below (see Section III.D). In a number of instances, protein or RNA synthesis do not appear to mediate these effects.

III. EFFECTS ON RNA SYNTHESIS IN VIVO

A. RNA Levels and Labeling Studies

In general, *hormones cause marked proliferation of the protein synthetic apparatus in target cells,* an effect which is manifest in terms of increased levels of ribosomes,[25-29] tRNA,[30,31] mRNA,[32,33] and membranes[25] in the cytoplasm and enhanced rates of initiation of translation.[34-36] This section briefly considers some of the relevant isotope-labeling studies indicating that many of these changes are mediated at the transcrip-tional level.

The early demonstration by Mueller et al.[37] that incorporation of precursors into RNA was stimulated by estrogen in rat uterus was confirmed by Means and Hamil-ton,[38] although in these cases, effects on precursor uptake by the uterus were not ana-lyzed. The latter topic subsequently became an area of intense research, since a knowl-edge of precursor pools preempted any interpretation of labeling data. A concise account of this work has been made by Spaziani,[18] and the following conclusions, pertinent to the rat uterus, can be made: (1) estrogen increases free nucleotide pool sizes 8 to 10 hr after treatment, but there is some disagreement on the pool size during the first 4 hr; (2) in the first 6 hr, purine nucleotide synthesis is enhanced; (3) estrogen has a very rapid and early effect on nucleoside transport. The latter phenomenon led two groups to conclude that increased precursor transport almost completely ac-counted for the higher specific activity of labeled uterine RNA during the first 4 to 5 hr of E treatment.[39-41] Secondly, since the RNA content of the uterus did not change, Miller[42] concluded that the RNA labeled at early times must turn over rapidly, i.e., it is probably not rRNA or tRNA.

Data obtained from another line of attack indicate that rRNA and tRNA synthesis is enhanced 1 to 3 hr after treatment with E. Munns and Katzman[43,44] administered hormone in vitro and measured the transfer of methyl groups from labeled methyl-methionine to rRNA and tRNA in organ culture. Precursor uptake or pool sizes were not affected by E, and since actinomycin D (AcD) blocked RNA methylation, labeling of RNA was considered to reflect the rate of RNA synthesis. (It should be noted that mRNA would also be methylated,[45] but only at 10 to 20% of the level seen for rRNA and tRNA, and that increased methylase activity, noted later by Luck and Hamilton[46] and by Munns et al.,[47] would overestimate apparent rates of RNA synthesis. The re-sults should be considered in this light.)

Recently, Catelli and Baulieu[48] obtained similar results by incorporating uridine in vivo, analyzing RNA labeling patterns on gels, and quantitating peak areas by planimetry. As shown in Figure 1A, E did not alter the radioactive RNA profile significantly, in agreement with other results in rat uterus[49] and also in chick oviduct.[31] But the data reveal a marked increase in the rate of rRNA synthesis, beginning within 1 hr of E treatment (Figure 1B). The results can be criticized since no correction was made for precursor uptake and pool size changes, although the authors found no correlation between the kinetics of RNA labeling and the acid-soluble uridine pool. Judging from the data, they may have overestimated rates of RNA synthesis, particularly at early time points.

Attempts to define the early effects of E on HnRNA synthesis have met with limited success. Knowler and Smellie[50] demonstrated an apparently marked increase (1 hr after E) in the labeling of a >45S fraction from rat uteri, as determined by its accumulation at the top of a polyacrylamide gel. But subsequent analysis on agarose gels[51] only provided slim evidence that (1) synthesis of this RNA was enhanced and (2) the latter preceded the activation of rRNA synthesis. Catelli and Baulieu[48] also find no early, specfic effect on HnRNA synthesis. Using double-label techniques, Baulieu[52] identified two distinct estrogen-induced peaks of labeled RNA (15S and 8S) when rat uterine RNA was resolved by electrophoresis, but Frolik and Gorski,[53] who recently performed similar double-label experiments and found no specific estrogen-induced RNAs, indicate that artifactual changes in isotope ratio could account for the original observation.

The general conclusion that *most hormones facilitate an increased rate of incorporation of exogenous precursors into all major RNA classes* is confirmed in other systems; for example, for C in rat liver,[54] vitamin D in rat intestine,[55] growth hormone in rat liver,[56] and aldosterone in toad bladder.[28,32] In all cases, sizes and precursor uptake were accounted for, and in one case, increased RNA labeling was seen despite a drop in the specific activity of the precursor pool. Unfortunately, assumptions have to be made in all these studies: (1) that nuclear pools approximate cytoplasmic pools and (2) the specific activity of uridine approximates that of UTP. Since RNA accumulation through stabilization seems unlikely *for rRNA and tRNA* due to their long halflife)[57,58] *enhanced precursor incorporation probably reflects the rate of synthesis.* (But note that there are some indications that hormones stabilize these molecules.[59]) *The picture is less clear for HnRNA synthesis,* since these species have relatively short halflives which can be rapidly modified in response to biological signals (see Section VIII.B). *All data are compatible with a hormone-mediated increase in rate of synthesis or decrease in degradation of these molecules or both.* As discussed below, hormonal effects on transcription for a few specific genes are better understood, and in all cases analyed to date, the rate of synthesis is accentuated (see Section VI).

B. Endogenous RNA Polymerases

A voluminous literature relates the fact that, *in general, hormones enhance endogenous RNA polymerase (Pol) activities in nuclei, nucleoli, and chromatin* isolated from target tissues. This section will attempt to summarize this work and point out the difficulties in interpretation in terms of defining hormone action.

Following reports from Mueller et al.,[37] Gorski,[60] and Hamilton et al.[61] stating that E enhanced RNA synthesis in crude preparations of uterine nuclei, the two major contributing enzyme activities were characterized in more detail[62] and shown to reside at specific locations in the nucleus.[63] Subsequent work by Hamilton and co-workers[29,64] suggested that Pol I activity was stimulated 1 hr after injection of E into ovariectomized rats, whereas Pol II was unaffected for about 12 hr. However, by rapidly isolating nuclei in 2.2 *M* sucrose buffer, resuspending them in a glycerol buffer, and performing assays at 15°C, Glasser et al.[65] demonstrated a marked biphasic response of Pol II to E. The initial peak of activity occurred at 1 hr, the second at 2 to 3 hr. The effect of Pol I was similar to that seen by Hamilton, but it occurred earlier. Borthwick and

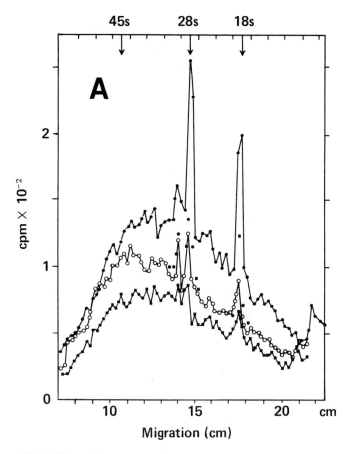

FIGURE 1.   Effect of estradiol on the labeling of rat uterine RNA by uridine in vivo. (A) Electrophoresis of total uterine RNA, labeled for 1 hr with (^{3}H)-uridine in vivo, at different times after E treatment: (x—x), controls; (0—0), after 1 hr E; (■—■), 1.5 hour E; (●—●), 3 hr E. For 1.5 hr-treated animals, only the rRNA peaks are plotted. In all cases, 70 μg of RNA were loaded onto the gel. (B) Effect of E on labeling of the different types of uterine RNA, as analyzed by planimetry of labeled RNA profiles of the kind shown in panel (A). Data were obtained from three experiments (except for the 6-hr points; two experiments), and the bars indicate the S.D. The increase in radioactivity was calculated and expressed as a percent of control levels. The different regions of the RNA profile examined were (△—△), 28S and 18S rRNA; (0—0), >45S HnRNA; (□—□), <28S heterodisperse RNA. (From Catelli, M. G. and Baulieu, E. E., *Mol. Cell. Endocrinol.*, 6, 129, 1976. With permission.)

Smellie[66] reported similar changes in rabbit uterine nuclei. The latter were isolated in 0.25 *M* sucrose buffer, centrifuged through 2.4 *M* sucrose buffer, and finally assayed at 37°C; this suggests that the Pol response is more refractory to "standard" isolation conditions than had previously been supposed. Using immature rats and yet another method for isolating nuclei (the hexylene glycol procedure developed by Wray[67]), Hardin et al.[68] reported even more dramatic effects of estrogens. Although response patterns were similar to those of Glasser et al.[65] the magnitude of the effects was enormous; that is, an 8- to 10-fold increase in Pol II activity after 1 hr of E and at least a 12-fold increase in Pol I activity after 4 hr. Results from three separate groups are, thus, fairly similar.

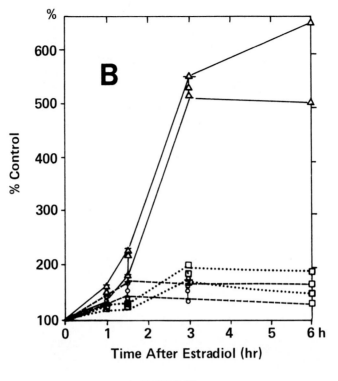

FIGURE 1B

On the other side of the coin, there is more recent, and apparently careful, work showing either no, or a comparatively minor, change in Pol II activity in response to E. Weil et al.,[69] using immature rats and the hexylene glycol method, saw no change in Pol II activity for at least 6 hr but did see marked effects on Pol I after 2 to 3 hr. Mn^{++} (but not Mg^{++}) ions were present in their assays, whereas Hardin et al.[68] included both. Other minor procedural differences do not appear to explain the variance between these two observations. The second report by Bouton et al.[70] describes a twofold increase in Pol II activity at early times (up to 2 hr) when using low-salt assays, but, in marked contrast to the findings of Glasser et al.[66] and Borthwick et al., there was no change in Pol II activity when nuclei were assayed in high salt. Again, an early increase in Pol I activity was seen, using either high- or low-salt assays. (Incidentally, Pol III activity is also accentuated by E in rat uterus.[69,71])

In chick oviduct, both estrogens and progesterone (P) elevate endogenous Pol activities.[72-76] Results using the former class of steroids are discussed later. While P apparently enhances Pol II activity in immature chick oviduct,[72] it does not have clear-cut effects when given to chicks pretreated with, and then withdrawn from, estrogen.[76] In other systems, steroids activate both Pol I and II; for example, these effects are achieved by E in chick liver,[77] by C and cortisone in rat liver,[78-80] by testosterone (T) in rat prostate,[81,82] by 1α,25-dihydroxyvitamin D_3 in chick intestine,[83] and by dexamethasone (Dex) in rat thymus cells.[84,85] In the latter two cases, no effect on Pol I is seen, and in thymus cells, the Pol II response is rapid (ten minutes after hormone). Growth hormone,[56,86] thyroid hormones[87,88] and insulin[89] also modulate RNA polymerases.

We must now consider these effect from a biological standpoint. RNA synthesis directed by Pol I or II in isolated nuclei is due primarily to elongation of preexisting RNA chains in either high- or low-salt conditions;[90-94] Pol III does initiate, but its activity is relatively low.[92] Thus, enhanced activity is attributable to more elongating enzymes or a greater rate (or extent) of elongation or both. In cases where these alternatives have been distinguished, greater elongation accounts for the effect. Barry and Gorski[95] analyzed endogenous RNA products in rat uterine nuclei by alkaline hydrolysis; they found no change in the number of labeled chains, judging by radioactivity incorporated into the 3′ ends, but a twofold increase in the extent of elongation was seen 2 hr after E treatment. Similar conclusions were reached by Fuhrman and Gill[96] with respect to ACTH action in guinea pig adrenal gland. In an illuminating discussion, they note that if these effects truly represent an action of the hormone at the level of elongation, then control Pol I activity should (given time) attain hormone-stimulated levels in the vitro assay. This does not occur; in fact, the average extent of elongation of Pol I in this system does not exceed 300 nucleotides. Thus, one can draw the important conclusion that *premature termination takes place in isolated nuclei.*

Effects of E on Pol II activity in chick oviduct are, in this author's experience, equally puzzling. When nuclei were assayed by Spelsberg and Cox at 15°C, a marked biphasic response was seen.[76] This author decided to analyze this response in detail by hydrolyzing the RNA product.[75] However, at 15°C, the amount of radioactivity incorporated into RNA was inadequate for the analysis, and secondly, rapidly prepared nuclei were contaminated with cytoplasm. The final choice was to use purified nuclei incubated at 37°C in the presence of heparin and high salt, to inhibit all initiation. Many controls were performed to establish that labeled uridine recovered was a faithful estimate of the number of 3′ termini in elongated RNA chains and, hence, of the number of participating Pol II enzymes. The results obtained (Figure 2) show very little or no change in the number of elongating Pol II molecules up to 6 hr after E treatment; that is, there were 11,000 to 14,000 active enzymes per diploid genome. Since transcription complexes are so resistant to solubilization,[97] selective loss of an "estrogen-dependent" fraction during the isolation of nuclei seems unlikely. Secondly, theoretical considerations[75] suggest that these nuclei contained a full complement of actively transcribing Pol II enzymes. Thus, a comparison of the data obtained by Spelsberg and this author suggests (indirectly) that the response of Pol II to E seen in nuclei reflects different degrees of elongation of a constant number of enzymes; also, as seen in guinea pig adrenal nuclei, the average extent of elongation is only a few hundred nucleotides.[75] However, as shown in Figure 2, the number of Pol I enzymes bound to chromatin template in chick oviduct does increase two- to threefold, implying that E enhances the rate of initiation of these enzymes on ribosomal genes.

Courvalin et al.[98] have also studied the early effect of E on the number of "tightly bound" Pol II enzymes in rat uterine nuclei using labeled α-amanitin, which binds specifically and stochiometrically to Pol II.[99] They found no change up to 6 hr after hormone treatment. But again, "tightly bound" Pol I did increase in response to hormone.

When viewed optimistically, an enhanced degree of elongation could reflect the appearance of factors which modulate either elongation or attenuation[100] (that is, release of a block in the ability of Pol to read through previously restricted segments of the genome). However, it is well known that the rate of elongation of Pol II is severely impaired in vitro: it is at least order of magnitude lower than that measured in vivo.[75,90] In view of the latter phenomenon, the diverse results obtained in rat uterus and chick oviduct, and the poor extent of elongation seen in vitro, *the proposal is made that the major fraction of the early steroid-induced change in Pol II activity is artifactual.* This is not to say that elongating polymerases are bound to sites other than those transcribed in vivo (see Section VI.D) but that in vitro activity at these sites may be misleading. It is suspected that proteins and RNA in transcriptionally active regions condense around

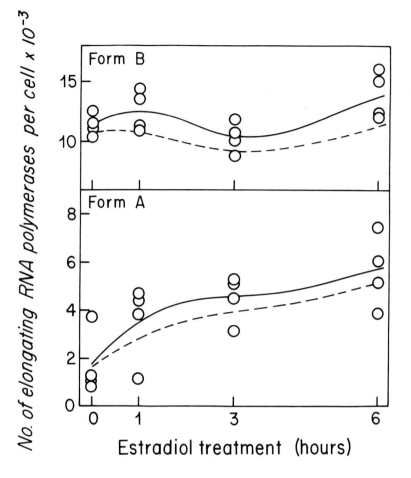

FIGURE 2.   Quantitation of elongating RNA polymerases in chick oviduct nuclei in response to estradiol in vivo. ³H-UTP incorporated into 3′ termini of endogenous RNA chains and released as uridine after alkaline hydrolysis was measured for Pol I (Form A) and Pol II (Form B) enzymes. From these data the number of elongating enzymes per oviduct cell was estimated from 16 separate nuclei preparations and plotted as a function of the time of E treatment in vivo. Average values for each group are indicated by the solid line. Average values obtained after making corrections for the generation of uridine by RNase and phosphatase activities are indicated by the dashed lines. (From Cox, R. F., *Cell*, 7, 455, 1976. With permission.)

the template nonspecifically when exposed to "isolation" buffers. Thus, the extent of elongation (particularly in low salt) could reflect the degree to which such condensation occurs for a given chromatin during its isolation. We know that hormones orchestrate rapid changes in chromatin structure, mobilize the transfer of degradative enzymes to the nucleus (see Section III.D), and alter the ability of nuclei to process RNA (see Section VIII.A). Any number of factors mediating such changes might modify the degree of template condensation and, hence, the extent of Pol II elongation in vitro. If this is the case, a hormonally induced transition from one aberrant type of in vitro elongation to another will bear little resemblance to the in vivo effect of hormone on Pol II transcription. Studies by Courvalin et al.[98] suggest that an increase in the overall rate of initiation of Pol II may occur at later times after steroid treatment, but because of the problems discussed above, it will be hard to assess if any part of the early response to steroids seen in vitro is due to a "real" effect on elongation or attenuation.

In at least two cases cited above,[75,98] steroids enhance the level of Pol I enzyme bound to chromatin, suggesting that in vitro assays do reflect (to some extent) in vivo changes. Activation of Pol I by steroids is also blocked by cycloheximide,[66,101] revealing an intrinsic difference between Pol I and II responses seen in vitro. In cultured fibroblasts, stimulation of growth by serum has marked effects on Pol I activity when assayed in ghost monolayers,[102] but there is little early effect on Pol II. *Thus, in some cases, steroids probably enhance the rate of initiation of Pol I on ribosomal RNA genes.* But as noted above, other authors see only elongation effects for Pol I, and again, it is suggested that nonspecific structural changes in isolated template could be the cause.

Finally, a technical note. Yu[103] has shown that nuclei contain ribohomopolymer polymerases. Titration with α-amanitin is the method of choice to determine Pol II and III activities,[69] but drug-resistant activity may have often been wrongly attributed to Pol I. The latter activity should, therefore, be defined by its sensitivity to AcD[104] and its dependence on all four RNA precursors in both control and steroid-treated nuclei.

C. Solubilized RNA Polymerases

A concensus of opinion on the effect of hormones on the levels and activities of solubilized Pol enzymes has by no means been reached. Provided here is the author's own assessment of the current situation in the hope that it will aid future attempts to illuminate this area.

When demand for DEAE-cellulose was only imminent, several groups had already analyzed hormonal effect on solubilized Pol enzymes. For example, it was found[81] that T (1 to 16 hr in vivo) could enhance "low-salt/Mg⁺⁺ Pol I" activity several-fold in rat prostrate, although "high-salt" activity was unchanged. In chick oviduct,[74] E (24 hr) enhanced solubilized Pol I activity fourfold and Pol II activity twofold. C also stimulated Pol I activity several-fold in rat liver,[105] and a similar response to E was seen in rooster liver.[106] Thus, a pattern emerged suggesting that whereas steroids had minor effects on Pol II, Pol I levels were dramatically increased. This pattern held for the actions of auxin,[107] growth hormone,[108] and phytohemagglutinin.[109]

The validity of this apparently clear-cut pattern was weakened by a report from Shields and Tata's laboratory[110] showing that the recovery of isolated enzymes from DEAE-Sephadex® columns varied with the hormonal status of the tissue. This discovery negated an earlier claim[108] that treatment of hyophysectomized rats with growth hormone enhanced Pol I levels. A second problem which emerged was that differential levels of nucleases or proteases coeluted with Pol enzymes,[110,111] resulting in partial inactivation of the latter or in degradation of the DNA template or RNA product in the final assay. (Incidentally, the problem of "void-volume" RNA polymerases described in earlier papers was also solved; it was attributed to column overloading.[110]) But the above criticisms did not alter the basic conclusions in some systems. For example, when chromatographic steps were omitted, and at least RNase activity was accounted for, Weckler and Gschwendt[112] still observed changes in solubilized Pol levels in chicken liver; after 1 day of E treatment, Pol II and Pol I and III (combined) activities were both elevated by 160%.

More recent work has shown that in some cases, little response is seen. Weil et al.[69] observed no change in Pol I, II, or III enzyme levels in rat uterine nuclei after 6 hr of E treatment in vivo. This was confirmed in rabbit uterus[66] and also for Pol I and II in rat uterus by Courvalin et al.,[98] who examined these levels at earlier timepoints as well. Furthermore, the latter authors made precise estimates of Pol II levels in total homogenates by binding labeled α-aminitin. Approximately 5000 and 8000 Pol II molecules were present per haploid genome in uteri from ovariectomized adult and immature rats, respectively, and little change was seen up to 12 hr after E. At later times, Pol I and II levels rose (by less than 50%).

In other cases, only Pol II levels are elevated. Zerwekh et al.[83] reported that $1\alpha,25$-dihydroxyvitamin D_3 administration to rachitic chicks enhanced this enzyme level two- to threefold in intestinal nuclei, a particularly marked effect since it occurred 2 hr after hormone treatment. And in yet other cases, the status of the hormonal effect is equivocal. Pol I levels have been variously reported to increase markedly[105,111] or to remain unchanged[113] in rat liver nuclei in response to C treatment in vivo. Since RNase (also activated by the steroid) has been shown[111] to coelute with these enzymes on Bio-Gel® (used instead of DEAE-cellulose), the true biological situation may not yet be revealed.

Where steroids have been shown to alter Pol levels, attempts to distinguish between enzyme activity and amount have been made using enzyme- or DNA-excess titration methods. Thus, Sajdel and Jacob[105] showed that "control" Pol I saturated DNA well before an equivalent amount of enzyme isolated after C treatment in vivo, and van den Berg et al.[106] showed that at saturating DNA, Pol I from estrogen-treated rooster liver was more active compared with controls. The general conclusion made by both groups, that steroid treatment accentuates the ability of Pol I to initiate, must be viewed with caution, since no account was taken of contaminating nuclease levels; for example, nicks introduced into DNA by endogenous DNases can easily account for enhanced transcriptional efficiency.[114] Such problems are compounded when constant DNA is titrated with increasing amounts of crude enzyme.

In addition to varying Pol levels, *hormones alter the chromatographic behavior and metal ion and salt-sensitives of Pol I and III enzymes.* Fuhrman and Gill[115] reported that administration of ACTH to guinea pigs increased Pol II and III levels extracted from adrenal gland nuclei. No effect on Pol I level was noted. However, after ACTH treatment, the salt-elution profile of this enzyme on DEAE-Sephadex® changes; that is, in controls all enzyme elutes at $0.17M$ ammonium sulfate, but after ACTH, 30% of the activity elutes with a distinct peak at $0.14M$ salt. A similar response was observed by Mauck.[116] After treating fibroblasts with serum, there was a fourfold increase in Pol I levels accompanied by a gradual shift in the salt-elution sensitivity from $0.15M$ in resting cells to $0.11M$ in growing cells. Separate peaks were not observed in this case, but conversion from one enzyme form to another best explains the data. Serum stimulation also changes the Mg^{++} and ammonium sulfate sensitivity of the modified Pol I enzyme.[116]

These changes may well be biologically significant. A report from Butterworth's group[117] indicates that two forms of Pol I exist, one of which is transcriptionally active. The latter (A II) is indeed eluted first on DEAE-Sephadex®. It is conceivable, then, that hormone treatment increases the efficiency of conversion of A I to A II, possibly via addition of a subunit. A similar shift in Pol I is seen in chick liver nuclei after E treatment[77], but again, there is no change in the level of Pol I. In rat uterus, E also alters the structure of Pol III, since there is a small shift from Pol IIIA to IIIB.[69]

The possibility that steroids modulate Pol activity by (1) direct phosphorylation or (2) synthesis of specific activating factors must also be considered. Steroids increase the rate of phosphorylation of nuclear proteins[118] and the activity of protein kinases in nuclei;[119] and phosphorylation of Pol accentuates its activity.[120,121] A closer link between these phenomena has been established in calf ovary. Jungmann et al.[122] indicate that Pol IA, IB, and II are selectively phosphorylated in isolated nuclei by a homologous protein kinase, yielding a three- to ninefold stimulation in activity. In separate experiments, ACTH promotes translocation of cytoplasmic kinase into the nucleus.[123] A direct relationship between these events has not, however, been demonstrated in vivo. Returning to steroid action, a report[124] that nucleolar RNA polymerase is activated via its association with phosphorylated estradiol-receptor complex has not been confirmed or substantiated. A number of factors have now been isolated which modify Pol activity,[125] and steroid-induced effects on Pol I may indeed be factor-mediated (see Section IX.B); but as yet, there is no evidence for modulation of Pol II at this level.

In summary, *steroids elevate the amount and/or the activity of Pol enzymes in general, but current data do not reveal a consistent pattern of events,* probably partly due to technical difficulties. Enzyme recoveries and contamination with degradative enzymes have not, in many cases, been adequately monitored. Also, enzyme activity is frequently measured per unit of crude protein, but per unit of nuclear DNA would be more meaningful if protein levels fluctuate in response to hormone. The cellular complexity of many target tissues is an added problem.

Although there is a general correlation between Pol I and II levels and the rate of growth and proliferation of tissues,[126] cellular rates of RNA synthesis are not always reflected by their RNA polymerase level.[127] For Pol II, modulation by template-bound factors is a more likely control site than modulation by enzyme concentration, in view of the effects of steroids on specific genes (see Section VI.C). At a second level, Pol II enzyme concentration may rise as a result of pleiotropic effects of hormones on cell metabolism. Indeed, mitogens have remarkable effects in this respect.[109] For Pol I and rRNA synthesis, at least two regulatory mechanisms may exist, and both could be steroid-sensitive. The first, studied in detail by Grummt and co-workers[20,128] involves regulation by ATP. It is independent of protein synthesis, and steroid effects on nucleotide precursor uptake and metabolism could conceivably mediate this kind of response. The rate of rRNA synthesis is also activated by amino acids;[19,129] (and in this case, incidentally, there is no change in Pol levels.[129]) The second mechanism, involving the synthesis of a Pol II-directed protein factor, is discussed below (see Section IX.B). It will be interesting to see if the change in chromatographic behavior of Pol I is caused by a hormone-mediated addition of an initiation factor to the molecule.

D. Template Capacity and Chromatin Structure

Considerable excitement accompanied demonstrations[130,131] that *chromatin from steroid-treated tissues is a more efficient (or "open") template for bacterial Pol enzyme,* since they were the first clues that steroids acted directly at the site of transcription. These effects have now been demonstrated in other systems. For example, E elevates chromatin template capacity in rat uterus[132] and chick oviduct,[76,133] and in the latter case, steroid-treated chromatin is also a better template for homologous Pol II.[74] Vitamin D activates template capacity in rat and chick intestine,[134,135] and chorionic gonadotropin triggers similar effects in rat ovary.[136]

An exhaustive series of studies in chick oviduct has been performed by O'Malley and co-workers[137-141] using two inhibitors of initiation, rifampicin and heparin. Since the rate of elongation was similar for all templates studied, RNA synthesis under conditions preventing reinitiation could be equated with the number of putative initiation sites. Template capacity (in terms of initiation sites) was thus determined by titrating a fixed amount of chromatin with increasing amounts of bacterial enzyme to achieve saturation. Using this assay, chromatin template capacity is enhanced two- to threefold after a secondary stimulation of estrogen for 2 hr[142] and of P for 1 hr.[143] Since plateau levels were rarely achieved in these experiments (suggesting contamination of *Escherichia coli* Pol with other polymerizing enzymes, or a modification of the chromatin structure as the enzyme protein level increases), the method of determing the "true" plateau value was accordingly somewhat arbitrary. Similar results were obtained using homologous Pol II enzyme,[139] and estrogen withdrawal also reduced template capacity two- to threefold.[142]

Accompanying these events are marked changes in the composition of chromatin. A trenchant example of the effects of mitogens on nuclear "activation" is the response of lymphocytes to concanavalin A;[144] 15 min after mitogen addition there is a massive migration of preexisting cytoplasmic proteins to the nucleus. Although the data in steroid-responsive tissues are less terse, they suggest that, at least for those steroids with mitogenic activity, comparable changes occur. After 4 hr of secondary stimulation with E, there is a three- to fourfold increase in nonhistone protein levels in chick oviduct nuclei[76] followed at later times by a two- to sixfold increase in amino acid incorporation into both histones and nonhistones.[145] A rapid effect of E on the synthesis and uptake of proteins by nuclei also occurs in chick liver and is accompanied by the synthesis of two nonhistone proteins.[146] Selective synthesis of nonhistone proteins is equally apparent in rat uterus after E treatment[147,148] and in liver in response to C.[149] Furthermore, it can be shown by reconstitution studies that steroid-mediated changes in the nonhistone content of chromatin do indeed enhance chromatin template capacity.[150]

The degree of protein phosphorylation also governs chromatin structure.[151] Not only can phosphorylated proteins stimulate transcription of Pol II on DNA,[152,153] but dephosphorylation reduces template capacity.[154] Its role in mediating steroid action is supported by studies on rat ventral prostate showing that T treatment for 30 min in vivo increased the rate of phosphorylation of nonhistone proteins,[118] and on rat uterus where E stimulates protein phosphorylation and protein kinase activity in concert.[155] The latter enzyme is also enhanced by E in chick oviduct.[119]

Steroids also mediate acetylation of chromatin proteins. An extremely early effect (within 5 min) in estrogen-primed rat uterus is the selective acetylation of histones H2-H4,[156] and in aldosterone-primed rat kidney, there is selective acetylation of histone H4 within the same time period.[157] In kidney, this modification is transient, since the acetylation rate returns to control levels after 20 min, but it is both tissue- and steroid-specific. McCarty and McCarty[158] illustrate the drastic change in chromatin structure which could ensue by altering (by acetylation) a single charge on a histone molecule. And Marushige[159] has shown that direct chemical acetylation of all five histones in chromatin increases its template capacity for bacterial enzyme, although the rate of elongation, not initiation, seems to be affected. Yet another steroid-induced modification is the rapid effect (within 15 to 30 min) of C on the thiol content of rat liver nuclear proteins,[160] a response which can be mimicked by mixing the hormone with nuclei in vitro.

Perhaps even more dramatic is the influx of catabolic enzymes into the nucleus. Szego et al.[161] claim that 2 min after E injection, the level of cathepsin B_1 (of lysosomal origin) is at least 20-fold higher in ultrapurified nuclei from rat preputial gland compared to controls. Since cathepsin B_1 possesses peptide transferase activity, a role for this enzyme in modifying chromatin structure is likely. The potential importance of such an event warrants similar analyses in other, better characterized target tissues, since proteases have been shown to mimic estrogen-mediated increases in template capacity in rat uterus.[162] Other lysosomal enzymes also invade the nucleus;[163] whereas control rat uterine nuclei contain little or no acid ribonuclease II, this activity is considerably enhanced 2 min after E treatment. The enzyme can be readily distinguished from nuclear alkaline ribonuclease by dint of its metal and hydrogen ion requirements and differential degradation of homopolymers. Its specificity on nuclear RNA would be worth investigating. Other reports indicate that chromatin isolated after steroid treatment contains elevated nuclease levels,[164] and in the author's experience,[165] secondary stimulation of chick oviduct with E increases the level of ribonuclease in isolated nuclei within 1 hr. This activity is capable of limited digestion of nascent RNA chains synthesized by endogenous Pol II enzyme.

A more critical assessment of the relationship between template capacity, chromatin structure, and hormone action is considered in Section V.

IV. EFFECTS ON RNA SYNTHESIS IN VITRO

Ultimately, hormonal effects on transcription will be analyzed in vitro, and a number of groups have taken the first steps in this line of attack. In some of the original work, it appeared that free steroid could modify transcription. For example, the addition of C to nuclei accentuated endogenous Pol activity,[166] and cortisol phosphate activated the template activity of rat liver chromatin.[167,168] However, maximal effects were seen only at hyperphysiological steroid concentrations. These results have not been subsequently corroborated, and their significance remains unclear.

Steroids associate with a receptor molecule prior to eliciting a respose in vitro. This was first indicated in calf uterus: cytoplasmic supernatant exerted an effect on nuclear RNA synthesis only after prior incubation with E.[169] This system was examined in more detail by Jensen and co-workers.[170-172] Transformation of cytosol receptor from a 4S to a 5S form was required to trigger a two- to threefold increase in endogenous Pol activity; the effect was E-dependent, tissue-specific (as shown by dose-response curves), and was accomanied by an increase in the G-C content of the RNA product. Other preliminary data indicate that estrogen-containing cytosol can enhance the template capacity of uterine chromatin for homologous enzymes.[171]

The work of Davies and Griffiths[173-176] on the effect of androgen-receptor on RNA synthesis in rat prostate nuclei alerted many skeptics in the field to the reality and apparent reproducibility of "in vitro" effects. In the presence of dihydrotestosterone (DHT), prostate cytosol accentuated endogenous Pol activity by 50 to 100% under low-salt conditions, but not in high-salt, in agreement with Jensen. A similar degree of enhancement was seen when a crude mixture of homologous Pol enzymes was used to transcribe prostate chromatin in the presence of cytosol hormone; the effect was tissue-specific with respect to the chromatin and cytosol, and the stimulated Pol activity was α-amanitin insensitive (at 0.12 $\mu g/m\ell$). In the same system, Mainwaring and Jones[82] have also reported an in vitro effect on chromatin template activity. Preincubation of chromatin with cytosol hormone effected an 80% increase using homologous Pol II enzyme; no effect was obtained with spleen cytosol/hormone mixtures or spleen chromatin. In this case, chromatin was preincubated in cytosol hormone and then collected by centrifugation prior to the enzyme assay, since, unlike Davies and Griffiths, they found that cytosol inhibited Pol activity.

In a study which convincingly demonstrates the steroid- and tissue-specificity of these in vitro effects, Zerwekh and co-workers[135] could mimic very closely in vitro the elevation in template capacity (12 to 20%) of intestinal chromatin isolated 2 hr after in vivo administration of $1\alpha,25$-dihydroxyvitamin D_3. In this case, nuclei were incubated with cytosol hormone prior to preparing chromatin, and statistically significant increases (12 to 24%) in template capacity were obtained. Neither similar concentrations of structurally related steroids nor kidney or liver cytosol could mediate the response. In other systems, antheridiol[177] and prolactin[178] can also modify RNA synthesis in vitro.

Considering the complexity of cytosol preparations in these reports, a direct role for steroid receptors in modulating template effects is questionable. However, due to the painstaking work of Kuhn and co-workers,[179] who succeeded in purifying chick oviduct progesterone receptor to homogeneity, it has been shown[143,180,181] that template effects can be mediated by the receptor per se. Preincubation of oviduct chromatin from withdrawn chicks with H-R complex enhances template capacity by 50%, measured using

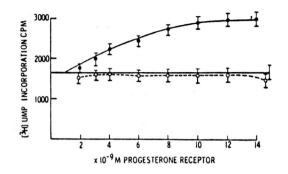

FIGURE 3.   Effect of purified progesterone-receptor complexes on chick oviduct chromatin template capacity in vitro. An ammonium sulfate "cut" of chick oviduct cytosol was divided into two parts. P was added to one half (0—0), and the other half was untreated (•—•). Both fractions were separately incubated with an affinity resin to purify the H-R complex. The eluted fraction which was pretreated with P did not contain receptors, whereas the untreated fraction did. Various amounts of these fractions were then added to withdrawn oviduct chromatin (5 μg DNA) and incubated at 22°C for 30 min. A saturating amount of *E. coli* Pol was then added, and the mixture was incubated for a further 30 min. RNA synthesis was then assayed in the presence of rifampicin and heparin, as described by Tsai et al.[137] The straight line represents the level of constitutive RNA synthesis in the absence of added receptors. (From O'Malley, B. W., Schwartz, R. J., and Schrader, W. T., *J. Steroid Biochem.*, 7, 1151, 1976. With permission.)

the rifampicin assay of Tsai et al.[137] (Figure 3). Half-maximal stimulation was observed with 5×10^{-9} *M* progesterone, which is similar to the value for the affinity of the H-R complex for chromatin. Very little effect was observed using liver or erythrocyte chromatins, and two useful controls were performed to substantiate the biological relevance of the result: (1) chromatin isolated from chicks pretreated with P in vivo was not stimulated by H-R complexes in vitro; (2) control assays contained "receptor" which was bound to, and eluted from, an affinity column in the presence of excess P. This fraction had no effect on template capacity, thus eliminating the possibility that minor contaminants (which were recovered from the column but had no specific affinity for P) elicited the response. However, some doubt remains as to the absolute requirement for P in the receptor-mediated effect. The response to receptor both free from, and bound to, P was measured, but the data were not directly compared with a reaction containing P but not receptor.[181]

In evaluating this work to date, *there seems to be some reluctance to define in vitro effects in precise biochemical terms,* particularly in work using crude cytosol preparations. An evaluation of the various subreactions of RNA synthesis and enzyme activities capable of modifying the chromatin DNA template or the RNA product is needed. Receptor preparations do contain ribonuclease activity.[182] In other cases, the nature of the enhanced activity requires further definition; for example, effects in the rat prostate system are α-amanitin insensitive,[176] but whether this represents Pol I, Pol III, or ribohomopolymer formation is not clear; as pointed out by Buller et al.,[183] contamination of receptor and enzyme preparations with nucleic acid synthetases is a real problem. Controls and subcontrols are not always satisfactory; in one report,[174] a statement to the effect that cytosol (without hormone) did not modify Pol activity is difficult to believe in the light of another report[82] indicating that cytoplasmic extracts per se inhibit RNA synthesis. Dose-response curves, data on reproducibility, and information on the state of the H-R complex during the incubation are also required. In the latter case, Davies and Griffiths[175] demonstrate the conversion of 8S receptor to 3S or 4 to 4.5S forms prior to association of the latter with chromatin; however, receptor dimers appear to be more effective in inducing in vitro responses in both chick oviduct[181] and rat prostate systems.[175]

One important, emerging aspect of this work is the apparent steroid and tissue specificity of the responses described to date. This alone is adequate justification for developing this line of attack, particularly when purified components are available. Whether H-R complexes are exerting a true biological effect in vitro and how this might relate to RNA synthesis in vivo is considered below.

V. BIOLOGICAL RELEVANCE OF TEMPLATE AND IN VITRO EFFECTS

Steroids induce gross changes in chromatin structure both in vivo and in vitro. Using AcD binding as an indicator of the availability of double-stranded DNA, E given in vivo triggers small increases (up to twofold) in this parameter when nuclei are analyzed in fixed preparations of rat uterine tissue,[184] but a several-fold increase in binding is observed when nuclei are preincubated with a mixture of E and uterine cytosol.[185] The proportion of the in vitro effect which is "real" is, therefore, a moot point, but for the initial discussion, it is assumed to be 100%. There is also considerable evidence against, and none to support, the contention that bacterial Pol enzymes (or eukaryotic Pol II, for that matter) initiate asymmetrically and only at DNA sequences recognized by eukaryotic Pol enzymes in vivo (see Section VI.B). Thus, titrating chromatin with excess exogenous enzyme probably yields little more information than that obtained by binding AcD to "open" DNA.

What biological, hormone-sensitive changes might alter the availability of DNA in chromatin? First, we must, of course, consider structural gene* transcription. The hypothesis that steroids generate large "active patches" in the vicinity of genes has been proposed by Yamamoto and Alberts[7] and is an extension of the puffing phenomenon observed in response to ecdysone or heat shock on dipteran polytene chromosomes. Although it is conceivable that hormones have similar effects on interphase chromatin, our recent experiments do not bear this out. Using cDNA to ovalbumin (Ov) mRNA as a probe, we find that the Ov gene is indeed more sensitive than the major chromatin DNA fraction to DNase digestion in chick oviduct nuclei, but this sensitivity is not altered after acute withdrawal of estrogen in vivo.[350] Palmiter et al.[186] reached similar conclusions using tamoxifen, a potent antiestrogen; the DNase sensitivity of the Ov gene was unaffected when tamoxifen was administered to estrogen-treated chicks under conditions known to block induction of Ov mRNA. Thus, it seems unlikely that at least the coding sequence of the Ov gene is "puffed" or "open" in the presence of steroid but covered with "repressor" proteins in its absence. Globin genes are also selectively DNase-sensitive long after transcription of this gene has ceased in erythrocytes.[187]

Other reports[142,188] imply that template capacity reflects the number of initiation sites on structural genes which are available or "open" for transcription in vivo. Two

---

* Structural gene = any gene containing a protein-encoding DNA sequence.

considerations suggest that this correlation is not yet justified. (1) There is no solid evidence that hormones trigger *de novo* the expression of large numbers of structural genes (see Section VII). (2) If more initiation sites for Pol II became available, one might expect to see an increased level of transcribing enzyme. This does not occur in chick oviduct or rat uterus (see Section III.B). Also, Pol II activity remains the same after serum stimulation of fibroblasts;[102] and in carcinoma cells, where Dex alters specific gene transcription, the overall rate of RNA synthesis is unaffected.[189] Thus, we do not see a situation in which more enzymes are transcribing more genes.

What other changes might potentiate increases in template capacity? The status of RNA processing and transport could partly account for template effects induced in vivo; more efficient packaging of RNA into ribonucleoprotein (RNP) or removal of RNP complexes from DNA could alter the availability of "open" DNA. Equally relevant is the recent demonstration that exogenous RNA Pol transcribe RNA templates (see Section VI.B); thus, enhanced RNA synthesis in vivo may raise the level of chromatin-associated RNA and, in turn, increase the available "template". Template capacity could also partly reflect the "activation" of ribosomal genes or even genes coding for regulatory RNA molecules. DNA replication or events leading up to it, is another possible candidate: the entire genome is responsive, modification of chromatin proteins is an intrinsic requirement,[190] and the process is steroid-sensitive.[191,192] These changes could also influence the way in which chromatin structure is modified during its isolation (see Section III.B). Whatever the cause, it is herein maintained that *it is premature to equate the major fraction of a given change in template capacity with alterations to structural genes or to increases in the number of these genes available for transcription.*

Finally, we do not know what fraction of a given template effect generated in vitro is artifactual. These changes seem to be steroid- and tissue-specific. But one might imagine a situation in vivo where H-R complexes activate factors or enzymes whose site of action is restricted by the subtle architecture of the chromatin, whereas in vitro, modifications to chromatin during isolation enable such components, when activated in vitro, to "broaden" their specificity. For example, if the membranes of lysosomes contaminating chromatin or cytosol were destabilized by H-R complexes,[23] released enzymes may exhibit a nonspecific action.

The proposal is made that template capacity changes elicited both in vivo and in vitro are, at best, a crude marker of hormonal effects on gene expression. They may, in part, reflect the latter and in part, a number of other complex events. Recently, O'Malley and co-workers[180] claimed that progesterone-receptor complex enhances the ability of bacterial Pol to transcribe Ov gene sequences in chromatin. If this result is corroborated and the criticisms outlined in Section VI.B. are met, it will obviously represent very strong evidence for the fidelity of the interaction between receptors and chromatin components in vitro.

VI. EFFECTS ON SPECIFIC GENE EXPRESSION

A. Induction of Protein and mRNA Levels

Knox and co-workers,[193] 20 years ago, pioneered the concept that hormones act by inducing specific proteins. Today, this idea has been confirmed unequivocally, and the essential step in modulating this effect has been defined: that is, *hormones regulate the cytoplasmic concentration of mRNA coding for these inducible proteins.*

The induction of Ov by E in chick oviduct is particularly well characterized. Oka and Schimke[194] were the first to demonstrate that a secondary stimulation of E elevated total protein synthesis 10-fold and Ov synthesis 100-fold, and this increase in the so-

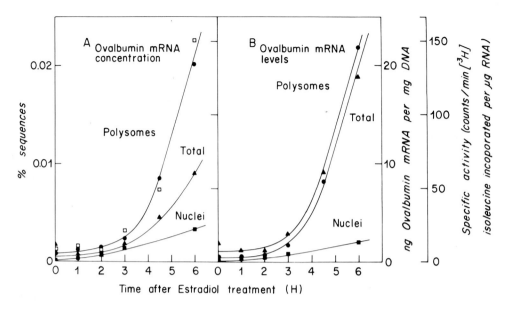

FIGURE 4. The appearance of Ov mRNA sequences in nuclear and polysomal RNA from chick oviduct in response to E. Values for (A) the percent of Ov mRNA sequences and (B) the content of Ov mRNA per unit DNA were calculated for nuclear (■—■), polysomal (●—●), and total (▲—▲) RNA samples after 0 to 6 hr treatment of withdrawn oviduct with 2 mg E. In addition, polysomal RNAs (10 to 60 μg) were assayed for their content of translatable Ov mRNA in a reticulocyte lysate. The specific activity of each RNA sample was then calculated, as shown (□—□) in panel (A). (From Cox, R. F., Haines, M. E., and Emtage, J. S., *Eur. J. Biochem.*, 49, 225, 1974. With permission.)

called relative rate of Ov synthesis was confirmed by Palmiter.[195] A direct correlation between the latter and the level of translatable Ov mRNA in total and polysomal RNA, as measured in a cell-free protein synthesizing system, led to the conclusion that either the level or the activity of Ov mRNA was altered in response to hormone.[196,197] However, selective translation of induced proteins in oviduct had already been tentatively ruled out by Palmiter.[35]

With the advent of techniques for obtaining complementary DNA copies (cDNA) of mRNA molecules, cDNA to Ov mRNA was synthesized, characterized, and hybridized to oviduct RNA.[198] As shown in Figure 4, we found a direct correlation between the actual amount of Ov mRNA in polysomal RNA and its translational activity. Coupled with the observation that Ov protein synthesis was induced in vivo with the same kinetics,[197] the data strongly indicated that E controls Ov mRNA levels in the cytoplasm and that this step is rate-limiting for the accumulation of Ov protein. Estrogen did not release a block in transport of Ov mRNA from nucleus to cytoplasm, since mRNA levels in withdrawn oviduct nuclei were very low.[198] Also, by comparison of results obtained for polysomal and total RNAs, it was clear that nearly all Ov mRNA was sequestered into polysomes. Later work[76,199,200] confirmed these findings and suggested that P regulates Ov mRNA in the same fashion.

More recently, many examples of hormonal effects on specific mRNA levels have been documented, but the results in chick oviduct typify the essential features of the response. A good correlation between specific protein and corresponding mRNA levels or activites has been shown for vitellogenin induction by E in *Xenopus* liver,[201] tryptophan oxygenase and tyrosine aminotransferase induction by C in rat liver,[202,203] casein induction during pregnancy in the rabbit or rat mammary gland,[204,205] α_{2u}-globulin induction by thyroid hormones or DHT in rat liver,[206,207] and growth hormone induction by thyroid hormone or Dex in cultured pituitary cells.[208]

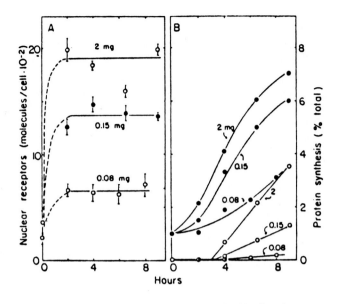

FIGURE 5.   Effect of estradiol benzoate on the kinetics of estrogen receptor appearance in chick oviduct nuclei and on ovalbumin and conalbumin induction. Various doses (0.08 to 2 mg per bird) of hormones were administered to withdrawn chicks and at various times chicks were killed. (A) Part of the oviduct was used to isolate nuclei and determine the level of specific estrogen receptors. (B) Part was incubated with (³H) leucine, and the percentage of total protein synthesis that was specifically immunoprecipitated by antiovalbumin (0—0) and anticonalbumin (•—•) was determined. (From Mulvihill, E. R. and Palmiter, R. D., *J. Biol. Chem.*, 252, 2060, 1977. With permission.)

Double-labeling techniques provide an indirect method of identifying induced proteins. E facilitates the rapid appearance (within 15 min) of "induced protein" (IP) either in vivo or when uteri are incubated in E-containing media in vitro,[209] and more recently,[210] this protein has been isolated and characterized. Double-label experiments[211] performed by translating polyadenylated (PolyA[+]) mRNA fractions in vitro and mixing the resulting labeled protein products have also yielded information on the androgen-induced proteins in rat prostate.

A number of studies[209,212-216] show a good correlation between biological response and the level of hormone or its specific receptor. In polytene chromosomes,[213] both early and late puffs are half-maximally induced by 1×10^{-7} M ecdysone. More specifically, IP induction in rat uterus parallels the amount of nuclear-bound E,[209] and the efficiency with which steroids induce tyrosine aminotransferase activity depends on their capacity to promote binding of the receptor to sites in the nucleus.[215] The most succinct correlation to date comes from Mulvihill and Palmiter[216] who show that the level of conalbumin mRNA in chick oviduct is directly proportional to the concentration of nuclear estrogen receptors. By comparison, a two- to threefold greater level of nuclear receptors is required to half-maximally induce Ov mRNA. The effect of graded doses of E on the rate of Ov and conalbumin induction is shown in Figure 5. Note that a dose of 2 mg E elicits maximal respose, both in terms of nuclear receptor levels and rates of specific protein synthesis; and for reasons which are not clear, Ov induction follows a 3-hr lag period, whereas conalbumin induction is immediate. *These results strongly implicate receptors in mediating steroid action in the nucleus and suggest that the rate of specific gene transcription is not simply an "on" or "off" phenomenon but is subject to fine control.*

To date, there is no documented exception to the emerging dogma that steroids elevate the level of a specific set of mRNA molecules which are, in most cases, derived from unique genes.[217,218] Some evidence that this is achieved, at least in part, at the level of transcription is considered below.

B. Chromatin Transcription In Vitro Using Exogenous Enzymes

Ever since the early claims[219,220] that *E. coli* Pol could recognize tissue-specific differences in isolated chromatins, in vitro transcription experiments have been viewed with a critical eye. In some cases, the fidelity of the cDNA probe has been questioned, but a major intangible factor, given the design of the experiments, was the inability to distinguish between endogenous and in vitro-synthesized RNA sequences. In reconstitution experiments in particular, claims[221-223] that nonhistone proteins are positive effectors for specific gene expression are undermined by the possibility that endogenous RNA sequences contaminate the protein fraction in question.

Recent work has amplified the confusion in this field, due, ironically, to development of a method to separate synthesized and endogenous RNA sequences.[224] This involves using mercurated nucleoside triphosphates as precursors for RNA synthesis and subsequent recovery of the RNA on sulphydryl-agarose columns. Unfortunately, Zasloff and Felsenfeld[225] have recently shown that *E. coli* Pol uses endogenous RNA in reticulocyte chromatin as a template in an AcD-resistant, but rifampicin-sensitive, process, with the consequence that 80 to 90% of the globin sequences recovered on sulphydryl-agarose (by virtue of their hydrogen bonding to the mercurated transcript) were endogenous contaminants of chromatin. Prelabeling of endogenous RNA sequences in vivo prior to chromatin isolation enabled Shih et al.[226] to reach similar conclusions, although they suggest that *E. coli* Pol elongates preexisting RNA chains. Reports that both *E. coli* and eukaryotic Pol II enzymes products synthesized on chromatin contain high levels of double-stranded RNA[227] and that considerable aggregation of endogenous RNA and in vitro-synthesized mercurated RNA (Hg-RNA) transcripts occurs[228] are all consistent with the above data.

These findings are directly relevant to a report from O'Malley's group[229] describing an analysis of Hg-RNA transcripts synthesized by bacterial RNA polymerase using chick oviduct chromatin as template. Their claim that *E. coli* enzyme recognizes tissue-specific differences in chromatin with respect to expression of Ov or globin genes is open to strong criticism since they may well be comparing the relative levels of contaminating endogenous mRNA sequences. Also, the apparent asymmetry of Ov gene transcription at low enzyme/chromatin levels could feasibly relate to a preference of bacterial enzyme for RNA template under the conditions used.

Earlier analyses made by this group[222,223,230] on RNA transcripts synthesized from chick oviduct chromatin are also hard to interpret. In these cases, isolated RNA contained both labeled transcripts and unlabeled endogenous RNA sequences. This author's experience has been that addition of bacterial enzyme to incubations containing oviduct chromatin invariably lowers the level of Ov mRNA recovered (as judged by hybridization to cDNA copies of Ov mRNA and calculated on the basis of mRNA sequences per unit chromatin DNA in the original reaction mixture). The results are consistent with symmetrical transcription (if any) of Ov genes and synthesis of anti-Ov mRNA copies on endogenous RNA, the later in effect lowering the amount of single-stranded Ov mRNA sequence available for interaction with cDNA. But Harris et al.[230] and Tsai et al.[222] recovered increased levels of Ov mRNA sequence in reactions containing bacterial enzyme. A partial explanation may relate to their method of analysis. In reactions containing no enzyme, carrier RNA (equivalent to the amount of RNA synthesized in the [+] enzyme reaction) is added. In view of the subsequent hybridization analysis in terms of RNA/cDNA ratio, addition of the correct amount of carrier is critical. However, differential recovery of labeled RNA and tRNA, as well as uncertainties in estimating precisely the amount of RNA synthesized in (+) enzyme reaction (e.g., contaminating RNA synthetase activities, problems of aliquoting due to clumping of chromatin), renders this approach technically difficult and could lead to "overdilution" of control RNA samples with carrier. Thus, direct comparison of hybridization kinetics (based on RNA/cDNA ratios) is tenuous.

Finally, aberrant transcription of eukaryotic genes in chromatin is problematic. In situations where eukaryotic Pol enzymes transcribe in vitro with high fidelity, *E. coli* enzyme copies 5S genes symetrically[231] and rRNA genes with low fidelity.[232] More specific answers to the question of whether bacterial enzyme transcribes at Pol II initiation sites on chromatin and, indeed, whether Pol II itself transcribes with any degree of fidelity await more critical analyses than are presently documented,[233-235] particularly in view of the RNA template problems described above. As yet, there is no convincing evidence that either enzyme transcribes chromatin DNA with high fidelity.

To conclude, *analysis of steroid action by measuring gene expression with exogenous enzymes in vitro has met with considerable technical difficulty.* In contrast, transcription artifacts of the kind discussed above are not significant when measuring endogenous enzyme activities in nuclei; in chick oviduct, RNA synthesized by Pol enzyme using mercurated precursors is both AcD- and RNase-sensitive,[236] and this has also been noted for erythroleukemic cell nuclei.[237]

C. Selective Transcription of Genes in Tumor Cell Lines

Considerable advances in our knowledge have been made by two groups[189,238] studying the control of glucocorticoids on viral gene expression in cloned mouse mammary tumor cells. The results are particularly striking because almost identical conclusions are obtained in two different cell lines using two different methods[239,240] to assay the rate of synthesis of viral gene sequences.

Young and co-workers[238] prelabeled cells for 15 min with ³H-uridine before addition of Dex (5µg/mℓ). Isolated RNA was then challenged with excess unlabeled cDNA to mouse mammary tumor viral RNA (MMTV RNA) which had been elongated with a stretch of poly(dC). The mixture was passed through a poly(I)-Sephadex® column, bound hybrid (retained by virtue of the poly[dC] tail on cDNA) was digested with RNase, and radioactive RNA, representing MMTV gene transcripts, was finally eluted and measured. As shown in Figure 6, Dex treatment (for 1 hr) increases the proportion of total labeled RNA represented by MMTV gene transcripts by about tenfold. In the absence of cDNA, very little RNA binds to the column (at least 40-fold lower than in its presence). In a second control, cells were superinfected with Moloney leukemia virus (MoMuLV) prior to Dex treatment. Using cDNA copies to this viral RNA, it was shown that hormone treatment had no effect on the rate of synthesis of this gene (Figure 6), suggesting that (1) Dex induction was specific and (2) induction of MMTV transcripts was unlikely to be caused by changes in UTP pools. To see if increased transcript stability accounted for the results, steady-state levels of MMTV RNA were measured in the presence of AcD. The sequences were less stable in the presence of hormone than in its absence, suggesting that MMTV RNA induction did, indeed, represent an increased rate of synthesis of this gene sequence.

Ringold et al.[189] labeled MMTV-infected cells for 15-min periods with ³H-uridine at various times before and after introduction of Dex to the medium. In this case, labeled RNA was challenged with excess "tailed duplex" DNA complementary to MMTV

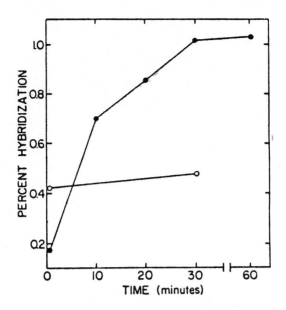

FIGURE 6. Kinetics of Dex stimulation of MMTV RNA synthesis in mammary tumor cells. After superinfection with Mo MuLV, cells were labeled with 200 μCi of (^{3}H)-uridine per milliliter, and Dex was added 15 min afterwards. At various times after Dex, RNA was extracted and hybridized for 18 hr with either MMTV poly (dC)-cDNA (•) or Mo MuLV poly (dC)-cDNA (O). RNA (25,000 to 75,000 cpm/μg; 200,000 cpm input) which hybridized was determined by Poly(I)-Sephadex® chromatography, and viral RNA content was corrected using ^{32}P-labeled 70S viral RNA as an internal standard. (From Young, H. A., Shih, T. Y., Scolnick, E. M., and Parks, W. P., *J. Virol.*, 21, 139, 1977. With permission.)

RNA. After hybridization and digestion with RNase, the mixture was passed through hydroxylapatite columns under conditions in which only cDNA (and hybridized RNA) was retained, by dint of its partially double-stranded structure. Bound radioactivity was, therefore, an estimate of the proportion of MMTV RNA sequences synthesized, as shown by a number of control experiments. Within 15 min of Dex treatment, a tenfold increase (0.05 to 0.5%) in the percentage of total synthesized RNA represented by MMTV RNA sequences was obtained, but total incorporation into RNA was not altered. Since steady-state levels also increased tenfold, this was probably entirely accounted for by effects on transcription, although effects on RNA degradation were not measured in this work. In contrast, the rate of MMTV RNA synthesis in infected lymphoma cells was not altered by Dex.

Since both groups have shown that effects of Dex on MMTV RNA synthesis are independent of DNA and protein synthesis,[241,242] *these data represent the most convincing evidence to date that steroids act by increasing the rate of transcription of specific genes.* Studies on viral RNA stability deserve further attention but are unlikely to invalidate the major conclusions. Although we cannot strictly extrapolate these conclusions directly to hormonal control of eukaryotic structural genes (since Dex may fortuitously interact with viral DNA sites which do not exist in uninfected target cells), it seems that the activated viral genes are all integrated into the host genome.[243]

Table 1

ESTIMATION OF RELATIVE
RATES OF MMTV RNA
SYNTHESIS IN WHOLE CELLS
AND ISOLATED NUCLEI IN
RESPONSE TO DEX

| | Percentage of total (^{3}H)-labeled RNA represented by MMTV-specific RNA sequences | | Ratio (+ Dex) |
System	−Dex	+ Dex	(− Dex)
Isolated nuclei	0.025	0.430	17
Whole cells	0.036	0.444	12

Note: Nuclei were isolated either from untreated cells, or from cultures which had been exposed to 1×10^{-6} *M* Dex for 30 min at 37°C and then incubated for 60 min at 25°C in reaction mixtures containing (^{3}H)CTP. Labeled MMTV RNA was then measured by hybridization to "tailed-duplex" cDNA and hydroxylapatite chromatography. Typical whole cell labeling data were obtained after incubating cells for 15 min at 37°C with (^{3}H)-uridine.

Modified from Yamamoto, K. R., Ivarie, R. D., Ring, J., Ringold, G. M., and Stallcup, M. R., *Biochemical Actions of Hormones,* Vol. 5, Litwack, G., Ed., Academic Press, New York, 1978, 373. With permission.

D. Selective Transcription in Isolated Nuclei

A number of reports[232,244,245] attest to the fidelity of transcription (with respect to the kinds of DNA sequences transcribed) which exists in isolated nuclei and nucleoli. RNA processing and transport also occur.[245,246] These conclusions have now been strengthened and extended by Yamamoto's group[247] who examined RNA synthesis in nuclei from control and Dex-treated cells. They find a remarkable correlation between the proportion of MMTV RNA sequences synthesized both in vivo and in vitro, as shown in Table 1. Furthermore, selective inhibition of Pol II activity blocks the synthesis of Dex-induced MMTV RNA almost completely, in agreement with previous indications[248] that Pol II enzyme mediates viral gene transcription. Since endogenous Pol II activity in isolated nuclei is due mainly to elongation (see Section III.B), *the data fit best with the idea that Dex enhances the rate of initiation of Pol II on viral genes in vivo, leading to an increased packing of Pol on these genes.* Elongation of nascent RNA in these transcription complexes thus provides a direct estimate of the relative degree of packing of Pol enzymes on different genes.

Rates of transcription of the Ov gene in chick and hen tissues have also been measured. Schutz et al.[249] used Hg-cDNA (copied from Ov mRNA) as a probe to estimate Ov mRNA sequences in RNA transcripts synthesized in vitro in chick oviduct nuclei. They found that in nuclei from hormone-withdrawn tissue, 0.0044% of the labeled transcript contained Ov mRNA sequence, compared with a value of 0.09% measured

6 hr after in vivo injection of estrogen; that is, there was a 20-fold increase in the apparent rate of Ov gene transcription.

Ov Gene transcription in hen tissues has recently been analyzed. In this case, Hg-RNA transcripts were synthesized in oviduct or spleen nuclei,[236] and the fraction of Ov gene copies was determined in hybridization reactions containing filters to which pOV$_{230}$ plasmid DNA (containing Ov gene sequences)[250] was affixed. As shown in Table 2, about 0.5% of the labeled transcript from oviduct nuclei was scored as Ov mRNA sequence, a 20- to 30-fold higher level than that seen in transcripts from spleen. Judging from the sensitivity of the assay, it is hard to say if the Ov gene in spleen nuclei is active or not. But the high level of Ov mRNA sequence in oviduct transcript is close to that found in total hen oviduct nuclear RNA (0.3 to 0.4%).[198] Based on the assumption that the Ov gene is only one of 13,000 different genes transcribed in hen oviduct,[251] it is clear that this gene is selectively transcribed. Nguyen-Huu and co-workers[252] and Bellard and co-workers[253] have reached similar conclusions and, in addition, have evidence that Pol II is responsible for Ov gene transcription. The data in Table 2 also show that Ov mRNA competes out 96% of the hen oviduct RNA hybridizing to pOV$_{230}$ DNA. Thus, in this case, transcription of a specific gene in isolated nuclei is essentially asymmetric; but note that Pol II does not copy asymmetrically in all cases, as evidenced by studies on viral gene transcription in transformed cells.[254] Although not directly related to hormone action, analysis of RNA synthesized in erythroleukemic cell nuclei[237] suggests that induction of globin synthesis by dimethylsulphoxide is also controlled at the transcriptional level.

The important implications of the above results augur well for future analyses of hormone action on responsive genes. It is clear that isolated nuclei retain certain features of their in vivo structure and activity, and it will be exciting to see if selective gene activation can be achieved in vitro by addition of purified H-R complexes. This task may be more formidable than meets the eye, since correct and efficient reinitiation of Pol II enzyme will be a primary requirement for such a system.

VII. EXPRESSION OF GENOTYPE

Due to recent technical advances,[255,256] a detailed analysis of hormonal effects on the spectrum of genes which are transcribed and translated can now be made. The author has recently analyzed[33] the effect of an acute withdrawal of estrogen (by removal of an estrogen-containing pellet) in chick oviduct on the complexity of cytoplasmic poly (A+) mRNA by synthesizing cDNA copies of each mRNA population and back-hybridizing to an excess of the original template. Quinlan and associates[257] then analyzed the reaction kinetics by computer which, by comparison with a standard reaction (globin mRNA and its cDNA), converted the data to a plot displaying the frequency distribution of mRNAs within the total population, as shown in Figure 7. Each peak represents a discrete mRNA frequency class, and the position of the peak on the abscissa indicates the number of mRNA sequences per cell for that class. A single component reaction, e.g., globin mRNA/cDNA, gives one peak spanning 1.5 log units using this analysis, so it follows that each mRNA class exhibits very little heterogeneity with respect to frequency. These plots yield a more graphic illustration of concentration groupings in mRNA populations than previously attained.

In the presence of estrogen, four mRNA frequency classes are apparent and peak 4 is predominantly Ov mRNA.[33] After withdrawal (for 24 hr), the Ov mRNA class (peak 4) disappears, and the mRNAs shift into two classes, a high-complexity class in which individual mRNAs are present at a concentration of one to three copies per cell (i.e., the same abundance as peak 1 prior to withdrawal) and a more abundant class (100

Table 2
ESTIMATION OF RELATIVE RATES OF OVALBUMIN GENE TRANSCRIPTION IN ISOLATED NUCLEI FROM HEN OVIDUCT AND SPLEEN

| Source of RNA transcripts | Filter | | | Hybrid (cpm) | Input (cpm) | % Hybridized | | | % Ovalbumin gene sequence in nuclear transcripts | | |
	pOV230	PMB9	OV mRNA[a]			Observed	Corrected[b]	Average	Total[c]	Negative strand[d]	Positive strand[e]
Hen oviduct	+			136	84,026	0.161	0.512	0.536	0.499		0.483
	+			148	84,026	0.176	0.560				
		+		12	84,026	0.014	0.030	0.037			
		+		18	84,026	0.021	0.045				
			+	20	95,416	0.020	0.063	0.053		0.016	
			+	14	95,416	0.014	0.044				
Hen spleen	+			145	142,151	0.102	0.324	0.341	0.017		0.017
	+			160	142,151	0.112	0.358				
		+		220	142,151	0.154	0.332	0.324			
		+		209	142,151	0.147	0.316				
			+	154	145,183	0.106	0.337	0.316		—	
			+	135	145,183	0.092	0.295				

Note: Transcription complexes in isolated nuclei were elongated in the presence of ^{3}H-GTP, Hg-UTP, 0.25 M ammonium sulfate and 1 mg/mℓ heparin as described previously.[236] Labeled Hg-RNA transcripts were then isolated on columns of SH-Sepharose® after pretreatment of Hg-RNA with *p*-hydroxymercuribenzoate. Only Hg-RNA which was retained on SH-Sepharose® at 70°C in the presence of 50% formamide-10 mM Tris-HCl (pH 7.5)-0.1 M NaCl-1 mM EDTA-0.1% SDS was used for hybridization (20 to 50% of the loaded cpm). This thermal retention procedure considerably reduced the recovery of nonmercurated endogenous nuclear RNA in the mercaptoethanol eluate. Prior to hybridization, labeled transcripts were demercurated by heating (107°C; 15 min), according to Zasloff and Felsenfeld,[225] and at least four different preparations of RNA (either from oviduct or spleen) were pooled.

The content of Ov gene transcripts was determined in DNA excess filter hybridization reactions using Hae III restriction endonuclease-cut pOV$_{230}$ plasmid DNA[250] (kindly provided by Doctors S.L.C. Woo and B. W. O'Malley). This recombinant plasmid contains the tetracycline-resistant plasmid PMB9 sequence, together with 95% of the DNA sequence complementary to Ov mRNA. Approximately 20 μg pOV$_{230}$ DNA was denatured and affixed to a 24-mm diameter nitrocellulose filter (Schleicher and Schuell®); the latter was dried *in vacuo* and cut into 0.8- × 4-mm strips containing 0.4 μg plasmid DNA. Control filter strips containing an equivalent amount of Hae III-cut PMB9 DNA were also prepared.

Hybridization mixtures containing ³H-RNA transcripts (100,000 to 200,000 cpm) and approximately 5 mg/mℓ *E. coli* tRNA in 50% formamide-2 × SSC (pH 7.0)-0.1% SDS were heat denatured (75°C; 5 min) and 2.5 μℓ aliquots were introduced into 50 lambda Dade® capillaries, each containing a DNA filter strip. The ends of the capillary were sealed with paraffin, and reactions were incubated at 41°C for 48 hr. After incubation, capillaries were bent in two places (to retain the filters) and flushed successively with chloroform, 50% formamide-2 × SSC, 2 × SSC (all at 40°C), then with 2 × SSC containing 2.5 μg/mℓ RNase A and 2.5 units/mℓ RNase T₁ (at 37°C), and finally with 2 × SSC (at 40°C). Filters were then removed and counted in toluene-based scintillation fluid.

Note that background levels for oviduct and spleen transcripts differ. Using PMB9 DNA filters, about 15 cpm of oviduct transcripts (0.017% of input) are retained, whereas about 200 cpm of spleen transcripts (0.14%) are recorded. The reason for this is not clear but may indicate some homology between PMB9 DNA sequences and spleen RNA.

ᵃ Where indicated, 0.6 μg Ov mRNA was present in the hybridization mixture.

ᵇ Observed values were corrected to 100% hybridization efficiency, as judged by the ability of ³H-cRNA to PMB9 plasmid DNA (synthesized using *E. coli* RNA polymerase) to hybridize to filters containing PMB9 or pOV₂₃₀ DNA. These standards were run in each experiment and, in this case, 31.4% and 46.5% of input ³H-cRNA hybridized to filters containing pOV₂₃₀ and PMB9 DNA, respectively. Considerable care was taken to remove DNA from the cRNA preparation.

ᶜ Obtained by subtracting the average value in line 3 from that in line 1.

ᵈ Obtained by subtracting the average value in line 3 from that in line 5.

ᵉ Obtained by subtracting the "negative strand" value from the "total strand" value.

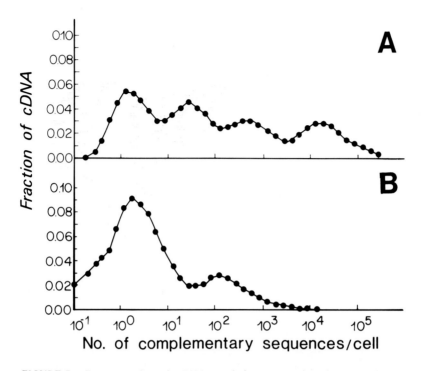

FIGURE 7.   Frequency plots of mRNA populations present in polysomal poly(A +) RNA isolated from chick oviduct (A) in the continuous presence of estrogen or (B) after withdrawal of steroid for 1 day. Hybridization data (taken from Cox[33]) were obtained by synthesizing cDNA copies of each poly(A +) RNA sample (using oligo[dT] as a primer for reverse transcriptase) and then back-hybridizing cDNA to the original RNA template. A computer program was used to fit the data to a number of pseudo-first-order reactions.[257] When the best fit had been obtained, the abscissa (Rot) was divided into equal intervals, and for each interval, the fraction of cDNA was determined and plotted on the ordinate. The number of complementary mRNA sequences per cell for a given cDNA fraction was calculated as described,[33] assuming 0.045 pg and 0.02 pg of poly(A +) mRNA per cell for estrogen-stimulated and 1 day estrogen-withdrawn tissues, respectively. Since a single component reaction gives one peak spanning 1.5 log units using this analysis (see text), values on the abscissa only strictly relate to the peak positions in these profiles.

copies per cell). However, further analysis[33] shows that all mRNA species present prior to withdrawal persist after withdrawal; that is, in both cases the same 10,000 to 12,000 individual mRNA types are present, but their abundance is altered in a notably discrete manner.

Assuming that the halflife of the average mRNA is several hours,[59] the results suggest that transcription of the majority of these mRNAs continues in the absence of steroid. It has also been shown by Hynes et al.[251] that withdrawn chick oviduct and hen oviduct tissues not only contain the same number (13,000) of individual polysomal poly(A +) mRNA sequences, but within the limits of detection, all sequences present in hen are present in withdrawn oviduct. Furthermore, in fibroblasts, serum stimulation produces at most a 3% increase in the number of cytoplasmic poly(A +) mRNA species.[258] All these results are consistent with the idea that, although rates of synthesis, processing, or transport may be modified, relatively few (if any) new mRNA species appear in the cytoplasm in response to hormones. Interestingly, Ivarie and O'Farrell[259] have examined phenotypic effects of Dex on HTC cells by two-dimensional electrophoresis of the cell proteins and conclude that less than 1% of the resolved protein spots change in intensity in response to hormone.

Extrapolation of these results might suggest that genotypic expression is not altered in response to hormones, but due to a notable lack of cross-hybridization data between nuclear RNAs and their respective cDNAs, such a conclusion is premature. Monahan et al.[188] have, indeed, compared the complexity of total poly(A+) mRNA from withdrawn and long-term estrogen-treated chick oviduct and conclude that the latter contains twice as many kinds of RNA sequences. But since estrogen may alter the spectrum of RNA species which are polyadenylated, this result should be considered tentative. In earlier work,[260,261] competition-hybridization and DNA saturation techniques were used to determine the spectrum of expressed RNA in chick oviduct. The results are in keeping with the idea that estrogen increases the number of genes expressed, but Rosen and O'Malley[262] note that the DNA saturation data are equivocal. Also, the rapid accumulation of a single cell type after estrogen treatment complicates a comparison of RNA species from immature and long-term estrogen-treated tissue. This objection is overruled in the cases where Hahn et al.[263] and O'Malley et al.[73] show that short-term P treatment of estrogen-stimulated chicks results in the appearance of new (albeit repetitive) RNA sequences in the oviduct.

Since steroids have minor effects on the complexity of mRNA and proteins in the cytoplasm, *it seems unlikely, a priori, that large hormone-mediated effects on the number of genes expressed would occur but not be transmitted to the cytoplasm.* Only further analyses will resolve this point.

VIII. CONTROL AT THE POSTTRANSCRIPTIONAL LEVEL

A. RNA Processing

Much progress has been made in defining the conversion of RNA transcript to mature mRNA.[264,265] *The role of hormones in these events is not understood, although in general, RNA processing appears to be enhanced, at least by steroids.* A series of papers by Luck and co-workers[266,267] convincingly demonstrates that E increases the rate of processing of newly synthesized rRNA by about fourfold in rat uterus, using labeled methyl-methionine as a precursor to monitor the conversion of 45S rRNA to mature rRNAs. Also, a larger percentage of newly synthesized rRNA becomes methylated,[267] in keeping with the demonstration that E enhances uterine methylase activities.[47] But whether this effect per se triggers subsequent processing events is not clear. Processing of rRNA precursors in rooster liver is also accentuated by E.[268]

A refreshingly concordant set of data, reviewed by Shields,[269] suggests that hormones enhance HnRNA processing (and/or transport of the product to the cytoplasm) in cultured fibroblasts. During the serum-stimulated transition from resting to growing states, the rate of HnRNA synthesis,[270] the proportion of HnRNA which is polyadenylated,[271] and the nuclear poly(A) content [271] remain virtually unchanged, but there is a twofold increase in the rate of transfer of labeled RNA to the cytoplasm within 3 hr of serum treatment.[270,271] Assuming that steroid hormones in serum induce these changes,[272] this work is good evidence for control at this level. By identifying mRNA on the basis of its poly(A) content, labeling studies[32,211] also show enhanced synthesis, processing, or transport of mRNA in response to hormone, but which of these pathways is activated is not clear. The level of cytoplasmic Poly(A+) mRNA is undoubtedly increased, as shown for aldosterone action in toad bladder[28,32] and for E in toad liver.[273] The reverse effect, withdrawal of hormone (estrogen) for 1 day, leads to a 50% reduction in polysomal Poly(A+) mRNA in chick oviduct.[33] Church and McCarthy[274] claim that E increases RNA transport in rabbit endometrium, although these experiments deal mainly with repetitive RNA sequences. Since Schumm and Webb[275] show a marked ATP-dependent release of RNA from nuclei in vitro, control of RNA transport by hormone-mediated changes in cellular ATP levels remains an interesting possibility.

A specific event in HnRNA processing, namely the sequestering of RNA transcripts into RNP particles, is apparently stimulated by E in rat uterus,[276] as judged by uridine labeling in vitro. Also, Tata and Baker[277] have shown a two- to tenfold increase in the poly(A) content of nuclear RNA in *Xenopus* liver in response to E. However, both reports are difficult to evaluate due to lack of data on precursor pool sizes. There appears to be no change in poly(A) polymerase activity in quail oviduct nuclei after estrogen treatment.[278] Finally, there is evidence[279-281] that hormones bind to nuclear RNP particules, but the significance of this event is unknown. In view of the accumulating evidence for mRNA precursors,[282,283] as well as the demonstration that discrete, time-dependent transitions in precursor size occur during maturation,[282] the outlook is optimistic for future research in this area.

B. mRNA Stability

There is now suggestive evidence that, in chick oviduct, estrogens stabilize Ov mRNA. Palmiter and Carey[284] first showed that translatable Ov mRNA activity in polysomes decayed rapidly after acute withdrawal of estrogen from the chick and concluded that estrogen produces a cellular environment in which egg-white protein mRNAs are relatively stable. These observations have recently been confirmed and extended[33] as outlined in Figure 8. In this case, translatable Ov mRNA activity is almost undetectable 24 hr after withdrawal, whereas total mRNA activity is only reduced by 40 to 50% after 4 days withdrawal (Figure 8A). Hybridization analysis with cDNA copies of Ov mRNA (Figure 8B) shows that loss of activity is caused by a depletion of Ov mRNA sequences in polysomes; this applies to total cell RNA as well. Selective loss of a limited number of mRNAs is also suggested[33] from an analysis of the peptides synthesized by polysomal RNA in a wheat germ assay; the Ov peak disappears after withdrawal, but otherwise the profiles are similar. Considering that in the presence of estrogen, Ov mRNA decays with a halflife of at least 24 hr[197] and under these conditions Ov mRNA is probably several-fold more stable than the average mRNA,[285] *some mechanism for selectively stabilizing this species relative to total mRNA must be operative in the presence of hormone.*

Control of gene expression by regulating mRNA stability is important in other systems. In HeLa cells, histone mRNA stability is directly coupled to DNA synthesis,[286] and Bastos and Aviv[287] have argued that destabilization of a large mRNA class is the best way to explain the rapid accumulation of globin mRNA during erythropoiesis; the latter mRNA is not stabilized per se during this process. Stiles and co-workers[288] note that in HTC cells, alanine aminotransferase mRNA stability is not altered by C, but some fascinating experiments by Warner et al.[289] indicate that there is a factor residing in rat hepatoma cell nuclei which specifically mediates the turnover of tyrosine aminotransferase activity. Clearly, no simple pattern of hormonal control of mRNA stability has yet emerged, but the impression is that the significance of these mechanisms in regulating gene expression is currently underrated.

C. Translation

Although hormones enhance translational efficiency, Lodish, in a recent review,[290] concludes that, in general, the translational apparatus has the same specificity towards all mRNAs. This is in agreement with Palmiter's findings in chick oviduct.[36] Furthermore, changes in protein synthetic activity per se do not seem to influence mRNA stability.[288] Thus, it seems that *mRNA synthesis, maturation, and degradation are the principle control levels through which hormones modulate the kinds and relative amounts of proteins synthesized in target cells.*

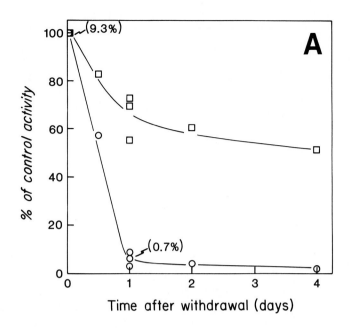

FIGURE 8. Effect of estrogen withdrawal on the translatable and hybridizable polysomal mRNA activities in chick oviduct. (A) Aliquots of polysomal RNA (0 to 10 μg) isolated at various stages of withdrawal were assayed in a wheat germ protein-synthesizing system. Total (□) and Ov (○) protein synthesis were measured and expressed as a percentage of non-withdrawn levels. Values in parentheses indicate the percent contribution of Ov protein synthesis to total protein synthesis. Three replicates of analysis (using separate animals) are shown for one day withdrawn RNA. (B) The kinetics of disappearance of Ov mRNA as measured by translation and hybridization. Estimates of the number of molecules of Ov mRNA in polysomal RNA per oviduct tubular gland cell (○) were made using cDNA copies of Ov mRNA. The level of translatable Ov mRNA in polysomes (□) was derived from the data in (A) and expressed as a percentage of non-withdrawn levels. (From Cox, R. F., *Biochemistry*, 16, 3433, 1977. With permission.)

IX. HORMONE ACTION AS DEDUCED FROM INHIBITOR STUDIES

A. Inhibitors

A certain hesitancy accompanies inferences based on inhibitor studies, particularly when using AcD. Anomalous effects of this drug have incited at least two groups[291,292] to implicate repressor molecules in the steroid-mediated control of mRNA levels, propositions which seem to be rapidly losing support.[293-296] In many cases, "superinduction" of mRNAs or their proteins can be explained on the basis of differential mRNA degradation in the presence of AcD and competition for rate-limiting translation factors.[297,298] In addition, AcD interferes with protein synthesis,[299,300] RNA processing,[301] and ATP pool sizes.[296] Cordycepin also affects protein synthesis,[300] and in view of its conversion to 3′ dATP and consequent inhibition of HnRNA synthesis,[302] the basis for inhibition of polyadenylation by this drug has been questioned. The drug α-amanitin probably retains its "specificity" in vivo, although it inhibits all nuclear RNA synthesis,[303,304] possibly because of the dependence of rRNA and tRNA synthesis on Pol II-directed RNA products.[303] Compared with AcD, cycloheximide boasts a better record of "specificity", but high concentrations may directly affect RNA synthesis.[305]

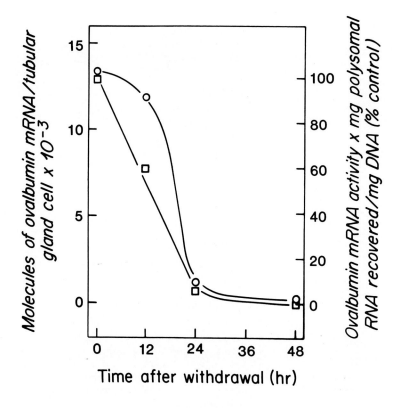

FIGURE 8B

The demonstration by Ernest et al.[306] that inhibitors of protein synthesis can selectively induce tyrosine aminotransferase mRNA levels in rat liver obviously complicates any straightforward interpretation of the action of these drugs. And finally, with all in vitro injection regimens, secondary effects of inhibiting protein synthesis in other endocrine glands are difficult to take into account.

Despite these obvious drawbacks, the attempt is made here to summarize the principle conclusions gleaned from the use of inhibitors to study effects of hormones at the level of transcription.

B. Factors and rRNA Synthesis

There is considerable suggestive evidence that steroids enhance rRNA synthesis via the production of Pol II-directed protein components. Gorski et al.[307] first showed that the E-mediated enhancement of "low-salt" Pol activity in isolated nuclei was blocked by giving puromycin in vivo, whereas control activity was unaffected. While examining the effect of cycloheximide in organ culture, Mueller and co-workers[308,309] also noted that maintenance of E-induced Pol activity (attained in vivo) was cycloheximide-sensitive, whereas control levels were not. Maintenance of E-induced activity was also inhibited by α-amanitin.[310] More recent and careful studies confirm and extend these observations. Nicolette and Babler[101] demonstrated the translation-dependent effect of E on Pol activity and showed that in vitro, the latter was DNA-dependent and α-amanitin-insensitive. Borthwick and Smellie[66] established that the steroid-induced rise in Pol I activity in nuclei was blocked by AcD, α-amanitin, and cycloheximide given in vivo. But if the latter two drugs were given 30 min after E, the rise in Pol I activity was unaffected. In both examples cited, control Pol I levels were again unaffected by α-amanitin or cycloheximide.

Two conclusions have been drawn from this work. (1) Steroid-induced activation of rRNA synthesis is mediated by protein synthesis which, in turn, requires Pol II-directed transcription; this is consistent with observations made in HeLa cells grown in the presence of serum,[311] where the rate of synthesis and processing of rRNA is translation-dependent; (2) In contrast, "constitutive" rRNA synthesis appears to be less dependent on continued protein synthesis.

Yu and Feigelson[80,312,313] extended these ideas with the claim that in rat liver, C enhances transcription of mRNA coding for a polypeptide moiety of Pol I. These authors first confirmed earlier work[78] showing that glucocorticoids enhanced Pol I activity in nuclei or nucleoli and showed, in addition, that "free" enzyme activity in isolated nucleoli, measured using poly d(AT) template in the presence of AcD, was also enhanced.[80] Subsequent work[312] using cycloheximide in vivo established that the drug considerably reduced both total and "free" Pol I enzyme in isolated nucleoli, although effects on template were not analyzed. The authors concluded that cycloheximide affected the catalytic activity of Pol I enzyme per se. In view of the report by Kellas et al.,[117] the interpretation of the AcD/poly d(AT) assays is somewhat questionable. However, in a third paper, Yu and Feigelson[313] showed that both α-amanitin and cycloheximide in vivo reduce Pol I activity in nucleoli to similar, low levels in both control and C-treated animals, implicating a Pol II-directed RNA product in the control of rRNA synthesis.

Subsequent work suggests that Pol I per se is not rapidly inactivated by cycloheximide. Benecke et al.[113] find unaltered Pol I levels in isolated nuclei up to 24 hr after injection of the drug, and in HeLa cells, Chesterton et al.[314] show that 3 hr after treatment with cycloheximide or puromycin, the level of Pol I is unexpectedly increased (1.9 × control). In addition, these authors show that Pol I is no longer bound to the chromatin template, implicating loss of a component which regulates its initiation.

To summarize, the data show that C may mediate its effect on rRNA synthesis via a Pol II-directed protein, possibly an initiation factor, but it is not clear whether this factor interacts with the enzyme or the template. Certainly Pol I retains catalytic activity in its absence. Furthermore, since control Pol I activity in nuclei is also reduced by cycloheximide,[313] it seems that "constitutive" control is also acutely dependent on protein mediators. Consequently, C may be augmenting a preexisting cellular control pathway. This does not seem to be the case for E action on Pol I activity in rat uterus, as discussed above.[66,101,307-310] It should be noted that the above conclusions rest, in part, on the assumption that increases in endogenous Pol I activity measured in vitro reflect a real steroid-mediated effect on the rate of initiation or elongation of Pol I in vivo; as discussed earlier, this may or may not be the case (see Section III.B), and the results should be considered in this light.

C. Induction of Specific Genes

The effects of inhibitors on the accumulation of IP in response to E are typical of those seen in other systems. Protein induction is blocked by AcD administered in vivo[209,315] but not by puromycin or cycloheximide in vivo if uteri are excised, washed, transferred to culture medium, and IP induction subsequently measured in the presence of AcD.[315] E can also induce IP in organ culture[209,316] but not in the presence of α-amanitin or AcD.[316] But if these drugs are introduced 15 min after E, IP is induced. Consequently, RNA synthesis is a prerequisite for protein induction, and protein synthesis is not required for mRNA accumulation. A similar heirarchy of events has been established in other systems; for example, in chick intestine for calcium-binding protein[317] and in mouse mammary gland for α-lactalbumin.[318] In chick oviduct, some doubt exists as to the requirement of Ov induction for protein synthesis,[319] since cycloheximide blocks induction by estrogen, but emetine (another inhibitor of protein synthesis) does not. Cycloheximide also blocks the induction of tyrosine aminotransferase by a combination of Dex and glucagon in suspensions of rat liver hepatocytes.[320]

Munck and co-workers[321,322] have defined the action of glucocorticoids on glucose transport in thymus cells by a series of steps: (1) an irreversible step in which C modifies glucocorticoid receptors; (2) an AcD-sensitive step, requiring at least 5 min of RNA synthesis; (3) a temperature-sensitive step, which influences the rapidity of the biological response; and (4) a cycloheximide-sensitive step. Using cordycepin, which in this case appears to block polyadenylation and not RNA synthesis, Young et al.[323] have confirmed the essential features of this response. Chu and Edelman[324] have also used cordycepin to show that in toad bladder, activation of sodium transport was mediated by RNA synthesis.

In summary, *RNA synthesis is essential for hormone-mediated induction of specific proteins,* but it is not known if transcription of the specific coding gene is the only requirement. *In some cases, protein synthesis appears not to be a prerequisite of gene activation, but in other cases it is.* The basis of this discrepancy may lie in the complexity of the action of these inhibitors on cellular mechanisms, of which we probably know very little.

X. MODELS FOR HORMONE ACTION

This section will discuss two relevant models: one to account for recent data describing "fine control" and multihormonal control of specific gene transcription, and the second, a current working model for steroid action in general. Transcription in relation to chromatin structure has not been considered since this is dealt with elsewhere.[325-327]

In the first model, it is assumed that induced levels of mRNA and protein directly reflect the efficiency of transcription of a given gene. Also, the idea is favored that in fully differentiated cells, steroids modulate structural gene expression, as opposed to activating genes *de novo* (see Section VII). It is not clear whether binding of H-R complexes to DNA or chromatin protein is the essential step in mediating steroid action, but Schrader et al.[328] have evidence that progesterone receptor subunits play a dual role in this respect. Cell-hybridization studies[329] reveal that glucocorticoid receptors may act by inactivating or competing with proteins which inhibit transcription of the tyrosine aminotransferase gene. And the biological consequence of the interaction between H-R complexes and the genome, as deduced from work on MMTV RNA and Ov mRNA induction (see Section VI.D) is probably an enhanced packing of Pol II enzymes on specific genes. The following proposals are consistent with the above data: (1) control of inducible structural genes may be direct or indirect, allowing for mediation by RNA[330-332] and protein molecules; (2) positive control is exerted at Pol II initiation sites or antiterminator (attenuator) sites on the gene.

The idea of negative control by hormones has received little attention considering the fascinating demonstration by Ashburner et al.[213] that, in polytene chromosomes, late puffs are prematurely induced after washing out ecdysone but regress when hormone is added back. It is difficult to find an alternative to Ashburner's proposition that ecdysone suppresses gene activity at some chromosomal sites. Clear-cut inhibitory effects of E on DHT-mediated expression of α_{2u}-globulin mRNA in rat liver[207,333] and of P on prolactin-mediated induction of casein mRNA in mammary gland[334] have also been described.

Presumably, in most target cells, a number of hormones (both steroid and nonsteroid)[335,336] interact with the genome at any given moment. Since transcription seems to be rate-limiting with respect to protein induction, it is pertinent to consider an interaction between hormone "effectors" at this level. Current models for transcriptional control adequately explain "all or none" induction of a gene product (coarse control) but not intermediate rate changes (fine control) nor additive and synergistic effects on mRNA and protein levels. For example, E and P induce conalbumin and conalbumin mRNA in chick oviduct when given alone but elicit synergism when administered together.[337,338] Thyroid hormone and C exert an additive effect on growth hormone synthesis in pituitary cells,[339] but only the former hormone is active alone. Also, there is a close correlation between the rate of specific mRNA synthesis and the level of nuclear estrogen receptors in chick oviduct (see Section VI.A).

It is conceptually difficult to envisage precise control of the rate of initiation of Pol II by multiple effectors at a single site. For this reason, *it is proposed that multiple initiation sites on specific genes could mediate control at this level,* and a possible mechanism is considered in Figure 9. In most cases, it is assumed that, once initiated, movement of Pol II along the DNA is unrestricted. RNA synthesis could begin at the site of initiation or after "rightward" movement of the enzyme to a "start site". Transcription from the initiation site is more feasible and implies heterogeneity in the length of the transcripts. It is also assumed that each initiation site is either "on" (available for rapid initiation) or "off" (accepting low rates of initiation). Low levels of "constitutive" mRNA transcription could occur at any of the multiple sites.

Multihormonal control and "fine control" are now conceptually simple, on the basis that H-R complexes activate different initiation sites and that, in some cases, two different H-R complexes are needed to activate the same site. An additional proviso is required to explain inhibitory effects and the interplay between cortisol-receptor and thyroid hormone-receptor complexes; in this case, Pol II initiating at a distal, C-sensitive site cannot traverse a more proximal site until the latter is activated by thyroid hormone; thus, control is achieved by a combination of initiation and attenuation effects. Single initiation sites on genes are, in fact, adequate to explain inhibitory or nonadditive effects of hormones, but multiple-site models are included in Figure 9 for the sake of completeness. Note that a direct action of hormones at inducible genes is not a stipulation of the model, and intermediates (for example, RNA primers)[330] could act as effector molecules.

The parallelism between nuclear receptor levels and the rate of conalbumin induction[216] can be explained by stepwise activation of a bank of estrogen-sensitive initiation sites, assuming (simplistically) a direct proportionality between the fraction of nuclear "acceptor sites" and the fraction of conalbumin gene initiation sites occupied by H-R complexes. Limited cooperative effects between H-R complexes at any single initiation site might also increase the sensitivity of fine control. As discussed previously,[216] the differential response of Ov and conalbumin mRNA production may be due to a variation in the affinity of the H-R complex for different control loci.

An equally feasible model to explain fine control would require a single initiation site per gene but multiple attenuator sites either distal to the mRNA coding region or in intervening sequences. Consider a high constitutive rate of initiation of Pol II on a gene with nine such attenuator sites, with passage of the enzyme through each site precipitating a 10% chance of premature termination. Few enzymes would complete transcription of the coding region. But stepwise activation of each site by H-R complexes, resulting in read-through of all Pol II enzymes at each activated locus, would provide fine control of the rate of transcription of the coding sequence. Variations on this theme could also explain multihormonal control, but they have intrinsically less latitude (capacity for a wide spectrum of response) than models with multiple initiation sites.

Additional hormonal actions would no doubt temper the end result in terms of cel-

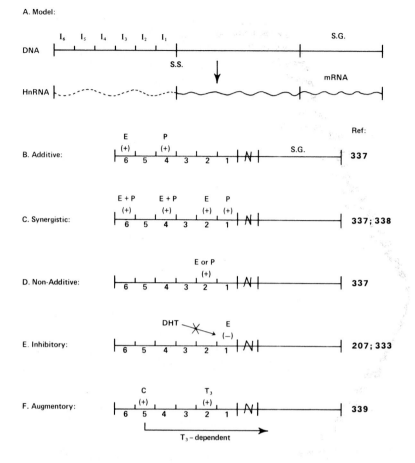

FIGURE 9.   Multiple initiation site model for hormonal control of specific gene transcription. (A) Schematic diagram of a hormone-sensitive gene and its RNA product. Six initiation sites for Pol II are depicted at the leftward end of the gene, but the number of sites in each bank would be variable for a given gene. Once initiated, Pol II would either traverse to a "start site" and begin RNA synthesis or, alternatively, begin transcription immediately after initiation. At present, there seems to be no evidence for or against the idea of multiple initiation sites on eukaryotic genes.[351] (B) to (F) Proposed mechanism for multihormonal control of the rate of initiation on specific genes. Each attempts to explain an effect on specific mRNA or protein levels described in the literature (see reference in figure). In all cases except (F), once Pol II has initiated, transcription is rightward and is unrestricted by any initiation site (whether active or inactive) it might traverse. (+) signifies full activation of, and (−) signifies no effect on "constitutive" initiation at that site. (B) *Additive.* P-receptor complex activates site 4 and E-receptor complex activates site 6, each giving rise to a similar, maximal rate of initiation; when both complexes are present, the rate of initiation is approximately doubled on this gene. (C) *Synergistic.* Sites 4 and 6 are only activated by two different H-R complexes, resulting in a synergistic effect of E and P on the rate of transcription. (D) *Nonadditive.* Either hormone can activate a common initiation site. (E) *Inhibitory.* Estrogen-receptor complex binds to site 1, but has no effect on initiation at that site; however, this blocks the binding of a potential activator, DHT-receptor complex. Other alternatives can explain inhibitory effects. (F) *Augmentory.* Pol II enzymes which have initiated at site 5 cannot traverse site 2 unless the latter is activated by a second H-R complex. I_1-I_6 or 1-6 signify banks of separate initiation sites; s.s. = "start site", assuming that polymerases can traverse to this point without synthesizing RNA; E, P, DHT, C, T_3 = hormone-receptor complexes containing estrogen, progesterone, dihydrotestosterone, cortisol, and thyroid hormones, respectively.

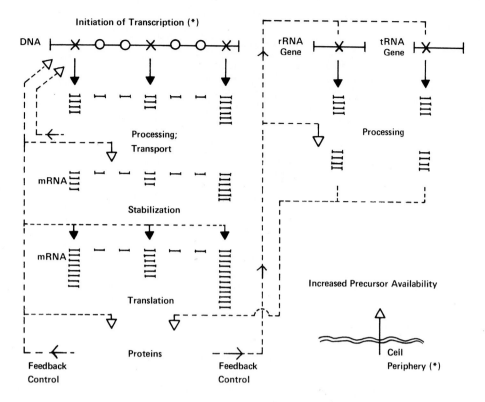

FIGURE 10. A working model for sex steroid action on RNA metabolism. (1) Two primary sites of action are proposed: one at the cell surface (see Section II) and one in the nucleus (see Section VI). The former interaction increases precursor uptake or availability; the latter enhances specific gene transcription. (2) Increased precursor availability activates rRNA synthesis (in view of the findings of Grummt and Grummt[20]) and HnRNA and tRNA synthesis as well. (3) In turn, elevated levels of rRNA (as ribosomes) and tRNA increase the efficiency of translation. (4) Positive feedback control by proteins or "regulatory RNAs" (small nuclear RNAs, intervening sequences in primary gene transcripts, etc.) activates HnRNA, rRNA (see Section IX.B) and tRNA synthesis. (5) It is proposed that one particular feedback pathway stabilizes specific mRNAs (see Section VIII.B). Thus, proliferation of cellular components potentiates the production of specific gene products. Negative feedback control of cell metabolism is not considered in this diagram. x = specific gene (steroid-sensitive); 0 = specific gene (insensitive); closed arrow denotes steroid-induced activation of a particular process for a specific gene; open arrow denotes steroid activation of a process for all genes; * = primary site of steroid action; 1—1 = RNA molecule; ——- = feedback control pathway.

lular mRNA or protein levels, and *the second model* (Figure 10) deals with control in broader terms. It also *serves as a summary of the data and viewpoints discussed in this article.* Strictly, it pertains to sex steroid acion, and more specifically to estradiol, since effects on both mRNA stability and precursor uptake have been incorporated. For other steroids, e.g., glucocorticoids, increased precursor uptake may not occur; in this case, mRNA production may not be accompanied by general anabolic effects. Our current understanding of steroid action on specific genes is fairly clear, but a comment is needed on HnRNA production. *There is only suggestive evidence that the rate of synthesis of HnRNA, in general, is increased by steroids* (see Section III.A). Secondly, this response is not a prerequisite for total mRNA accumulation; a decreased rate of degradation of mRNA or an increase in the efficiency of utilization of mRNA sequences in HnRNA (in terms of the fraction of protein-encoded sequences processed and transported to the cytoplasm) will also elevate steady-state levels of mRNA. The contribution made by each of these mechanisms is unknown, but Figure 10 assumes

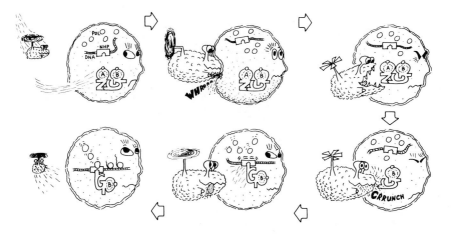

FIGURE 11. Mitochondrion-eye view of an unsuccessful gambit by a progesterone-receptor complex to elude the attentions of a voracious lysosome. Refuge in the nucleus is to no avail. The lysosome proceeds to devour the particularly juicy "A" subunit. Fortuitously, the "B" subunit now "locks in" to an initiation site on the ovalbumin gene and activates transcription.

that steroids have only secondary effects on the synthesis and on the efficiency of processing and transport of structural gene products in general.

The role of lysosomal enzymes has not been considered in the above models, but these proteins may well have important effects on the structure of chromatin, RNA processing, and even in mediating steroid-receptor action. It is hoped that the interrelationship shown in Figure 11 will guide future research in this area and will encourage collaboration between groups [24,181] with conflicting viewpoints.

XI. PERSPECTIVES

Considerable progress has been made recently in our understanding of steroid action at the level of specific gene expression. There is now convincing evidence that glucocorticoids and estrogens enhance the rate of initiation of RNA polymerases on specific genes, and it is likely that this will prove to be a general feature of the action of all steroids.

In contrast, efforts to define effects of steroids on RNA synthesis in general, particularly by analyzing isolated nuclei and chromatin fractions, have met with some difficulty, probably for a number of reasons. First, although steroids seem to have at least one common site of action (that is, at the level of transcription), each hormone may control a defined set of additional mechanisms. For example, E might act at the cell surface, on DNA synthesis, at the lysosomal membrane, and possibly at the level of RNA processing. This multiplicity of action is likely to confound any attempt to relate a given experimental effect to a particular control level. Secondly, the complexity of cell types in most target tissues magnifies this problem. And third, the contribution of artifacts to the experimental results obtained in vitro has not been realistically evaluated.

To avoid at least some of these problems in interpretation, those entering the field should take extra care in their choice of a biological system. For example, the action of aldosterone on toad bladder is a comparatively "simple" system since the hormone does not induce hypertrophy and hyperplasia and has the added advantage that blader tissue is responsive in organ culture. Other "ideal" systems are currently being exploited. For example, vitellogenin induction by E in *Xenopus* liver[340,341] and growth hormone induction by thyroid hormones in pituitary cells.[339,342] Both responses are elicited in tissue culture, and the regulation of specific gene products is intrinsic to each. Induction of viral gene expression in culture cells[238] will no doubt continue to yield important information, and the response of fungal hyphae to the steroid antheridiol deserves some attention.[343] The merits of analyzing hormone action in cell culture and using cell-cell hybridization techniques and genetic approaches have recently been discussed.[344-346]

Currently, steroid-sensitive genes are being isolated[347] and will no doubt be used as a framework upon which to reconstruct hormone action in vitro. Also, the striking discovery [348,349] that DNA sequences coding for Ov mRNA are separated in the natural gene by at least six intervening sequences has created much excitement. Both of these advances will help to allay our virtual ignorance of the events occurring between the binding of H-R complexes to nuclear components and the rise in cellular mRNA levels. For this reason alone, there is undoubtedly a bright future ahead for our efforts to dissect hormone action.

ABBREVIATIONS

AcD	Actinomycin D
C	Cortisol or hydrocortisone
cDNA	Complementary DNA
Dex	Dexamethasone
DHT	Dihydrotestosterone
DNase	Deoxyribonuclease
E	Estradiol
Hg-RNA	Mercurated RNA
HnRNA	Heterogneous nuclear RNA
H-R complex	Hormone-receptor complex
IP	Induced protein
Mo MuLV	Moloney leukemia virus
mRNA	Messenger RNA
Ov	Ovalbumin
P	Progesterone
Pol	RNA polymerase
Pol I, II, and III	RNA polymerases I (or A), II (or B), and III (or C)
Poly(A +)	Polyadenylated
RNase	Ribonuclease
RNP	Ribonucleoprotein
rRNA	Ribsomal RNA
T	Testosterone
tRNA	Transfer RNA

REFERENCES

1. **King, R. J. B. and Mainwaring, W. I. P.,** *Steroid-Cell Interactions,* University Park Press, Baltimore, 1974.
2. **Baulieu, E.-E., Atger, M., Best-Belpomme, M., Corvol, P., Courvalin, J., Mester, J., Milgrom, E., Robel, P., Rochefort, H., and de Catalogne, D.,** Steroid hormone receptors, *Vitam. Horm. (NY),* 33, 649, 1975.
3. **Gorski, J. and Ganon, F.,** Current models of steroid hormone action: a critique, *Annu. Rev. Physiol.,* 38, 425, 1976.
4. **Gannon, F., Katzenellenbogen, B., Stancel, G., and Gorski, J.,** Estrogen receptor movement to the nucleus: discussion of a cytoplasmic exclusion hypothesis, in *The Molecular Biology of Hormone Action,* Papaconstantinou, J. P., Ed., Academic Press, New York, 1976, 137.
5. **Rousseau, G. G.,** Interaction of steroids with hepatoma cells: molecular mechanisms of glucocorticoid hormone action, *J. Steroid Biochem.,* 6, 75, 1975.
6. **Yamamoto, K. R., Gehring, U., Stampfer, M. R., and Sibley, C. H.,** Genetic approaches to steroid hormone action, *Recent Prog. Horm. Res.,* 32, 3, 1976.
7. **Yamamoto, K. R. and Alberts, B. M.,** Steroid receptors: elements for modulation of eukaryotic transcription, *Annu. Rev. Biochem.,* 45, 721, 1976.
8. **Buller, R. E. and O'Malley, B. W.,** The biology and mechanism of steroid hormone receptor interaction with the eukaryotic nucleus, *Biochem. Pharmacol.,* 25, 1, 1976.
9. **Milgrom E. and Atger, M.,** Receptor translocation inhibitor and apparent saturability of the nuclear acceptor, *J. Steroid Biochem.,* 6, 487, 1975.
10. **Buller, R. E., Schrader, W. T., and O'Malley, B. W.,** Progesterone-binding components of chick oviduct. IX. The kinetics of nuclear binding, *J. Biol. Chem.,* 250, 809, 1975.
11. **Clark, J. H., Eriksson, H. A., and Hardin, J. W.,** Uterine receptor-estradiol complexes and their interaction with nuclear binding sites, *J. Steroid Biochem.,* 7, 1039, 1976.
12. **Puca, G. A., Nola, E., Hibner, U., Cicala, G., and Sica, V.,** Interaction of the estradiol receptor from calf uterus with its nuclear acceptor sites, *J. Biol. Chem.,* 250, 6452, 1975.
13. **Spelsberg, T. C., Webster, R. W., Pikler, G., Thrall, C., and Wells, D.,** Role of nuclear proteins as high affinity sites ("acceptors") for progesterone in the avian oviduct, *J. Steroid Biochem.,* 7, 1091, 1976.
14. **Jackson, V. and Chalkley, R.,** The binding of estradiol-17β to the bovine endometrial nuclear membrane, *J. Biol. Chem.,* 249, 1615, 1974.
15. **Stumpf, W. E. and Sar, M.,** Autoradiographic localization of estrogen, androgen, progestin, and glucorticosteroid in "target tissues" and "nontarget tissues", in *Receptors and Mechanisms of Action of Steroid Hormones, Part I,* Pasqualini, J. R., Ed., Marcel Dekker, New York, 1976, 41.
16. **Spaziani, E. and Szego, C. M.,** Further evidence for mediation by histamine of estrogenic stimulation of the rat uterus, *Endocrinology,* 64, 713, 1959.
17. **Spaziani, E. and Szego, C. M.,** The influence of estradiol and cortisol on uterine histamine of the ovariectomized rat, *Endocrinology,* 63, 669, 1958.
18. **Spaziani, E.,** Accessory reproductive organs in mammals: control of cell and tissue transport by sex hormones, *Pharmacol. Rev.,* 77, 207, 1975.
19. **Grummt, I., Smith, V. A., and Grummt, F.,** Amino acid starvation affects the initiation frequency of nucleolar RNA polymerase, *Cell,* 7, 439, 1976.
20. **Grummt, F. and Grummt, I.,** Control of nucleolar RNA synthesis by the intracellular pool sizes of ATP and GTP, *Cell,* 7, 447, 1976.
21. **Peitras, R. J. and Szego, C. M.,** Specific binding sites for oestrogen at the outer surfaces of isolated endometrial cells, *Nature (London),* 265, 69, 1977.
22. **Munck, A. and Leung, K.,** Glucocorticoid receptors and mechanisms of action, in *Receptors and Mechanism of Action of Steroid Hormones, Part II,* Pasqualini, J. R., Ed., Marcel Dekker, New York, 1977, 311.
23. **Szego, C. M.,** The lysozomal membrane complex as a proximate target for steroid hormone action, in *The Sex Steroids,* McKerns, H. W., Ed., Appleton-Century-Crofts, Englewood Cliffs, N. J., 1971, 1.
24. **Szego, C. M.,** The lysozome as a mediator of hormone action, *Recent Prog. Horm. Res.,* 30, 171, 1974.
25. **Tata, J. R.,** The formation, distribution and function of ribosomes and microsomal membranes during induced amphibian metamorphosis, *Biochem. J.,* 105, 783, 1967.
26. **Palmiter, R. D., Christensen, A. K., and Schimke, R. T.,** Organization of polysomes from preexisting ribosomes in chick oviduct by a secondary administration of either estradiol or progesterone, *J. Biol. Chem.,* 245, 833, 1970.

27. **Means, A. R., Abrass, I. B., and O'Malley, B. W.,** Protein biosynthesis on chick oviduct polyribosomes, *Biochemistry,* 10, 1561, 1971.
28. **Wilce, P. A., Rossier, B. C., and Edelman, I. S.,** Actions of aldosterone on rRNA and Na⁺ transport in the toad bladder, *Biochemistry,* 15, 4286, 1976.
29. **Hamilton, T. H.,** Control by estrogen of genetic transcription and translation, *Science,* 161, 649, 1968.
30. **O'Malley, B. W., Aronow, A., Peacock, A. C., and Dingman, C. W.,** Estrogen-dependent increase in transfer RNA during differentiation of the chick oviduct, *Science,* 162, 567, 1968.
31. **Dingman, C. W., Aronow, A., Bunting, S. L., Peacock, A. C., and O'Malley, B. W.,** Changes in chick oviduct ribonucleic acid following hormonal stimulation, *Biochemistry,* 8, 489, 1969.
32. **Wilce, P. A., Rossier, B. C., and Edelman, I. S.,** Actions of aldosterone on polyadenylated ribonucleic acid and Na⁺ transport in the toad bladder, *Biochemistry,* 15, 4279, 1976.
33. **Cox, R. F.,** Estrogen withdrawal in chick oviduct: selective loss of high abundance classes of polyadenylated messenger RNA, *Biochemistry,* 16, 3433, 1977.
34. **Rudland, P. S., Weil, S., and Hunter, A. R.,** Changes in RNA metabolism and accumulation of presumptive messenger RNA during transition from the growing to the quiescent state of cultured mouse fibroblasts, *J. Mol. Biol.,* 96, 745, 1975.
35. **Palmiter, R. D.,** Regulation of protein synthesis in chick oviduct. II. Modulation of polypeptide elongation and initiation rates by estrogen and progesterone, *J. Biol. Chem.,* 247, 6770, 1972.
36. **Palmiter, R. D.,** Quantitation of parameters that determine the rate of ovalbumin systesis, *Cell,* 4, 189, 1975.
37. **Mueller, G. C., Herranen, A. M., and Jervell, K. F.,** Studies on the mechanism of action of estrogens, *Recent Prog. Horm. Res.,* 14, 95, 1958.
38. **Means, A. R. and Hamilton, T. H.,** Early estrogen action: concomitant stimulations within two minutes of nuclear RNA synthesis and uptake of RNA precursor by the uterus, *Proc. Natl. Acad. Sci. U.S.A.,* 56, 1594, 1966.
39. **Billing, R. J., Barbiroli, B., and Smellie, R. M. S.,** The mode of action of oestradiol. I. The transport of RNA precursors into the uterus, *Biochem. Biophys. Acta,* 190, 52, 1969.
40. **Billing, R. J., Barbiroli, B., and Smellie, R. M. S.,** The mode of action of oestradiol. II. The synthesis of RNA, *Biochem. Biophys. Acta,* 190, 60, 1969.
41. **Miller, B. B. and Baggett, B.,** The effects of 17β-estradiol on the rate of synthesis of RNA in the uterus, *Biochim. Biophys. Acta,* 281, 353, 1972.
42. **Miller, B. G.,** Rate of synthesis of non-ribosomal RNA in castrate uterus after oestradiol-17β stimulation, *Nature (London) New Biol.,* 237, 109, 1972.
43. **Munns, T. W. and Katzman, P. A.,** Effects of estradiol on uterine ribonucleic acid metabolism. I. In vitro uptake and incorporation of ribonucleic acid precursors, *Biochemistry,* 10, 4941, 1971.
44. **Munns, T. W. and Katzman, P. A.,** Effects of estradiol on uterine ribonucleic acid metabolism. II. Methylation of ribosomal ribonucleic acid and transfer ribonucleic acid, *Biochemistry,* 10, 4949, 1971.
45. **Perry, R. P. and Kelley, D. E.,** Existence of methylated messenger RNA in mouse L cells, *Cell,* 1, 37, 1974.
46. **Luck, D. N. and Hamilton, T. H.,** Early estrogen action: stimulation of the synthesis of methylated ribosomal and transfer RNAs, *Biochim. Biophys. Acta,* 383, 23, 1975.
47. **Munns, T. W., Sims, H. F., and Katzman, P. A.,** Effects of estradiol on uterine ribonucleic acid metabolism, *Biochemistry,* 14, 4758, 1975.
48. **Catelli, M. G. and Baulieu, E. E.,** Estrogen-induced changes of ribonucleic cid in the rat uterus, *Mol. Cell. Endocrinol.,* 6, 129, 1976.
49. **Joel, P. B. and Hagerman, D. D.,** Extraction of RNA from rat uterus, *Biochim. Biophys. Acta,* 195, 328, 1969.
50. **Knowler, J. T. and Smellie, R. M. S.,** The synthesis of ribonucleic acid in immature rat uterus responding to oestradiol-17β, *Biochem. J.,* 125, 605, 1971.
51. **Knowler, J. T. and Smellie, R. M. S.,** The oestrogen-stimulated synthesis of heterogeneous nuclear ribonucleic acid in the uterus of immature rats, *Biochem. J.,* 131, 689, 1973.
52. **Baulieu, E. E.,** A 1972 survey of the model of action of steroid hormones in *Excerpta Medica,* Int. Cong. Series, 273, Scow, R. O., Ed., American Elsevier, New York, 1973, 30.
53. **Frolik, C. A. and Gorski, J.,** Quantitative isolation of ribonucleic acid from the immature rat uterus — examination of ribonucleic acid synthesis following in vivo 17β-estradiol administration, *J. Steroid Biochem.,* 8, 713, 1977.
54. **Kenny, F. T., Wicks, W. D., and Greenman, D. L.,** Hydrocortisone stimulation of RNA synthesis in induction of hepatic enzymes, *J. Cell. Comp. Physiol.,* 66 (Suppl.), 125, 1965.
55. **Stohs, S. J., Zull, J. E., and DeLuca, H. F.,** Vitamin D stimulation of [³H]orotic acid incorporation into ribonucleic acid of rat intestinal mucosa, *Biochemistry,* 6, 1304, 1967.

56. **Salaman, D. F., Betteridge, S., and Korner, A.,** Early effects of growth hormone on nucleolar and nucleoplasmic RNA synthesis and RNA polymerase activity in normal rat liver, *Biochim. Biophys. Acta,* 272, 382, 1972.

57. **Hadjiolov, A. A.,** Studies on the turnover and messenger activity of rat liver ribonucleic acids, *Biochim. Biophys. Acta,* 119, 547, 1966.

58. **Burdon, R. H.,** Ribonucleic acid maturation in animal cells, *Prog. Nucleic Acid Res. Mol. Biol,* 11, 33, 1971.

59. **Abelson, H. T., Johnson, L. F., Penman, S., and Green, H.,** Changes in RNA in relation to growth of the fibroblast. II. The lifetime of mRNA, rRNA and tRNA in resting and growing cells, *Cell,* 1, 161, 1974.

60. **Gorski, J.,** Early estrogen effects on the activity of uterine ribonucleic acid polymerase, *J. Biol. Chem.,* 239, 889, 1964.

61. **Hamilton, T. H., Widnell, C. C., and Tata, J. R.,** Sequential stimulation by oestrogen of nuclear RNA synthesis and DNA-dependent RNA polymerase in rat uterus, *Biochim. Biophys. Acta,* 108, 168, 1965.

62. **Widnell, C. C. and Tata, J. R.,** Studies on the stimulation by ammonium sulphate of the DNA-dependent RNA polymerase of isolated rat-liver nuclei, *Biochim. Biophys. Acta,* 123, 478, 1966.

63. **Maul, G. G. and Hamilton, T. H.,** The intranuclear localization of two DNA-dependent RNA polymerase activities, *Proc. Natl. Acad. Sci. U.S.A.,* 57, 1371, 1967.

64. **Hamilton, T. H., Widnell, C. C., and Tata, J. R.,** Synthesis of ribonucleic acid during early estrogen action, *J. Biol. Chem.,* 243, 408, 1968.

65. **Glasser, S. R., Chytil, F., and Spelsberg, T. C.,** Early effects of oestradiol-17β on the chromatin and activity of the deoxyribonucleic acid-dependent ribonucleic acid polymerases (I and II) of the rat uterus, *Biochem. J.,* 130, 947, 1972.

66. **Borthwick, N. M. and Smellie, R. M. S.,** The effects of oestradiol-17β on the ribonucleic acid polymerases of immature rabbit uterus, *Biochem. J.,* 147, 91, 1975.

67. **Wray, W.,** Parallel isolation procedures for metaphase chromosomes, mitotic apparatus, and nuclei, in *Methods in Enzymology,* Vol. 40, O'Malley, B. W. and Hardman, J. G., Eds., Academic Press, New York, 1975, 75.

68. **Hardin, J. W., Clark, J. H., Glasser, S. R., and Peck, E. J., Jr.,** RNA polymerase activity and uterine growth: differential stimulation by estradiol, estriol, and nafoxidine, *Biochemistry,* 15, 1370, 1976.

69. **Weil, P. A., Sidikaro, J., Stancel, G. M., and Blatti, S. P.,** Hormonal control of transcription in the rat uterus, *J. Biol. Chem.,* 252, 1092, 1977.

70. **Bouton, M.-M., Courvalin, J.-C., and Baulieu, E.-E.,** Effect of estradiol on rat uterus DNA-dependent RNA polymerases, *J. Biol. Chem.,* 252, 4607, 1977.

71. **Webster, R. A. and Hamilton, T. H.,** Comparative effects of estradiol-17β and estriol on uterine RNA polymerases I, II, and III in vivo, *Biochem. Biophys. Res. Commun.,* 69, 737, 1976.

72. **McGuire, W. L. and O'Malley, B. W.,** Ribonucleic acid polymerase activity of the chick oviduct during steroid-induced synthesis of a specific protein, *Biochim. Biophys. Acta,* 157, 187, 1968.

73. **O'Malley, B. W., McGuire, W. L., Kohler, P. O., and Korenman, S. G.,** Studies on the mechanism of steroid hormone regulation of synthesis of specific proteins, *Recent Prog. Horm. Res.,* 25, 105, 1969.

74. **Cox, R. F., Haines, M. E., and Carey, N. H.,** Modification of the template capacity of chick oviduct chromatin for form B RNA polymerase by estradiol, *Eur. J. Biochem.,* 32, 513, 1973.

75. **Cox, R. F.,** Quantitation of elongating form A and B RNA polymerases in chick oviduct nuclei and effects of estradiol, *Cell,* 7, 455, 1976.

76. **Spelsberg, T. C. and Cox, R. F.,** Effects of estrogen and progesterone on transcription, chromatin and ovalbumin gene expression in the chick oviduct, *Biochim. Biophys. Acta,* 435, 376, 1976.

77. **Bieri-Bonniot, F. and Dierks-Ventling, C.,** Multiple forms of DNA-dependent RNA polymerase I from immature chick liver, *Eur. J. Biochem.,* 73, 507, 1977.

78. **Jacob, S. T., Sajdel, E. M., and Munro, H. N.,** Regulation of nucleolar RNA metabolism by hydrocortisone, *Eur. J. Biochem.,* 7, 449, 1969.

79. **Schmidt, W. and Sekeris, C. E.,** Sequential stimulation of extranucleolar and nucleolar RNA synthesis in rat liver by cortisol, *FEBS Lett.,* 26, 109, 1972.

80. **Yu, F.-L. and Feigelson, P.,** Cortisone stimulation of nucleolar RNA polymerase activity, *Proc. Natl. Acad. Sci. U.S.A.,* 68, 2177, 1971.

81. **Mainwaring, W. I. P., Mangan, F. R., and Peterken, B. M.,** Studies on the solubilized ribonucleic acid polymerase from rat ventral prostate gland, *Biochem. J.,* 123, 619, 1971.

82. **Mainwaring, W. I. P. and Jones, D. M.,** Influence of receptor complexes on the properties of prostate chromatin, including its transcription by RNA polymerase, *J. Steroid Biochem.,* 6, 475, 1975.

83. **Zerwekh, J. E., Haussler, M. R., and Lindell, T. J.**, Rapid enhancement of chick intestinal DNA-dependent RNA polymerase II activity by 1α,25-dihydroxyvitamin D₃ in vivo, *Proc. Natl. Acad. Sci. U.S.A.*, 71, 2377, 1974.

84. **Borthwick, N. M. and Bell, P. A.**, Early glucocorticoid-dependent stimulation of RNA polymerase B in rat thymus cells, *FEBS Lett.*, 60, 396, 1975.

85. **Bell, P. A. and Borthwick, N. M.**, Glucocorticoid effects on DNA-dependent RNA polymerase activity in rat thymus cells, *J. Steroid Biochem.*, 7, 1174, 1976.

86. **Widnell, C. C. and Tata, J. R.**, Additive effects of thyroid hormone, growth hormone, and testosterone on deoxyribonucleic acid-dependent ribonucleic acid polymerase in rat-liver nuclei, *Biochem. J.*, 98, 621, 1966.

87. **Tata, J. R. and Widnell, C. C.**, Ribonucleic acid synthesis during the early action of thyroid hormones, *Biochem. J.*, 98, 604, 1966.

88. **Jothy, S., Bilodeau, J. L., Champsaur, H., and Simpkins, H.**, The early enhancement of rat liver deoxyribonucleic acid-dependent ribonucleic acid polymerase II activity by tri-iodothyronine, *Biochem. J.*, 150, 133, 1975.

89. **Turkington, R. W. and Riddle, M.**, Hormone-dependent phosphorylation of nuclear proteins during mammary gland differentiation in vitro, *J. Biol. Chem.*, 244, 6040, 1969.

90. **Cox, R. F.**, Transcription of high-molecular-weight RNA from hen-oviduct chromatin by bacterial and endogenous form-B RNA polymerases, *Eur. J. Biochem.*, 39, 49, 1973.

91. **Jacobson, A., Firtel, R. A., and Lodish, H. F.**, Synthesis of messenger and ribosomal RNA precursors in isolatd nuclei of the cellular slime mold *Dictyostelium discoideum*, *J. Mol. Biol.*, 82, 213, 1974.

92. **Marzluff, W. F., Jr. and Huang, R. C. C.**, Chromatin directed transcription of 5S and tRNA genes, *Proc. Natl. Acad. Sci. U.S.A.*, 72, 1082, 1975.

93. **Ferencz, A. and Seifart, K. H.**, Comparative effect of heparin on RNA synthesis of isolated rat-liver nucleoli and purified RNA polymerase A, *Eur. J. Biochem.*, 53, 605, 1975.

94. **Udvardy, A. and Seifart, K. H.**, Transcription of specific genes in isolated nuclei from HeLa cells in vitro, *Eur. J. Biochem.*, 62, 353, 1976.

95. **Barry, J. and Gorski, J.**, Uterine ribonucleic acid polymerase. Effect of estrogen on nucleotide incorporation into 3′ chain termini, *Biochemistry*, 10, 2384, 1971.

96. **Furhman, S. A. and Gill, G. N.**, Adrenocorticotropic hormone stimulation of adrenal RNA polymerase I and III activities. Nucleotide incorporation into internal positions and 3′ chain termini, *Biochemistry*, 14, 2925, 1975.

97. **Roeder, R. G. and Rutter, W. J.**, Specific nucleolar and nucleoplasmic RNA polymerases, *Proc. Natl. Acad. Sci. U.S.A.*, 65, 675, 1970.

98. **Courvalin, J.-C., Bouton, M.-M., and Baulieu, E.-E.**, Effect of estradiol on rat uterus DNA-dependent RNA polymerases, *J. Biol. Chem.*, 251, 4843, 1976.

99. **Cochet-Meilhac, M. and Chambon, P.**, Animal DNA-dependent RNA polymerases. II. Mechanism of the inhibition of RNA polymerases by amatoxins, *Biochim. Biophys. Acta*, 353, 160, 1974.

100. **Bertrand, K., Korn, L., Lee, F., Platt, T., Squires, C. L., Squires, C., and Yanofsky, C.**, New features of the regulation of the tryptophan operon, *Science*, 189, 22, 1975.

101. **Nicolette, J. A. and Babler, M.**, The role of protein in the estrogen-stimulated in vitro RNA synthesis of isolated rat uterine nucleoli, *Arch. Biochem. Biophys.*, 163, 263, 1974.

102. **Mauck, J. C. and Green, H.**, Regulation of RNA synthesis in fibroblasts during transition from resting to growing state, *Proc. Natl. Acad. Sci. U.S.A.*, 70, 2819, 1973.

103. **Yu, F.-L.**, Ribohomopolymer formation as a source of error in the radioactive precursor incorporation studies of nuclear DNA-dependent RNA synthesis, *Life Sci.*, 18, 1171, 1976.

104. **Biswas, D. K., Martin, T. F. J., and Tashjian, A. H., Jr.**, Extended RNA synthesis in isolated nuclei from rat pituitary tumor cells, *Biochemistry*, 15, 3270, 1976.

105. **Sajdel, E. M. and Jacob, S. T.**, Mechanism of early effect of hydrocortisone on the transcriptional process; stimulation of the activities of purified rat liver nucleolar RNA polymerases, *Biochem. Biophys. Res. Commun.*, 45, 707, 1971.

106. **van den Berg, J. A., Kooistra, T., Geert, A. B., and Gruber, M.**, Effect of estradiol on the RNA content and the activity of nucleolar RNA polymerase from rooster liver, *Biochem. Biophys. Res. Commun.*, 61, 367, 1974.

107. **Guilfoyle, T. J., Lin, C. Y., Chen, Y. M., Nagao, R. T., and Key, J. L.**, Enhancement of soybean RNA polymerase I by auxin, *Proc. Natl. Acad. Sci. U.S.A.*, 72, 69, 1975.

108. **Smuckler, E. A. and Tata, J. R.**, Changes in hepatic nuclear DNA-dependent RNA polymerase caused by growth hormone and triiodothyronine, *Nature (London)*, 234, 37, 1971.

109. **Jaehning, J. A., Stewart, C. C., and Roeder, R. G.**, DNA-dependent RNA polymerase levels during the response of human peripheral lymphocytes to phytohemagglutinin, *Cell*, 4, 51, 1975.

110. **Shields, D. and Tata, J. R.**, Variable stabilities and recoveries of rat-liver RNA polymerases A and B according to growth status of the tissue, *Eur. J. Biochem.*, 64, 471, 1976.

111. **Schmid, W. and Sekeris, C. E.,** Nucleolar RNA synthesis in the liver of partially hepatectomized and cortisol-treated rats, *Biochim. Biophys. Acta*, 402, 244, 1975.

112. **Weckler, C. and Gschwendt, M.,** The effect of estradiol on the activity of the nucleolar and nucleoplasmic RNA polymerases from chicken liver, *FEBS Lett.*, 65, 220, 1976.

113. **Benecke, B. J., Ferencz, A., and Seifart, K. H.,** Resistance of hepatic RNA polymerases to compounds effecting RNA and protein synthesis in vivo, *FEBS Lett.*, 31, 53, 1973.

114. **Butterworth, P. H. W., Flint, S. J., and Chesterton, C. J.,** Template integrity and the activity of eukaryotic deoxyribonucleic acid-dependent ribonucleic acid polymerase in vitro, *Biochem. Soc. Trans.*, 1, 650, 1973.

115. **Fuhrman, S. A. and Gill, G. N.,** Adrenocorticotropic hormone regulation of adrenal RNA polymerases. Stimulation of nuclear RNA polymerase III, *Biochemistry*, 15, 5520, 1976.

116. **Mauck, J. C.,** Solubilized DNA-dependent RNA polymerase activities in resting and growing fibroblasts, *Biochemistry*, 16, 793, 1977.

117. **Kellas, B. L., Austoker, J. L., Beebee, J. C., and Butterworth, P. H. W.,** Forms A1 and A11 DNA-dependent RNA polymerases as components of two defined pools of polymerase activity in mammalian cells, *Eur. J. Biochem.*, 72, 583, 1977.

118. **Ahmed, K. and Ishida, H.,** Effect of testosterone on nuclear phosphoproteins of rat ventral prostate, *Mol. Pharmacol.*, 7, 323, 1971.

119. **Keller, R. K., Chandra, T., Schrader, W. T., and O'Malley, B. W.,** Protein kinases of the chick oviduct: a study of the cytoplasmic and nuclear enzymes, *Biochemistry*, 15, 1958, 1976.

120. **Dahmus, M. E.,** Stimulation of ascites tumor RNA polymerase II by protein kinase, *Biochemistry*, 15, 1821, 1976.

121. **Hirsch, J. and Martelo, O. J.,** Phosphorylation of rat liver ribonucleic acid polymerase I by nuclear protein kinases, *J. Biol. Chem.*, 251, 5408, 1976.

122. **Jungmann, R. A., Hiestand, P. C., and Schweppe, J. S.,** Adenosine 3':5'-monophosphate-dependent protein kinase and the stimulation of ovarian nuclear ribonucleic acid polymerase activities, *J. Biol. Chem.*, 249, 5444, 1974.

123. **Jungmann, R. A., Hiestand, P. C., and Schweppe, J. S.,** Mechanism of action of gonadotropin, *Endocrinology*, 94, 168, 1974.

124. **Arnaud, M., Beziat, Y., Borgna, J. L., Guilleux, J. C., and Mousseron-Canet, M.,** Le récepteur de l'oestradiol, l'amp cyclique et la RNA polymérase nucléolaire dans l'utérus de génisse. Stimulation de la biosynthèse de RNA in vitro, *Biochim. Biophys. Acta*, 254, 241, 1971.

125. **Biswas, B. B., Ganguly, A., and Das, A.,** Eukaryotic RNA polymerases and the factors that control them, *Prog. Nucleic Acid Res. Mol. Biol.*, 15, 145, 1975.

126. **Schwartz, L. B., Sklar, V. E. F., Jaehning, J. A., Weinmann, R., and Roeder, R. G.,** Isolation and partial characterization of the multiple forms of deoxyribonucleic acid-dependent ribonucleic acid polymerase in the mouse myeloma, MOPC 315, *J. Biol. Chem.*, 249, 5889, 1974.

127. **Roeder, R. G.,** Multiple forms of deoxyribonucleic acid-dependent ribonucleic acid polymerase in *Xenopus laevis, J. Biol. Chem.*, 249, 1974.

128. **Grummt, F., Paul, D., and Grummt, I.,** Regulation of ATP pools, rRNA and DNA synthesis in 3T3 cells in response to serum or hypoxanthine, *Eur. J. Biochem.*, 76, 7, 1977.

129. **Gross, K. J. and Pogo, A. O.,** The effect of amino acid and glucose starvation and cycloheximide on yeast deoxyribonucleic acid-dependent ribonucleic acid polymerases, *J. Biol. Chem.*, 249, 568, 1974.

130. **Dahmus, M. E. and Bonner, J.,** Increased template activity of liver chromatin, a result of hydrocortisone administration, *Proc. Natl. Acad. Sci. U.S.A.*, 54, 1370, 1965.

131. **Barker, K. L. and Warren, J. C.,** Template capacity of uterine chromatin: control by estradiol, *Proc. Natl. Acad. Sci. U.S.A.*, 56, 1298, 1966.

132. **Teng, C. S. and Hamilton, T. H.,** The role of chromatin in estrogen action in the uterus, *Proc. Natl. Acad. Sci. U.S.A.*, 60, 1410, 1968.

133. **Spelsberg, T. C., Steggles, A. W., and O'Malley, B. W.,** Changes in chromatin composition and hormone binding during chick oviduct development, *Biochim. Biophys. Acta*, 254, 129, 1971.

134. **Hallic, R. B. and DeLuca, H. F.,** Vitamin D₃-stimulated template activity of chromatin from rat intestine, *Proc. Natl. Acad. Sci. U.S.A.*, 63, 528, 1969.

135. **Zerwekh, J. E., Lindell, T. J., and Haussler, M. R.,** Increased intestinal chromatin template activity. Influences of 1α,25-dihydroxyvitamin D₃ and hormone-receptor complexes, *J. Biol. Chem.*, 251, 2388, 1976.

136. **Jungmann, R. A. and Schweppe, J. S.,** Control of ovarian nuclear ribonucleic acid polymerase activity and chromatin template capacity, *J. Biol. Chem.*, 247, 5543, 1972.

137. **Tsai, M.-J., Schwartz, R. J., Tsai, S. Y., and O'Malley, B. W.,** Effects of estrogen on gene expression in the chick oviduct. IV. Initiation of RNA synthesis on DNA and chromatin, *J. Bio Chem.*, 250, 5165, 1975.

138. **Schwartz, R. J., Tsai, M.-J., Tsai, S. Y., and O'Malley, B. W.,** Effect of estrogen on gene expression in the chick oviduct. V. Changes in the number of RNA polymerase binding and initiation sites in chromatin, *J. Biol. Chem.,* 250, 5175, 1975.

139. **Tsai, M.-J., Towle, H. C., Harris, S. E., and O'Malley, B. W.,** Effect of estrogen on gene expression in chick oviduct. Comparative aspects of RNA chain initiation in chromatin using homologous vs. *Escherichia coli* RNA polymerase, *J. Biol. Chem.,* 251, 1960, 1976.

140. **Hirose, M., Tsai, M.-J., and O'Malley, B. W.,** Effect of estrogen on gene expression in the chick oviduct, *J. Biol. Chem.,* 251, 1137, 1976.

141. **Tsai, M.-J., Tsai, S. Y., Towle, H. C., and O'Malley, B. W.,** Effect of estrogen on gene expression in the chick oviduct, *J. Biol. Chem.,* 251, 5565, 1976.

142. **Tsai, S. Y., Tsai, M.-J., Schwartz, R., Kalimi, M., Clark, J. H., and O'Malley, B. W.,** Effects of estrogen on gene expression in chick oviduct: nuclear receptor levels and initiation of transcription, *Proc. Natl. Acad. Sci. U.S.A.,* 72, 4228, 1975.

143. **Schwartz, R. J., Kuhn, R. W., Buller, R. E., Schrader, W. T., and O'Malley, B. W.,** In vitro effect of purified hormone-receptor complexes on the initiation of RNA synthesis in chromatin, *J. Biol. Chem.,* 251, 5166, 1976.

144. **Johnson, E. M., Karn, J., and Allfrey, V. G.,** Effect of concanavalin A on the phosphorylation and distribution of non-histone chromatin proteins, *J. Biol. Chem.,* 249, 4990, 1974.

145. **Hemminki, K. and Bolund, L.,** Synthesis of oviduct nuclear and chromatin proteins during steroid-induced differentiation, *Cell Differ.,* 3, 347, 1975.

146. **Dierks-Ventling, C. and Jost, J. P.,** Effect of 17β-estradiol on the synthesis of non-histone nuclear proteins in chick liver, *Eur. J. Biochem.,* 50, 33, 1974.

147. **Barker, K. L.,** Estrogen-induced synthesis of histones and a specific nonhistone protein in the uterus, *Biochemistry,* 10, 284, 1971.

148. **Cohen, M. E. and Hamilton, T. H.,** Effect of estradiol-17β on the synthesis of specific uterine non-histone chromosomal proteins, *Proc. Natl. Acad. Sci. U.S.A.,* 72, 4346, 1975

149. **Shelton, K. R. and Allfrey, V. G.,** Selective synthesis of a nuclear acidic protein in liver cells stimulated by cortisol, *Nature (London),* 228, 132, 1970.

150. **Nyberg, L. M. and Wang, T. Y.,** The role of the androgen-binding nonhistone proteins in the transcription of prostatic chromatin, *J. Steroid Biochem.,* 7, 267, 1976.

151. **Kleinsmith, L. J.,** Phosphorylation of non-histone proteins in the regulation of chromosome structure and function, *J. Cell Physiol.,* 85, 459, 1975.

152. **Shea, M. and Kleinsmith, L. J.,** Template-specific stimulation of RNA synthesis by phosphorylated non-histone chromatin proteins, *Biochem. Biophys. Res. Commun.,* 50, 473, 1973.

153. **Kostraba, N. C., Montagna, R. A. and Wang, T. Y.,** Stimulation of deoxyribonucleic acid-templated ribonucleic acid synthesis by a specific deoxyribonucleic acid-binding phosphoprotein fraction, *J. Biol. Chem.,* 250, 1548, 1975.

154. **Kleinsmith, L. J., Stein, J., and Stein, G.,** Dephosphorylation of nonhistone proteins specifically alters the pattern of gene transcription in reconstituted chromatin, *Proc. Natl. Acad. Sci. U.S.A.,* 73, 1174, 1976.

155. **Cohen, M. E. and Kleinsmith, L. J.,** Stimulation of uterine nonhistone protein phosphorylation and nuclear protein kinase activity by estradiol-17β, *Biochim. Biophys. Acta,* 435, 159, 1976.

156. **Libby, P. R.,** Early effects of oestradiol-17β on histone acetylation in rat uterus, *Biochem. J.,* 130, 663, 1972.

157. **Libby, P. R.,** Early effects of aldosterone on histone acetylation in rat kidney, *Biochem. J.,* 134, 907, 1973.

158. **McCarty, K. S. and McCarty, K. S., Jr.,** Hormonal induction of postsynthetic modifications of chromosomal proteins in mammary neoplasia, in *Control Mechanisms in Cancer,* Criss, W. E., Ono, T., and Sabine, J. R., Eds., Raven Press, New York, 1976, 37.

159. **Marushige, K.,** Activation of chromatin by acetylation of histone side chains, *Proc. Natl. Acad. Sci. U.S.A.,* 73, 3937, 1976.

160. **Doenecke, D., Beato, M., Congote, L. F., and Sekeris, C. E.,** Effect of cortisol on the thiol content of rat liver nuclear proteins, *Biochem. J.,* 126, 1171, 1972.

161. **Szego, C. M., Seeler, B. J., and Smith, R. E.,** Lysosomal cathepsin B1: partial characterization in rat preputial gland and recompartmentation in response to estradiol-17β, *Eur. J. Biochem.,* 69, 463, 1976.

162. **Katz, J., Krone, P., Troll, W., Blaustein, A., and Levitz, M.,** Effect of proteases on in vitro RNA synthesis by rat uteri in different hormonal states, *Endocrinology,* 90, 1147, 1972.

163. **Szego, C. M., Steadman, R. A., and Seeler, B. J.,** Intranuclear concentration of lysosomal hydrolases in steroid target cells, *Eur. J. Biochem.,* 46, 377, 1974.

164. **Dati, F. A. and Maurer, H. R.,** Estradiol-mediated template activity of mouse and rat uterine chromatin: an unsolved problem, *Biochim. Biophys. Acta,* 246, 589, 1971.

165. **Cox, R. F.**, Chromatin-associated ribonucleases are activated by estradiol in chick oviduct, *J. Steroid Biochem.*, 9, 697, 1978.

166. **Lukacs, I. and Sekeris, C. E.**, On the mechanism of hormone action. IX. Stimulation of RNA polymerase activity of rat liver nuclei by cortisol in vitro, *Biochim. Biophys. Acta*, 134, 85, 1967.

167. **Stackhouse, H. L., Chetsanga, C. J., and Tan, C. H.**, The effect of cortisol on genetic transcription in rat-liver chromatin, *Biochim. Biophys. Acta*, 155, 159, 1968.

168. **Beato, M., Seifart, K. H., and Sekeris, C. E.**, The effect of cortisol on the binding of actinomycin D to and on the template activity of isolated rat liver chromatin, *Arch. Biochem. Biophys.*, 138, 272, 1970.

169. **Raynaud-Jammet, C. and Baulieu, E.-E.**, Action de l'estradiol in vitro: augmentation de la biosynthèse d'acide ribonucléique dan les noyaux utérins, *C. R. Acad. Sci. Ser. D*, 268, 3211, 1969.

170. **Mohla, S., DeSombre, E. R., and Jensen, E. V.**, Tissue-specific stimulation of RNA synthesis by transformed estradiol-receptor complex, *Biochem. Biophys. Res. Commun.*, 46, 661, 1972.

171. **Jensen, E. V., Mohla, S., Gorell, T. A., and DeSombre, E. R.**, The role of estrophilin in estrogen action, *Vitam. Horm. (NY).*, 32, 89, 1974.

172. **DeSombre, E. R., Mohla, S., and Jensen, E. V.**, Receptor transformation, the key to estrogen action, *J. Steroid Biochem.*, 6, 469, 1975.

173. **Davies, P. and Griffiths, K.**, Stimulation in vitro of prostatic ribonucleic acid polymerase by 5α-dihydrotestosterone-receptor complexes, *Biochem. Biophys. Res. Commun.*, 53, 373, 1973.

174. **Davies, P. and Griffiths, K.**, Stimulation of ribonucleic acid polymerase activity in vitro by prostatic steroid-protein receptor complexes, *Biochem. J.*, 136, 611, 1973.

175. **Davies, P. and Griffiths, K.**, Further studies on the stimulation of prostatic ribonucleic acid polymerase by 5α-dihydrotestosterone-receptor complexes, *J. Endocrinol.*, 62, 385, 1974.

176. **Davies, P. and Griffiths, K.**, Effects of α-amanitin on the stimulation of prostatic ribonucleic acid polymerase by prostatic steroid-protein receptor complexes, *Biochem. J.*, 140, 565, 1974.

177. **Horgen, P. A.**, Cytosol-hormone stimulation of transcription in the aquatic fungus, *Achlya ambisexualis*, *Biochem. Biophys. Res. Commun.*, 75, 1022, 977.

178. **Chomczynski, P. and Topper, Y. J.**, A direct effect of prolactin and placental lactogen on mammary epithelial nuclei, *Biochem. Biophys. Res. Commun.*, 60, 56, 1974.

179. **Kuhn, R. W., Schrader, W. T., Smith, R. G., and O'Malley, B. W.**, Progesterone binding components of chick oviduct. X. Purification by affinity chromatography, *J. Biol. Chem.*, 250, 4220, 1975.

180. **O'Malley, B. W., Schwartz, R. J., and Schrader, W. T.**, A review of regulation of gene expression by steroid hormone receptors, *J. Steroid Biochem.*, 7, 1151, 1976.

181. **Buller, R. E., Schwartz, R. J., Schrader, W. T., and O'Malley, B. W.**, Progesterone-binding components of chick oviduct. In vitro effect of receptor subunits on gene transcription, *J. Biol. Chem.*, 251, 5178, 1976.

182. **Dierks-Ventling, C. and Bieri-Bonniot, F.**, Stimulation of RNA-polymerase I and II activities by 17β-estradiol receptor on chick liver chromatin, *Nucleic Acids Res.*, 4, 381, 1977.

183. **Buller, R. E., Schwartz, R. J., and O'Malley, B. W.**, Steroid hormone receptor fraction stimulation of RNA synthesis: a caution, *Biochem. Biophys. Res. Commun.*, 69, 106, 1976.

184. **Leroy, F., Preumont, A. M., Galand, P., and Brachet, J.**, Increased chromatin acid lability and actinomycin-D binding in endometrial cells under the action of sex steroids, *J. Endocrinol.*, 52, 525, 1972.

185. **Leclercq, G., Hulin, N., and Heuson, J. C.**, Interaction of activated estradiol-receptor complex and chromatin in isolated uterine nuclei, *Eur. J. Cancer*, 9, 681, 1973.

186. **Palmiter, R. D., Mulvihill, E. R., McNight, G. S., and Senear, A. W.**, Regulation of gene expression in the chick oviduct by steroid hormones, *Cold Spring Harbor Symp. Quant. Biol.*, 42, 639, 1978.

187. **Weintraub, H. and Groudine, M.**, Chromosomal subunits in active genes have an altered conformation, *Science*, 193, 848, 1976.

188. **Monahan, J. J., Harris, S. E., and O'Malley, B. W.**, Effect of estrogen on the sequence and population complexity of chick oviduct poly(A)-containing RNA, *J. Biol. Chem.*, 251, 3738, 1976.

189. **Ringold, G. M., Yamamoto, K. R., Bishop, J. M., and Varmus, H. E.**, Glucocorticoid-stimulated accumulation of mouse mammary tumor virus RNA: increased rate of synthesis of viral RNA, *Proc. Natl. Acad. Sci. U.S.A.*, 74, 2879, 1977.

190. **Bradbury, E. M., Inglis, R. J., and Matthews, H. R.**, Molecular basis of control of mitotic cell division in eukaryotes, *Nature (London)*, 249, 553, 1974.

191. **Kaye, A. M., Sheratzk, D., and Lindner, H. R.**, Kinetics of DNA synthesis in immature rat uterus: age dependence and estradiol stimulation, *Biochim. Biophys. Acta*, 261, 475, 1972.

192. **Lippman, M., Bolan, G., Monaco, M., Pinkus, L., and Engel, L.**, Model systems for the study of estrogen action in tissue culture, *J. Steroid Biochem.*, 7, 1045, 1976.

193. **Knox, W. E., Auerbach, V. H., and Lin, E. C. C.**, Enzymatic and metabolic adaptations in animals, *Physiol. Rev.*, 36, 164, 1956.

194. **Oka, T. and Schimke, R. T.,** Effects of estrogen and progesterone on tubular gland cell function, *J. Cell Biol.*, 43, 123, 1969.

195. **Palmiter, R. D.,** Regulation of protein synthesis in chick oviduct. I. Independent regulation of ovalbumin, conalbumin, ovomucoid, and lysozyme induction, *J. Biol. Chem.*, 247, 6450, 1972.

196. **Chan, L., Means, A. R., and O'Malley, B. W.,** Rates of induction of specific translatable messenger RNAs for ovalbumin and avidin by steroid hormones, *Proc. Natl. Acad. Sci. U.S.A.*, 70, 1870, 1973.

197. **Palmiter, R. D.,** Rate of ovalbumin messenger ribonucleic acid synthesis in the oviduct of estrogen-primed chicks, *J. Biol. Chem.*, 248, 8260, 1973.

198. **Cox, R. F., Haines, M. E., and Emtage, J. S.,** Quantitation of ovalbumin mRNA in hen and chick oviduct by hybridization to complementary DNA, *Eur. J. Biochem.*, 49, 225, 1974.

199. **Harris, S. E., Rosen, J. M., Means, A. R., and O'Malley, B. W.,** Use of a specific probe for ovalbumin messenger RNA to quantitate estrogen-induced gene transcripts, *Biochemistry*, 14, 2072, 1975.

200. **McKnight, G. S., Pennequin, P., and Schimke, R. T.,** Induction of ovalbumin mRNA sequences by estrogen and progesterone in chick oviduct as measured by hybridization to complementary DNA, *J. Biol. Chem.*, 250, 8105, 1975.

201. **Shapiro, D. J., Baker, H. J., and Stitt, D. T.,** In vitro translation and estradiol-17β induction of *Xenopus laevis* vitellogenin messenger RNA, *J. Biol. Chem.*, 251, 3105, 1976.

202. **Schutz, G., Killewich, L., Chen, G., and Feigelson, P.,** Control of the mRNA for hepatic tryptophan oxygenase during hormonal and substrate induction, *Proc. Natl. Acad. Sci. U.S.A.*, 72, 1017, 1975.

203. **Roewekamp, W. G., Hofer, E., and Sekeris, C. E.,** Translation of mRNA from rat-liver polysomes into tyrosine aminotransferase and tryptophan oxygenase in a protein-synthesizing system from wheat germ, *Eur. J. Biochem.*, 70, 259, 204.

204. **Shuster, R. C., Houdebine, L. M., and Gaye, P.,** Studies on the synthesis of casein messenger RNA during pregnancy in the rabbit, *Eur. J. Biochem.*, 71, 193, 1976.

205. **Rosen, J. M., Woo, S. L. C., and Comstock, J. P.,** Regulation of casein messenger RNA during the development of the rat mammary gland, *Biochemistry*, 14, 2895, 1975.

206. **Kurtz, D. T., Sippel, A. E., and Feigelson, P.,** Effect of thyroid hormones on the level of the hepatic mRNA for α_{2u} globulin, *Biochemistry*, 15, 1031, 1976.

207. **Kurtz, D. T., Sippel, A. E., Ansah-Yiadom, R., and Feigelson, P.,** Effects of sex hormones on the level of the messenger RNA for the rat hepatic protein α_{2u} globulin, *J. Biol. Chem.*, 251, 3594, 1976.

208. **Martial, J. A., Baxter, J. W., Goodman, H. M., and Seeburg, P. H.,** Regulation of growth hormone messenger RNA by thyroid and glucocorticoid hormones, *Proc. Natl. Acad Sci. U.S.A.*, 74, 1816, 1977.

209. **Katzenellenbogen, B. and Gorski, J.,** Estrogen action in vitro. Induction of the synthesis of a specific uterine protein, *J. Biol. Chem.*, 247, 1299, 1972.

210. **Iacobelli, S., King, R. J. B., and Vokaer, A.,** Antibody to estrogen-induced protein (IP) and quantification of the protein in rat uterus by a radioimmunoassay, *Biochem. Biophys. Res. Commun.*, 76, 1230, 1977.

211. **Mainwaring, W. I. P., Wilce, P. A., and Smith, A. E.,** Studies on the form and synthesis of messenger ribonucleic acid in the rat ventral prostate gland, including its tissue-specific stimulation by androgens, *Biochem. J.*, 137, 513, 1974.

212. **Tomkins, G. M., Martin, D. W., Jr., Stellwagen, R. H., Baxter, J. D., Mamont, P., and Levinson, B. B.,** Regulation of specific protein synthesis in eucaryotic cells, *Cold Spring Harbor Symp. Quant. Biol.*, 35, 635, 1970.

213. **Ashburner, M., Chihara, C., Meltzer, P., and Richards, G.,** Temporal control of puffing activity in polytene chromosomes, *Cold Spring Harbor Symp. Quant. Biol.*, 38, 655, 1973.

214. **Clark, J. H., Anderson, J. N., and Peck, E. J.,** Nuclear receptor-estrogen complexes of rat uteri, *Adv. Exp. Med. Biol.*, 36, 15, 1973.

215. **Rousseau, G. G., Baxter, J. D., Higgins, S. J., and Tomkins, G. M.,** Steroid-induced nuclear binding of glucocorticoid receptors in intact hepatoma cells, *J. Mol. Biol.*, 79, 539, 1973.

216. **Mulvihill, E. R. and Palmiter, R. D.,** Relationship of nuclear estrogen receptor levels to induction of ovalbumin and conalbumin mRNA in chick oviduct, *J. Biol. Chem.*, 252, 2060, 1977.

217. **Harris, S. E., Means, A. R., Mitchell, W. M., and O'Malley, B. W.** Synthesis of [³H] DNA complementary to ovalbumin messenger RNA: evidence for limited copies of the ovalbumin gene in chick oviduct, *Proc. Natl. Acad. Sci. U.S.A.*, 70, 3776, 1973.

218. **Rosen, J. M. and Barker, S. W.,** Quantitation of casein messenger ribonucleic acid sequences using a specific complementary DNA hybridization probe, *Biochemistry*, 15, 5272, 1976.

219. **Gilmour, R. S. and Paul, J.,** Tissue-specific transcription of the globin gene in isolated chromatin, *Proc. Natl. Acad. Sci. U.S.A.*, 70, 3440, 1973.

220. **Axel, R., Cedar, H., and Felsenfeld, G.,** Synthesis of globin ribonucleic acid from duck-reticulocyte chromatin in vitro, *Proc. Natl. Acad. Sci. U.S.A.*, 70, 2029, 1973.

221. **Barrett, T., Maryanka, D., Hamlyn, P. H., and Gould, H. J.,** Nonhistone proteins control gene expression in reconstituted chromatin, *Proc. Natl. Acad. Sci. U.S.A.*, 71, 5057, 1974.

222. **Tsai, S. Y., Harris, S. E., Tsai, M.-J., and O'Malley, B. W.,** Effects of estrogen on gene expression in chick oviduct. The role of chromatin proteins in regulating transcription of the ovalbumin gene, *J. Biol.Chem.*, 251, 4713, 1976.

223. **Tsai, S. Y., Tsai, M.-J., Harris, S. E., and O'Malley, B. W.,** Effects of estrogen on gene expression in the chick oviduct, *J. Biol. Chem.*, 251, 6475, 1976.

224. **Dale, R. M. K. and Ward, D. C.,** Mercurated polynucleotides: new probes for hybridization and selective polymer fractionation, *Biochemistry*, 14, 2458, 1975.

225. **Zasloff, M. and Felsenfeld, G.,** Analysis of in vitro transcription of duck reticulocyte chromatin using mercury-substituted ribonucleoside triphosphates, *Biochemistry*, 16, 5135, 1977.

226. **Shih, T. Y., Young, H. A., Parks, W. P., and Scolnick, E. M.,** In vitro transcription of Moloney leukemia virus genes in infected cell nuclei and chromatin elongation of chromatin associated ribonucleic acid by *Escherichia coli* ribonucleic acid polymerase, *Biochemistry*, 16, 1795, 1977.

227. **Pays, E.,** Double-stranded RNA in chromatin transcripts formed by exogenous RNA polymerase, *Proc. Natl. Acad. Sci. U.S.A.*, 73, 1121, 1976.

228. **Konkel, D. A. and Ingram, V. M.,** RNA aggregation during sulfhydryl-agarose chromatography of mercurated RNA, *Nucleic Acid Res.*, 4, 1979, 1977.

229. **Towle, H. C., Tsai, M.-J., Tsai, S. Y., and O'Malley, B. W.,** Effect of estrogen on gene expression in the chick oviduct. Preferential initiation and asymmetrical transcription of specific chromatin genes, *J. Biol. Chem.*, 252, 2396, 1977.

230. **Harris, S. E., Schwartz, R. J., Tsai, M.-J., and O'Malley, B. W.,** Effect of estrogen on gene expression in the chick oviduct. In vitro transcription of the ovalbumin gene in chromatin, *J. Biol. Chem.*, 251, 524, 1976.

231. **Parker, C. S. and Roeder, R. G.,** Selective and accurate transcription of the *Xenopus laevis* 5S RNA genes in isolated chromatin by purified RNA polymerase III, *Proc. Natl. Acad. Sci. U.S.A.*, 74, 44, 1977.

232. **Ballal, N. R., Choi, Y. C., Mouche, R., and Busch, H.,** Fidelity of synthesis of preribosomal RNA in isolated nucleoli and nucleolar chromatin, *Proc Natl. Acad. Sci. U.S.A.*, 74, 2446, 1977.

233. **Butterworth, P. H. W., Cox, R. F., and Chesterton, C. J.,** Transcription of mammalian chromatin by mammalian DNA-dependent RNA polymerases, *Eur. J. Biochem.*, 23, 229, 1971.

234. **Cedar, H.,** Transcription of DNA and chromatin with calf thymus RNA polymerase B in vitro, *J. Mol. Biol.*, 95, 257, 1975.

235. **Henner, D., Kelley, R. I., and Furth, J. J.,** Transcription of fractionated calf thymus chromatin by RNA polymerase of calf thymus and *Escherichia coli, Biochemistry*, 14, 4764, 1975.

236. **Mizuno, S., Tallman, N. A., and Cox, R. F.,** Estrogen withdrawal in chick oviduct: characterization of RNA synthesized in isolated nuclei using a mercurated precursor, *Biochim. Biophys. Acta*, 520, 184, 1978.

237. **Orkin, S. H. and Swerdlow, P. S.,** Globin RNA synthesis in vitro by isolated erythroleukemic cell nuclei: direct evidence for increased transcription during erythroid cell differentiation, *Proc. Natl. Acad. Sci. U.S.A.*, 74, 2475, 1977.

238. **Young, H. A., Shih, T. Y., Scolnick, E. M., and Parks, W. P.,** Steroid induction of mouse mammary tumor virus: effect upon synthesis and degradation of viral RNA, *J. Virol.*, 21, 139, 1977.

239. **Stavnezer, E. and Bishop, J. M.,** in press.

240. **Coffin, J. M., Parsons, J. T., Rymo, L., Haroz, R. K., and Weissmann, C.,** A new approach to the isolation of RNA-DNA hybrids and its application to the quantitative determination of labeled tumor virus RNA, *J. Mol. Biol.*, 86, 373, 1974.

241. **Scolnick, E. M., Young, H. A., and Parks, W. P.,** Biochemical and physiological mechanisms in glucocorticoid hormone induction of mouse mammary tumor virus, *Virology*, 60, 148, 1976.

242. **Ringold, G. M., Yamamoto, K. R., Tomkins, G. M., Bishop, J. M., and Varmus, H. E.,** Dexamethasone-mediated induction of mouse mammary tumor virus RNA: a system for studying glucocorticoid action, *Cell*, 6, 299, 1975.

243. **Yamamoto, K. R. and Ringold, G. M.,** Glucocorticoid regulation of mammary tumor virus gene expression, in *Hormone Receptors*, Vol. 1. *Steroid Hormones*, Academic Press, New York, 1977, in press.

244. **Gilboa, E. and Aviv, H.,** Preferential synthsis of viral late RNA by nuclei isolated from SV40 lytically infected cells, *Cell*, 7, 567, 1976.

245. **Venstrom, B. and Philipson, L.,** Fidelity of adenovirus RNA transcription in isolated HeLa cell nuclei, *J. Virol.*, 22, 290, 1977.

246. **Winicov, I. and Perry, R. P.,** Synthesis, methylation, and capping of nuclear RNA by a subcellular system, *Biochemistry*, 15, 5039, 1976.

247. **Yamamoto, K. R., Ivarie, R. D., Ring, J., Ringold, G. M., and Stallcup, M. R.,** Integrated mammary tumor virus genes: transcriptional regulation by glucocorticoids and specific effects on host gene expression, in *Biochemical Actions of Hormones*, Vol. 5, Litwack, G., Ed., Academic Press, New York, 1978, 373.

248. **Rymo, L., Parsons, J. T., Coffin, J. M., and Weissmann, C.,** In vitro synthesis of Rous sarcoma virus-specific RNA is catalyzed by a DNA-dependent RNA polymerase, *Proc. Natl. Acad. Sci. U.S.A.,* 71, 2782, 1974.

249. **Schutz, G., Nguyen-Huu, M. C., Gieseke, K., Hynes, N. E., Groner, B., Wurtz, T., and Sippel, A. E.,** Hormonal control of egg white protein messenger RNA synthesis in the chicken oviduct, *Cold Spring Harbor Symp. Quant. Biol.,* 42, 617, 1978.

250. **McReynolds, L. A., Catterall, J. F., and O'Malley, B. W.,** The ovalbumin gene: cloning of a complete ds-cDNA in a bacterial plasmid, *Gene,* 2, 217, 1977.

251. **Hynes, N. E., Groner, B., Sippel, A. E., Nguyen-Huu, M. C., and Schutz, G.,** mRNA complexity and egg white protein mRNA content in mature and hormone-withdrawn oviduct, *Cell,* 11, 923, 1977.

252. **Nguyen-Huu, M. C., Sippel, A. E., Hynes, N. E., Groner, B., and Schutz, G.,** Preferential transcription of the ovalbumin gene in isolated hen oviduct nuclei by RNA polymerase B, *Proc. Natl. Acad. Sci. U.S.A.,* 75, 686, 1978.

253. **Bellard, M., Gannon, F., and Chambon, P.,** Nucleosome structure. III. The structure and transcriptional activity of the chromatin containing the ovalbumin and globin genes in chick oviduct nuclei, *Cold Spring Harbor Symp. Quant. Biol.,* 42, 779, 1978.

254. **Bitter, G. A. and Roeder, R. G.,** Transcription of viral genes by RNA polymerase II in nuclei isolated from adenovirus 2 transformed cells, *Biochemistry,* 17, 2198, 1978.

255. **Ross, J., Aviv, H., Scolnick, E., and Leder, P.,** In vitro synthesis of DNA complementary to purified rabbit globin mRNA, *Proc. Natl. Acad. Sci. U.S.A.,* 69, 264, 1972.

256. **Bishop, J. O., Morton, J. G., Rosbash, M., and Richardson, M.,** Three abundance classes in HeLa cell messenger RNA, *Nature (London),* 250, 199, 1974.

257. **Quinlan, T. J., Beeler, G. W., Cox, R. F., Elder, P. K., Moses, H. L., and Getz, M. J.,** The concept of mRNA abundance classes: a critical reevaluation, *Nucleic Acids Res.,* 5, 1611, 1978.

258. **Williams, J. G. and Penman, S.,** The messenger RNA sequences in growing and resting mouse fibroblasts, *Cell,* 6, 197, 1975.

259. **Ivarie, R. D. and O'Farrell, P. H.,** The glucocorticoid domain: steroid-mediated changes in the rate of synthesis of rat hepatoma proteins, *Cell,* 13, 41, 1978.

260. **O'Malley, B. W. and McGuire, W. L.,** Studies on the mechanism of estrogen-mediated tissue differentiation: regulation of nuclear transcription and induction of new RNA species, *Proc. Natl. Acad. Sci. U.S.A.,* 60, 1527, 1968.

261. **Liarakos, C. D., Rosen, J. M., and O'Malley, B. W.,** Transcription of chick tritiated unique deoxyribonucleic acid as measured by hybridization in ribonucleic acid excess, *Biochemistry,* 12, 2809, 1973.

262. **Rosen, J. M. and O'Malley, B. W.,** Hormonal regulation of specific gene expression in the chick oviduct, in *Biochemical Action of Hormones,* Vol. 3, Litwack, G., Ed., Academic Press, New York, 1975, 271.

263. **Hahn, W. E., Church, R. B., Gorbman, A., and Wilmot, L.,** Estrone- and progesterone-induced synthesis of new RNA species in the chick oviduct, *Gen. Comp. Endocrinol.,* 10, 438, 1968.

264. **Perry, R. P.,** Processing of RNA, *Annu. Rev. Biochem.,* 45, 605, 1976.

265. **Molloy, G. and Puckett, L.,** The metabolism of heterogeneous nuclear RNA and the formation of cytoplasmic messenger RNA in animal cells, *Prog. Biophys. Mol. Biol.,* 31, 1, 1976.

266. **Luck, D. N. and Hamilton, T. H.,** Early estrogen action: stimulation of the metabolism of high molecular weight and ribosomal RNAs, *Proc. Natl. Acad. Sci. U.S.A.,* 69, 157, 1972.

267. **Knecht, D. A. and Luck, D. N.,** Synthesis and processing of ribosomal RNA by the uterus of the ovariectomised adult rat during early oestrogen action, *Nature (London),* 266, 563, 1977.

268. **van den Berg, J. A., Gruber, M., and Ab, G.,** Estradiol-induced enhancement of the processing of the 32S ribosomal precursor in rooster liver, *FEBS Lett.,* 63, 65, 1976.

269. **Shields, R.,** Fibroblast model for hormone effects, *Nature (London),* 258, 194, 1975.

270. **Johnson, L. F., Levis, R., Abelson, H. T., Green, H., and Penman, S.,** Alterations in the production and processing of mRNA and rRNA in resting and growing cells, *J. Cell Biol.,* 71, 933, 1976.

271. **Johnson, L. F., Williams, J. G., Abelson, H. T., Green, H., and Penman, S.,** Changes in RNA in relation to growth of the fibroblast. III. Posttranscriptional regulation of mRNA formation in resting and growing cells, *Cell,* 4, 69, 1975.

272. **Milo, G. E., Malarkey, W. B., Powell, J. E., Blakesley, J. R., and Yohn, D. S.,** Effects of steroid hormones in fetal bovine serum on plating and cloning of human cells in vitro, *In Vitro,* 12, 23, 1976.

273. **Lanclos, K. D. and Hamilton, T. H.,** Translation of hormone-induced messenger RNA in amphibian oocytes. I. Induction by estrogen of messenger RNA encoded for vittelogenic protein in the liver of the male African clawed toad *(Xenopus laevis), Proc. Natl. Acad. Sci. U.S.A.,* 72, 3934, 1975.

274. **Church, R. B. and McCarthy, B. J.,** Unstable nuclear RNA synthesis following estrogen stimulation, *Biochim. Biophys. Acta,* 199, 103, 1970.

275. **Schumm, D. E. and Webb, T. E.,** Differential effect of ATP on RNA and DNA release from nuclei of normal and neoplastic liver, *Biochem. Biophys. Res. Commun.,* 67, 706, 1975.

276. **Knowler, J. T.,** The incorporation of newly synthesized RNA into nuclear ribonucleoprotein particles after oestrogen administration to immature rats, *Eur. J. Biochem.,* 64, 161, 1976.

277. **Tata, J. R. and Baker, B.,** Differential subnuclear distribution of polyadenylate-rich ribonucleic acid during induction of egg-yolk protein synthesis in male *Xenopus* liver by oestradiol-17β, *Biochem. J.,* 150, 345, 1975.

278. **Muller, W. E. G., Totsuka, A., Kroll, M., Nusser, I., and Zahn, R. K.,** Poly(A) polymerase in quail oviduct. Changes during estrogen induction, *Biochim. Biophys. Acta,* 383, 147, 1975.

279. **Liang, T. and Liao, S.,** Association of the uterine 17β-estradiol-receptor complex with ribonucleoprotein in vitro and in vivo, *J. Biol. Chem.,* 249, 4671, 1974.

280. **Rustow, B., Weihe, A., and Lindigkeit, R.,** Effect of RNA synthesis on the binding of ³H-cortisol to nuclear ribonucleoprotein particles from rat liver carrying DNA-like RNA in vivo, *Nucleic Acid. Res.,* 2, 2257, 1975.

281. **Defer, N., Sabatier, M. M., and Kruh, J.,** Glucocorticoid and thyroid hormone-binding to nuclear ribonucleoprotein particles, *FEBS Lett.,* 76, 320, 1977.

282. **Bastos, R. N. and Aviv, H.,** Globin RNA precursor molecules: biosynthesis and processing in erythroid cells, *Cell,* 11, 641, 1977.

283. **Melli, M., Spinelli, G., Wyssling, H., and Arnold, E.,** Histone mRNA sequences in high molecular weight RNA of HeLa cells, *Cell,* 11, 651, 1977.

284. **Palmiter, R. D. and Carey, N. H.,** Rapid inactivation of ovalbumin messenger ribonucleic acid after acute withdrawal of estrogen, *Proc. Natl. Acad. Sci. U.S.A.,* 71, 2357, 1974.

285. **Kafatos, F. C. and Gelinas, R.,** mRNA stability and the control of specific protein synthesis in the highly differentiated cells, in *Biochemistry of Cell Differentiation,* Paul, J., Ed., Butterworths, London, 1974, 223.

286. **Gallwitz, D.,** Kinetics of inactivation of histone mRNA in the cytoplasm after inhibition of DNA replication in synchronized HeLa cells, *Nature (London),* 257, 247, 1975.

287. **Bastos, R. N. and Aviv, H.,** Theoretical analysis of a model for globin messenger RNA accumulation during erythropoiesis, *J. Mol. Biol.,* 110, 205, 1977.

288. **Stiles, C. D., Lee, K.-L., and Kenney, F. T.,** Differential degradation of messenger RNAs in mammalian cells, *Proc. Natl. Acad. Sci. U.S.A.,* 73, 2634, 1976.

289. **Warner, W. J., Fan, W., Ivarie, R. D., and Levinson, B. B.,** Nucleus-dependent regulation of tyrosine aminotransferase degradation in hepatoma tissue culture cells, *J. Biol. Chem.,* 252, 7834, 1977.

290. **Lodish, H. F.,** Translational control of protein synthesis, *Annu. Rev. Biochem.,* 45, 39, 1976.

291. **Tomkins, G. M., Gelehrter, T. D., Granner, D., Martin, D., Jr., Samuels, H. H., and Thompson, E. B.,** Control of specific gene expression in higher organisms, *Science,* 166, 1474, 1969.

292. **Moscona, A. A., Moscona, M. H., and Saenz, N.,** Enzyme induction in embryonic retina: the role of transcription and translation, *Proc. Natl. Acad. Sci. U.S.A.,* 61, 160, 1968.

293. **Kenney, F. T., Lane, S. E., Lee, K., and Ihle, J. N.,** Glucocorticoid control of gene expression, in *Control Mechanisms in Cancer,* Criss, W. E., Ono, T., and Sabine, J. R., Eds., Raven Press, New York, 1976, 25.

294. **Steinberg, R. A., Levinson, B. B., and Tomkins, G. M.,** Kinetics of steroid induction and deinduction of tyrosine aminotransferase synthesis in cultured hepatoma cells, *Proc. Natl. Acad. Sci. U.S.A.,* 72, 2007, 1975.

295. **Killewich, L., Schutz, G., and Feigelson, P.,** Functional level of rat liver tryptophan 2,3-dioxygenase messenger RNA during superinduction of enzyme with actinomycin-D, *Proc. Natl. Acad. Sci. U.S.A.,* 72, 4285, 1975.

296. **Schwartz, R. J.,** Control of glutamine synthetase synthesis in the embryonic chick neural retina. A caution in the use of actinomycin D, *J. Biol. Chem.,* 248, 6426, 1973.

297. **Singer, R. H. and Penman, S.,** Messenger RNA in HeLa cells: kinetics of formation and decay, *J. Mol. Biol.,* 78, 321, 1973.

298. **Palmiter, R. D. and Schimke, R. T.,** Regulation of protein synthesis in chick oviduct. III. Mechanism of ovalbumin "superinduction" by actinomycin D, *J. Biol. Chem.,* 248, 1503, 1973.

299. **Singer, R. H. and Penman, S.,** Stability of HeLa cell mRNA in actinomycin, *Nature (London),* 240, 100, 1972.

300. **Leinwand, L. and Ruddle, F. H.,** Stimulation of in vitro translation of messenger RNA by actinomycin D and cordycepin, *Science,* 197, 381, 1977.

301. **Egyhazi, E.,** Actinomycin D and RNA transport, *Nature (London),* 250, 221, 1974.

302. **Maale, G., Stein, G., and Mans, R.,** Effects of cordycepin and cordycepin-triphosphate on polyadenylic and ribonucleic acid-synthesizing enzymes from eukaryotes, *Nature (London),* 255, 80, 1975.

303. **Jacob, S. T., Muecke, W., Sajdel, E. M., and Munro, H. N.,** Evidence for extranucleolar control of RNA synthesis in the nucleolus, *Biochem. Biophys. Res. Commun.,* 40, 334, 1970.

304. **Tata, J. R., Hamilton, M. J., and Shields, D.,** Effects of α-amanitin in vivo on RNA polymerase and nuclear RNA synthesis, *Nature (London) New Biol.,* 238, 161, 1972.

305. **Farber, J. L. and Farmar, R.,** Differential effects of cycloheximide on protein and RNA synthesis as a function of dose, *Biochem. Biophys. Res. Commun.,* 51, 626, 1973.

306. **Ernest, M. J., Delap, L., and Feigelson, P.,** Induction of hepatic tyrosine aminotransferase mRNA by protein synthesis inhibitors, *J. Biol. Chem.,* 253, 2895, 1978.

307. **Gorski, J., Noteboom, W. D., and Nicolette, J. A.,** Estrogen control of the synthesis of RNA and protein in the uterus, *J. Cell. Comp. Physiol.,* 66 (Suppl.), 91, 1965.

308. **Nicolette, J. A., Lemahieu, M. A., and Mueller, G. C.,** A role of estrogens in the regulation of RNA polymerase in surviving rat uteri, *Biochim. Biophys. Acta,* 166, 403, 1968.

309. **Mueller, G. C., Vonderhaar, B., Kim, U. H., and Mahieu, M. L.,** Estrogen action: an inroad to cell biology, *Recent Prog. Horm. Res.,* 28, 1, 1972.

310. **Raynaud-Jammet, C., Catelli, M. G., and Baulieu, E.-E,** Inhibition by α-amanitin of the oestradiol-induced increase in α-amanitin sensitive RNA polymerase in immature rat uterus, *FEBS Lett.,* 22, 93, 1972.

311. **Maden, B. E. H., Vaughan, M. H., Warner, J. R., and Darnell, J. E.,** Effects of valine deprivation on ribosome formation in HeLa cells, *J. Mol. Biol.,* 45, 265, 1969.

312. **Yu, F.-L., and Feigelson, P.,** The rapid turnover of RNA polymerase of rat liver nucleolus, and of its messenger RNA, *Proc. Natl. Acad. Sci. U.S.A.,* 69, 2833, 1972.

313. **Yu, F.-L., and Feigelson, P.,** A proposed model for the glucocorticoidal regulation of rat hepatic ribosomal RNA synthesis, *Biochem. Biophys. Res. Commun.,* 53, 754, 1973.

314. **Chesterton, C. J., Coupar, E. H., Butterworth, P. H. W., Buss, J., and Green, M. H.,** Studies on the control of ribosomal RNA synthesis in HeLa cells, *Eur. J. Biochem.,* 57, 79, 1975.

315. **DeAngelo, A. B. and Gorski, J.,** Role of RNA synthesis in the estrogen induction of a specific uterine protein, *Proc. Natl. Acad. Sci. U.S.A.,* 66, 693, 1970.

316. **Baulieu, E.-E.,** Some aspects of the mechanism of action of steroid hormones, *Mol. Cell. Biochem.,* 7, 157, 1975.

317. **Corradino, R. A.,** 1,25-Dihydroxycholecalciferol: inhibition of action in organ-cultured intestine by actinomycin D and α-amanitin, *Nature (London),* 243, 41, 1973.

318. **Vonderhaar, B. K.,** Studies on the mechanism by which thyroid hormones enhance α-lactalbumin activity in explants from mouse mammary glands, *Endocrinology,* 100, 1423, 1977.

319. **Palmiter, R. D., Moore, P. B., and Mulvihill, E. R.,** A significant lag in the induction of ovalbumin messenger RNA by steroid hormones: a receptor translocation hypothesis, *Cell,* 8, 557, 1976.

320. **Ernest, M. J., Chen, C., and Feigelson, P.,** Induction of tyrosine aminotransferase in isolated liver cell suspensions, *J. Biol. Chem.,* 252, 6783, 1977.

321. **Mosher, K. M., Young, D. A., and Munck, A.,** Evidence for irreversible, actinomycin D-sensitive, and temperature-sensitive steps following binding of cortisol to glucocorticoid receptors and preceding effects on glucose metabolism in rat thymus cells, *J. Biol. Chem.,* 246, 654, 1971.

322. **Munck, A.,** Glucocorticoid inhibition of glucose uptake by peripheral tissues: old and new evidence, molecular mechanisms and physiological significance, *Perspect. Biol. Med.,* 14, 265, 1971.

323. **Young, D. A., Barnard, T., Mendelsohn, S., and Giddings, S.,** An early cordycepin-sensitive event in the action of glucocorticoid hormones on rat thymus cells in vitro: evidence that synthesis of new mRNA initiates the earliest metabolic effects of steroid hormones, *Endocr. Res. Commun.,* 1, 63, 1974.

324. **Chu, L. H. and Edelman, I. S.,** Cordycepin and α-amanitin: inhibitors of transcription as probes of aldosterone action, *J. Membr. Biol.,* 10, 291, 1972.

325. **Georgiev, G. P.,** On the structural organization of the operon and the regulation of RNA synthesis in animal cells, *J. Theor. Biol.,* 25, 473, 1969.

326. **Paul, J.,** General theory of chromosome structure and gene activation in eukaryotes, *Nature (London),* 238, 444, 1975.

327. **MacLean, N. and Hilder, V. A.,** Mechanisms of chromatin activation and repression, in *International Review of Cytology,* Vol. 48, Bourne, G. H. and Danielli, J. F., Eds., Academic Press, New York, 1977, 1.

328. **Schrader, W. T., Toft, D. O., and O'Malley, B. W.,** Interaction of purified progesterone-receptor components with nuclear constituents, *J. Biol.Chem.,* 247, 2401, 1972.

329. **Thompson, E. B. and Gelehrter, T. D.,** Expression of tyrosine aminotransferase activity in somatic-cell heterokaryons: evidence for negative contol of enzyme expression, *Proc. Natl. Acad. Sci. U.S.A.,* 68, 2589, 1971.

330. **Brawerman, G.,** A model for the control of transcription during development, *Cancer Res.,* 36, 4278, 1976.

331. **Dickson, E. and Robertson, H. D.,** Potential regulatory roles for RNA in cellular development, *Cancer Res.,* 36, 3387, 1976.

332. **Goldstein, L.,** Role for small nuclear RNAs in "programming" chromosomal information?, *Nature (London),* 261, 519, 1976.

333. **Roy, A. K., Dowbenko, D. J., and Schiop, M. J.,** Studies on the mode of oestrogenic inhibition of hepatic synthesis of α_{2u}-globulin and its corresponding messenger ribonucleic acid in rat liver, *Biochem. J.,* 164, 91, 1977.

334. **Houdebine, L. M.,** Effect of prolactin and progesterone on expression of casein genes. Titration of casein mRNA by hybridization with complementary DNA, *Eur. J. Biochem.,* 68, 219, 1976.

335. **Levy, B. and Baxter, J. D.,** Distribution of thyroid and glucocorticoid hormone receptors in transcriptionally active and inactive chromatin, *Biochem. Biophys. Res. Commun.,* 68, 1045, 1976.

336. **Goldfine, I. D., Smith, G. J., Wong, K. Y., and Jones, A. L.,** Cellular uptake and nuclear binding of insulin in human cultured lymphocytes: evidence for potential intracellular sites of insulin action, *Proc. Natl. Acad. Sci. U.S.A.,* 74, 1368, 1977.

337. **Palmiter, R. D., Catlin, G. H., and Cox, R. F.,** Chromatin-associated receptors for estrogen, progesterone, and dihydrotestosterone and the induction of egg white protein synthesis in chick magnum, *Cell Differ.,* 2, 163, 1973.

338. **Palmiter, R. D. and Smith, L. T.,** Synergistic effects of oestrogen and progesterone on ovomucoid and conalbumin mRNA synthesis in chick oviduct, *Nature (London) New Biol.,* 246, 74, 1973.

339. **Samuels, H. H., Horwitz, Z. D., Stanley, F., Casanova, J., and Shapiro, L. E.,** Thyroid hormone controls glucocorticoid action in cultured GH_1 cells, *Nature (London),* 268, 254, 1977.

340. **Wangh, L. J. and Knowland, J.,** Synthesis of vitellogenin in cultures of male and female frog liver regulated by estradiol treatment in vitro, *Proc. Natl. Acad. Sci. U.S.A.,* 72, 3172, 1975.

341. **Green, C. D. and Tata, J. R.,** Direct induction by estradiol of vitellogenin synthesis in organ cultures of male *Xenopus laevis* liver, *Cell,* 7, 131, 1976.

342. **Seo, H., Vassart, G., Brocas, H., and Refetoff, S.,** Triiodothyronine stimulates specifically growth hormone mRNA in rat pituitary tumor cells, *Proc. Natl. Acad. Sci. U.S.A.,* 74, 2054, 1977.

343. **Groner, B., Hynes, N., Sippel, A. E., and Schutz, G.,** Induction of specific proteins in hyphae of *Achlya ambisexualis* by the steroid hormone antheridiol, *Nature (London),* 261, 599, 1976.

344. **MacIntyre, E. H.,** Cell culture in the study of the mechanism of hormone action, in *Biochemistry of Hormones,* Rickenberg, H. V., Ed., Butterworths, London, 1974, 305.

345. **Croce, C. M. and Litwack, G.,** Genetic approaches to enzyme induction in mammalian cells and hybrids in culture, in *Biochemical Actions of Hormones,* Vol. 3, Litwack, G., Ed., Academic Press, New York, 1975, 23.

346. **Thompson, E. B., Norman, M. R., and Lippman, M. E.,** Steroid hormone actions in tissue culture cells and cell hybrids, *Recent Prog. Horm. Res.,* 33, 571, 1977.

347. **Woo, S. L. C., Monahan, J. J., and O'Malley, B. W.,** The ovalbumin gene: purification of the anticoding strand, *J. Biol. Chem.,* 252, 5789, 1977.

348. **Mandel, J. L., Breathnach, R., Gerlinger, P., LeMeur, M., Gannon, F., and Chambon, P.,** Organization of coding and intervening sequences in the chicken ovalbumin split gene, *Cell,* 14, 641, 1978.

349. **Dugaiczyk, A., Woo, S. L. C., Lai, E. C., Mace, M. L., McReynolds, L., and O'Malley, B. W.,** The natural ovalbumin gene contains seven intervening sequences, *Nature (London),* 274, 328, 1978.

350. **Cox, R. F. and Mizuno, S.,** unpublished observations.

351. **Miller, O. L.,** personal communication.

INDEX

E

Echinoderms, sperm-histones of, II: 68
Escherichia coli
  histones lacking in, II: 60
  RNA polymerase
    transcription following phage infection, II: 3
    use in in vitro transcription, I: 6, 7, 12, 20;
      II: 197

F

Fish, histone pattern changes in spermatogenesis,
  II: 69
Fungi, histones in, II: 61

G

Genes
  antiterminator sites on, II: 210
  coding sequences, II: 45
  control of expression at RNA polymerase level,
    II: 2, 12, 41
  definition, I: 101, 121
  de-repression
    assays of, I: 134
    of host cells by donated RNA, I: 139
    process, I: 132
  dispersion, I: 101
  existence in genome, I: 102
  histone, clustering of, II: 85
  in DNA, I: 102
  intervening sequences, II: 215
  "jumping", I: 44
  multiple initiation sites, mediation of control,
    II: 211
  numbers in prokaryotic and eukaryotic
    systems, I: 81
  primer hypothesis of control, I: 149
  repetitive, I: 42
  specific expression, hormones affecting, II: 196
  structural organization, I: 43, 47
Genome defined, I: 74

H

Histones
  acetylation, II: 77, 88
  association with cell differentiation
    development, II: 65
  conformation, II: 74
  crosslinking, implications of, II: 84
  distribution during DNA replication, II: 86
  during embryonic development, II: 70
  effects on nonhistone chromosomal protein
    phosphorylation, II: 137

  evolution, II: 64
  function, II: 117
  gene transcription, II: 141
  history, II: 64
  in animals, II: 63
  in different species, II: 60
  informational role, II: 92
  in male gametes, II: 67
  in plants, II: 64
  in prokaryotes, lack of, II: 60
  interactions among, II: 75
  interaction with DNA, II: 75
  in tumors, II: 72
  isohistones, II: 63
  lysine-rich, specificity, II: 67
  major species, II: 61, 63
  methylation, II: 78
  mRNA synthesis, II: 71
  nonstructural function, II: 92
  nucleosomal, II: 66
  packing of DNA, role in, II: 80, 90
  phosphorylation, II: 76, 87
  poly-ADP-ribosylation, II: 78
  precursors, II: 65
  presence at transcription sites, II: 86
  role in chromatin structure, II: 79—84
  sperm-histones, II: 67
  structural role II: 90
  structure, II: 72
  synthesis, II: 85
  tissue specificity, II: 66
  variants, II: 63, 84
Hormones
  action at cell surface, II: 180
  effect on RNA polymerase activity, II: 26, 182
  induction of proteins, II: 194
  inhibitors, II: 207
  in vitro effects, relevance of, II: 193, 197
  modulation of cell metabolism, II: 180
  modulation of protein synthesis, II: 206
  multihormonal control of transcription, II: 210
  negative control by, II: 210
  receptors, role in mediating action in nucleus,
    II: 196, 210, 214
  regulation of mRNA stability, II: 206
  RNA primers as effector molecules, II: 211
  role in RNA processing, II: 205
  role in RNA synthesis, II: 181—215
  tissue specificity, II: 193

I

Immune response, role of gene de-repression in,
  I: 132
Insects, histones in spermatozoa of, II: 68
In vitro transcription, see Transcription

L

Liver cells, regeneration, II: 22, 42

UNIVERSITY LIBRARY
LOMA LINDA, CALIFORNIA

V

Y